Epilepsy

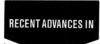

RECENT ADVANCES IN

Epilepsy

Edited by

T. A. Pedley MD

Professor and Vice-Chairman,
Department of Neurology,
College of Physicians and Surgeons of Columbia University;
Director, Columbia Comprehensive Epilepsy Center, New York, USA

B. S. Meldrum MA MB BChir PhD

Professor of Experimental Neurology,
Department of Neurology,
Institute of Psychiatry, London, UK

NUMBER SIX

CHURCHILL LIVINGSTONE
EDINBURGH LONDON MADRID MELBOURNE NEW YORK AND TOKYO 1995

CHURCHILL LIVINGSTONE
Medical Division of Pearson Professional Limited

Distributed in the United States of America by
Churchill Livingstone Inc., 650 Avenue of the Americas, New York,
N.Y. 10011, and by associated companies, branches and
representatives throughout the world.

First published 1995

ISBN 0–443–05125–9
ISSN 0264–7400

British Library Cataloguing in Publication Data
A catalogue record for this book is available from the British
Library

Library of Congress Cataloguing in Publication Data
A catalogue record for this book is available from the Library
of Congress

The
publisher's
policy is to use
**paper manufactured
from sustainable forests**

Produced by Longman Singapore Publishers Pte Ltd
Printed in Singapore

Contents

Preface

This is volume six of a continuing series that first appeared in 1983. The purpose now, as then, is to provide, at regular intervals, authoritative reviews of issues of immediate importance to physicians treating patients with epilepsy. The ongoing, even accelerating, advances in research into basic mechanisms of epileptogenesis, new or refined diagnostic procedures, improved medical and surgical therapies, and the importance of psychosocial measures mean that some of the information contained in this book will soon be outdated, incomplete, or simply wrong. It is therefore likely that given the continued support of the staff of Churchill Livingstone, as well as the generous participation of our many distinguished colleagues, a seventh volume can be anticipated in about two years.

The contributions here present, firstly, a status report on how greater understanding of excitatory neurotransmission is affecting antiepileptic drug development. Five chapters address new or updated diagnostic or investigative procedures. Several of these, e.g. chapters on MR spectroscopy, in vivo human microdialysis, and cortical localization of cognitive functions, illustrate how blurred can be the distinction between what is practice and what is clinical research that also illuminates brain function. Selected issues in medical and surgical therapy are covered in three chapters. The remaining chapters provide critical updates on diverse topics including Rasmussen's syndrome, language disorders and epilepsy, endocrine aspects of epilepsy in men and women, seizures in the elderly, and mortality relared to seizures and epilepsy.

In assembling this volume, we have tried to provide "state of the art" assessments that balance theoretical and scientific concerns with practical needs and guidance. We hope that the many unanswered questions contained in almost every chapter will further stimulate the spirit of inquiry.

As always, we thank our eminent contributors for their excellent and concise reviews and for their willingness to conform to editorial arbitrariness and deadlines. We thank our patients for their continuing inspiration and example.

T. A. Pedley   1995
B. S. Meldrum

Contributors

Frederick Andermann MD
Professor of Neurology, Montreal Neurological Institute, McGill
University, Montreal, Quebec, Canada

Karen Ballaban-Gil MD
Assistant Professor of Neurology and Pediatrics, Albert Einstein College of
Medicine, Bronx, New York, USA

Samuel F. Berkovic MD FRACP
Neurologist, Comprehensive Epilepsy Program, Austin Hospital,
Melbourne, Victoria, Australia

Astrid G. Chapman PhD
Senior Lecturer, Department of Neurology, Institute of Psychiatry,
London, UK

Alan Connelly PhD
Senior Lecturer, Institute of Child Health, Hospital for Sick Children
(Great Ormond Street), London, UK

John Duncan MA DM FRCP
Senior Lecturer in Neurology, Institute of Neurology; Honorary
Consultant Neurologist, National Hospital for Neurology and
Neurosurgery (Queen Square), London, UK

Matthew J. During MBChB FRACP FACP
Associate Professor of Medicine and Surgery, Yale University School of
Medicine, New Haven, Connecticut, USA

Christian E. Elger MD PhD
Director, University Clinic of Epileptology, University of Bonn, Bonn,
Germany

Antonio Gil-Nagel MD
Assistant Professor, MINCEP, University of Minnesota, Minneapolis, USA

Thomas Grunwald MD PhD
University Clinic of Epileptology, University of Bonn, Bonn, Germany

Marla J. Hamberger PhD
Assistant Professor of Clinical Neuropsychology, Columbia University, Neurological Institute, New York, USA

Yvonne M. Hart MD MRCP
Consultant Neurologist, Atkinson Morley's Hospital, London, and Kingston Hospital, Surrey, UK

Christoph Helmstaedter PhD
University Clinic of Epileptology, University of Bonn, Bonn, Germany

Andrew G. Herzog MD MSc
Associate Professor of Neurology, Harvard Medical School; Director, Neuroendocrine Unit, Beth Israel Hospital, Boston, Massachusetts, USA

Fenella J. Kirkham MRCP
Senior Lecturer in Paediatric Neurology, Neurosciences Unit, Institute of Child Health, London, UK

Martin Kurthen MD
Lecturer in Neuropsychology, Department of Epileptology, University of Bonn, Bonn, Germany

Ilo E. Leppik MD
Director of Research, MINCEP; Clinical Professor of Neurology and Pharmacy, University of Minnesota, Minneapolis, USA

Lina Nashef MBChB MRCP
Research Fellow, Epilepsy Research Group, Institute of Neurology, London, and National Society for Epilepsy, Chalfont Centre for Epilepsy, Chalfont St Peter, Buckinghamshire, UK

Mark R. Newton MD FRACP
Neurologist, Austin Hospital, Melbourne, Victoria, Australia

Theodore Rasmussen BS MB MD MS FRCS (Can)
Emeritus Professor of Neurosurgery, Montreal Neurological Institute, McGill University, Montreal, Quebec, Canada

J. W. A. S. Sander MD PhD
Associate Specialist in Neurology, Chalfont Centre for Epilepsy, Chalfont St Peter, Buckinshire, and National Hospital for Neurology and Neurosurgery (Queen Square), London, UK

Mark L. Scheuer MD
Assistant Professor of Neurology, College of Physicians and Surgeons of
Columbia University, and Columbia Comprehensive Epilepsy Center,
Neurological Institute, New York, USA

W. Donald Shields MD
Professor of Neurology and Pediatrics, Head, Division of Pediatric
Neurology, University of California, Los Angeles, California, USA

Simon Shorvon MA MD FRCP
Reader in Neurology, Institute of Neurology, London; Consultant
Neurologist, National Hospital for Neurology and Neurosurgery (Queen
Square), London; Medical Director, National Society for Epilepsy, UK

Thaddeus S. Walczak MD
Assistant Professor of Neurology, Columbia University; Director, Epilepsy
Monitoring Unit, Columbia Presbyterian Medical Center, New York, USA

Excitatory neurotransmission and antiepileptic drug development: a status report

A. G. Chapman

The extensive research efforts during the past 10–15 years devoted to deciphering the excitatory amino acid (EAA) neurotransmitter system have yielded invaluable information concerning the basic mechanisms of neuronal activation, the pharmacological diversity of EAA receptors, and the genetic and molecular basis for this diversity.

It has been shown that EAA neurotransmission is directly or indirectly involved in a host of neurophysiological or systemic processes, ranging from memory, learning and cognition to endocrine physiology and pain perception. Glutamate receptors are clearly involved in the initiation and spread of seizure activity and seizure-related neuropathology. However, despite high and sustained expectations, so far no EAA antagonist has been introduced into clinical use as a safe and effective antiepileptic drug (AED), although some of the drugs investigated are currently being evaluated as neuroprotective agents in stroke and head injury in several centres (Stewart et al 1993, Steinberg et al 1994).

The identification of potential AEDs among compounds affecting EAA neurotransmission has been approached from two angles:

1. By systematic screening of all new EAA antagonists and other EAA-related drugs as they become available in experimental animal models of epilepsy.
2. By testing novel experimental or clinical AEDs of unknown mechanism of action for affinity for EAA receptors, or for other forms of interaction with the EAA transmitter system.

The former approach has identified a number of compounds (mostly N-methyl-D-aspartate (NMDA) antagonists and α-amino-3-hydroxy-5-methyl-4-isoxazolepropionate (AMPA)/kainate antagonists) with reasonable therapeutic indices and potent anticonvulsant activities in several animal models of generalized convulsive epilepsy. Clinical experience with NMDA antagonists has been limited to small groups of patients with refractory complex partial seizures, and has not been favourable, either with respect to seizure control at the doses tested, or to the behavioural side-effects observed in these patients (Troupin et al 1986, Fisher et al 1990, Rogawski & Porter 1990, Sveinbjornsdottir et al 1993).

The second approach has revealed that some of the novel AEDs undergoing clinical trials or in current (or recent) clinical use (e.g. felbamate, lamotrigine, remacemide) interact with the EAA transmitter system (Miller et al 1986, Palmer et al 1992; McCabe et al 1993, Palmer & McTavish 1993, Meldrum & Leach 1994). There have been numerous reviews about the anticonvulsant properties and therapeutic prospects of EAA antagonists (Dingledine et al 1990, Wood et al 1990; Chapman 1991, Rogawski 1992, 1993, Chapman & Meldrum 1993, Lipton 1993, Meldrum 1994, Meldrum & Chapman 1994). This chapter — after providing brief background information about the role of glutamatergic transmission in epilepsy — is intended as an update of the experimental EAA antagonist anticonvulsant literature, and as an evaluation of the therapeutic potential of the different classes of EAA antagonists and compounds acting at other sites of EAA neurotransmission.

GLUTAMATERGIC NEUROTRANSMISSION AND EPILEPSY

EAA receptors

Glutamate and aspartate (and possibly related endogenous sulfur-containing carboxylic acids) are the major excitatory neurotransmitters in the central nervous system. Glutamatergic or EAA neurotransmission is mediated via ionotropic EAA receptors (NMDA and AMPA and kainate receptors, named after selective, potent receptor agonists and gating sodium and, under certain conditions, calcium currents) or via a diverse family of G-protein-coupled metabotropic glutamate receptors, linked to second messenger systems (phosphoinositide hydrolysis or adenyl cyclase). The original identification of the three distinct ionotropic EAA receptor subtypes (NMDA, AMPA and kainate; Watkins & Evans 1981) was based on electrophysiological and pharmacological criteria. The molecular basis for these categories has subsequently been established and elaborated further using the tools of molecular biology (Nakanishi 1992, Seeburg 1993, Hollmann & Heinemann 1994, Westbrook 1994). Each ionotropic EAA receptor class (NMDA receptors, AMPA/kainate receptors, and specific kainate receptors, for which little pharmacology is known) consists of a family of closely related subunits that can be expressed homomerically or heteromerically within the same family (Fig. 1.1). The recombinant subunits share many properties within the same family (and with the respective native EAA receptors), but there are also important distinctions between the subunits with respect to distribution, developmental profile, response to pathophysiological conditions, pharmacological properties and ion conductance.

There have been preliminary suggestions that certain classes of NMDA antagonists are selective for specific subunit combinations (Yamakura et al 1993, Buller et al 1993, Hollmann & Heinemann 1994, Laurie & Seeburg 1994, Lynch et al 1994). This is an area with promising scope for pharmacological exploitation by, for instance, designing antagonists that are

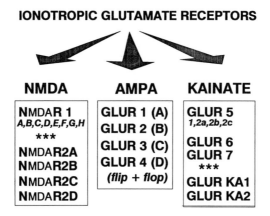

Fig. 1.1   Ionotropic glutamate receptor subunits. NMDA = *N*-methyl-D-aspartate;
AMPA = α-amino-3-hydroxy-5-methyl-4-isoxazolepropionate.

selective for subunit combinations that might show an increased expression
during epileptogenesis. Such selective antagonists would be expected to have
fewer undesired side-effects through lack of interaction with EAA receptors
involved in cerebral functions other than seizure generation.

Glutamate release and synaptic action

A simplified glutamatergic synapse with associated glutamatergic receptors
and transporters is shown in Figure 1.2.

During low-frequency transmission the excitatory synaptic response is
mainly mediated via AMPA/kainate receptors. Following electrical or chemical synaptic activation, the AMPA-mediated sodium and calcium influx and
resulting transient depolarization permit activation of the NMDA receptors.
Both AMPA/kainate (fast component of paroxysmal depolarization shift; PDS)
and NMDA (slow component of PDS) receptor activation contribute directly
to the generation of PDSs and associated action potential bursts, which are
considered to be the cellular equivalent of interictal spikes (Dingledine et al
1990). During synaptic activation there is a concomitant increase in calcium-
dependent glutamate (and aspartate) release, which, in turn, causes further
activation of postsynaptic NMDA and AMPA/kainate receptors. Glutamate
release is modulated by ionic conductance changes (calcium, potassium,
sodium, chloride) and by presynaptic receptors, including a glutamatergic
metabotropic receptor activated by 2-amino-4-phosphonobutyric acid (AP4) or
endogenous glutamate (Nicholls & Attwell 1990). Other neurotransmitters
(γ-aminobutyrate B-receptor) (GABA$_B$) agonists, adenosine A1 agonists, κ-
opioid agonists, muscarinic agonists) can modulate EAA neurotransmission via
presynaptic inhibition of glutamate release (Meldrum et al 1992). The action
of glutamate on NMDA and AMPA/kainate receptors (colocalized at most
excitatory synapses on dendritic spines; Westbrook 1994) can be terminated by:

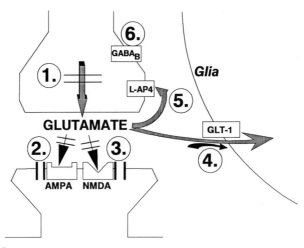

1. Inhibition of glutamate release (eg Ca^{++}; Na$^+$ channels)
2. Inhibition by AMPA/Kainate antagonists
3. Inhibition by NMDA antagonists
4. Facilitation of glutamate reuptake via glial transporter (GLT-1)
5. Feedback inhibition of glutamate release via L-AP4 activation
6. Activation of inhibitory transmitter systems

Fig. 1.2 Glutamate release, postsynaptic action and reuptake; sites for potential inhibition of glutamatergic transmission. AMPA = α-amino-3-hydroxy-5-methyl-4-isoxazole propionate NMDA = N-methyl-D-aspartate; GLT = glutamate; L-AP4 = 2-amino-4-phosphonobutyrate GABA$_B$ = γ-aminobutyrate B-receptor.

1. EAA antagonist binding.
2. AMPA receptor desensitization (Patneau & Mayer 1991).
3. Diffusion combined with glutamate reuptake, mediated by a family of glial or neuronal glutamate/aspartate transporters (Danbolt et al 1992, Amara & Kuhar 1993, Kanai et al 1994).
4. Feedback inhibition of glutamate release mediated via an inhibitory activation of presynaptic metabotropic AP4 receptor (Saugstad et al 1994).
5. Inhibitory action of other transmitter systems, such as GABA$_A$ or GABA$_B$.

Figure 1.2 summarizes the sites where potential anticonvulsant drugs may act to inhibit glutamatergic neurotransmission.

Epilepsy-related changes within the EAA system

Most of the information available concerning EAA-related neurochemical changes in human epilepsy has been obtained from patients with refractory complex partial epilepsy, from studies on resected tissue following temporal lobectomy, from in situ intraoperative studies, or from in situ microdialysis studies in ambulatory telemetry patients during depth electrode assessment of epileptic focus location. In general, observations made in humans with complex partial seizures are paralleled by similar findings in experimental focal seizure models in rodents, such as fully amygdala-kindled seizures in rats.

The onset of a partial seizure in humans is associated with a transient increased focal release of glutamate and aspartate. This has been demonstrated (using hippocampal microdialysis probes incorporated into standard-depth electroencephalogram electrodes) both during spontaneous seizures in ambulatory patients (During & Spencer 1993) and during spontaneous or evoked seizures during surgery (Do et al 1991; Ronne-Engström et al 1992).

Amygdala-kindled rats also exhibit an enhancement of evoked hippocampal glutamate release compared to control rats (Zhang et al 1991, Minamoto et al 1992). The molecular basis for enhanced glutamate release is not fully understood. It has been shown that kindled rats have an enhanced hippocampal response to NMDA (assessed by calcium influx). In control rats the NMDA-evoked calcium influx is predominantly in the pyramidal cell layer of CA1, while in kindled rats the NMDA response is widely extended to include the dendritic layer of CA1 (Mody & Heinemann 1987; McNamara 1994). A similar enlargement of the area showing enhanced susceptibility to NMDA has been demonstrated in human cortical epileptic tissue (Louvel & Pumain 1991). Resected temporal lobe tissue from patients with complex partial seizures also shows altered levels of EAA receptors, mainly increased kainate binding in the parahippocampal gyrus and increased AMPA binding in the dentate gyrus (Meldrum 1994).

ANTICONVULSANT ACTION OF GLUTAMATERGIC DRUGS

Generalized convulsive seizures in animals

Many of the animal seizure models used for screening novel antiepileptic drugs represent generalized convulsive epilepsy, either reflex-induced seizures in genetically seizure-susceptible strains of animals, or seizures induced by electroshock or chemical convulsants. Essentially all the anticonvulsant information concerns suppression of evoked, acute seizures following either acute or chronic drug administration. Maximal electroshock (MES) in rodents is the traditional screening model claimed to predict anticonvulsant efficacy in focal epilepsy and primary or secondary generalized tonic–clonic seizures. Audiogenic generalized seizures in mice (dilute brown agouti (DBA)/2) or rats (genetically epilepsy prone rat (GEPR)), or photically induced seizures in genetically photically sensitive baboons (*Papio papio*) have been used extensively in our own laboratory for demonstrating the activity of glutamatergic drugs against generalized convulsive seizures (Chapman 1991, Chapman & Meldrum 1993). Generalized tonic–clonic seizures induced by chemical convulsants such as bicuculline, β-carbolines, picrotoxin or high doses of pentylenetetrazol (PTZ) have also been assessed for response to glutamatergic drugs.

Competitive NMDA antagonists

AP7 (2-amino-7-phosphonoheptanoic acid) and AP5 (2-amino-5-phosphonovaleric acid) belong to the first generation of selective competitive NMDA antagonists and were shown in 1982 to suppress sound-induced seizures in DBA/2 mice following intracerebroventricular (i.c.v.) and intraperitoneal (i.p.) administration (Croucher et al 1982). AP7 and AP5 are structural analogs of glutamate and aspartate, where the carboxylic acid residues of the amino acid side-chains have been replaced by ω-phosphono or tetrazol residues in the antagonists. AP7 and AP5 have subsequently been succeeded by much more potent (50–100-fold more active than NMDA antagonists and anticonvulsants) selective competitive NMDA antagonists. These have all been close structural analogs of the parent compounds. The most potent members of the group, D-CPPene, CGS 19755, CGP 40116 (D-form of racemic CGP 37849), CGP 43487 (D-form of racemic CGP 39551), and LY 274614, have antiepileptic potencies falling within the same range (0.3–3 mg/kg, i.p.) in models of generalized convulsant epilepsy (sound-induced seizures in DBA/2 mice, NMDA-induced seizures or electroshock-induced seizures), or at somewhat higher doses (10–40 mg/kg, intravenously; i.v.) in photically induced myoclonic seizures in baboons (for reviews, see Chapman 1991, Rogawski 1992, Meldrum & Chapman 1994). The anticonvulsant activities reside with the D-enantiomers in all the above competitive NMDA antagonists (even though the agonists, aspartate and glutamate, are active in their L-forms), and they share many pharmacological properties:

1. All the antagonists tested are orally active (at doses 2–10-fold higher than what is required i.p. or i.v.).
2. They have a prolonged time-course of anticonvulsant action (an acute dose of CGP 39551 or D-CPPene provides protection for 2 days or more in baboons).
3. Their therapeutic indices (TI values) following acute administration in rodents (TI = 4–20, assessed by rotarod performance; Chapman 1991) are within the range of those obtained for established antiepileptic drugs (TI = 3–60; Macdonald 1983).
4. Chronic administration of D-CPPene or CGS 19755 does not appear to lead to diminished anticonvulsant efficacy in rodents (Chapman 1991, Smith & Chapman 1993).
5. Their acute cognitive and neurochemical side-effects appear relatively minor in control rodents and primates.

Very recently, a novel substituted ω-phosphono-2-amino-carboxylic acid, SDZ EAB 515, has joined the ranks of competitive NMDA antagonists with potent oral (p.o.) anticonvulsant activity (ED_{50} values against clonic seizures in DBA/2 mice: 4.7 mg/kg i.p. 1 h; 3.6 mg/kg p.o. 3 h). Interestingly, despite the similarity in structure to the other competitive NMDA antagonists, the

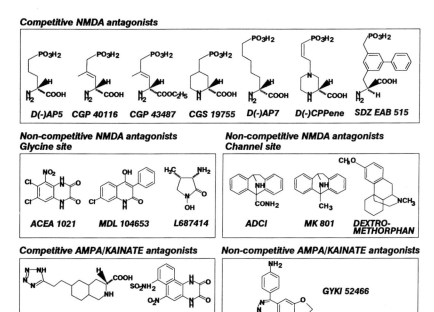

Fig. 1.3   Structures of different classes of *N*-methyl-D-aspartate (NMDA) and
α-amino-3-hydroxy-5-methyl-4-isoxazolepropionate. (AMPA) kainate antagonists.
D(−)AP5 = D(−)2-amino-5-phosphonopentanoic acid;
CGP 40116 = D(−)2-amino-4-methyl-5-phosphono-3-pentenoic acid;
CGP 43897 = D(−)2-amino-4-methyl-5-phosphono-3-pentenoate-1-ethyl ester;
CGS 19755 = cis-4-phosphonomethyl-2-piperidine-carboxylic acid;
D(−)AP7 = D(−)2-amino-7-phosphonoheptanoic acid;
D(−)CPPene = 3-)2-carboxypiperazin-4-yl)propenyl-1-phosphonic acid;
SDZ EAB 515 = *S*-α-amino-5-(phosphonomethyl)[1,1'-biphenyl]-3-propanoic acid.
   ACEA 1021 = 5-nitro-6,7-dichloroquinoxalinedione;
MDL 104653 = 3-phenyl-4-hydroxy-7-chloro-qinolin-2(1H)-one;
L687414 = R-(+)-cis-β-methyl-3-amino-1-hydroxypyrrolidin-2-one;
ADCI = 5-aminocarbonyl-10, 11-dihydro-5H-dibenzo[a,d]cycloheptene-5, 10-imine;
MK 801 (dizocilpine) = (+)-5-methyl-10,11-dihydroxy-5H-dibenzo(a,d)cyclohepten-5,10-imine.
   LY293558: (3S,4αR,6R,8αR)-6-[2(1H-tetrazol-5-yl)ethyl]decahydro-isoquinoline-3-carboxylic
acid; NBQX = 2,3-dihydroxy-6-nitro-7-sulphamoyl-benzo(F)quinoxaline;
GYKI 52466 = 1-(a-aminophenyl)-4-methyl-7,8-methylenedioxy-5H-2,3-benzodiazepine.

active enantiomer in this case is the L-form, while the D-form (SDZ 214 514)
is 20-fold less active, both as NMDA antagonist and as an anticonvulsant
(Chapman et al 1995a). The structure of this compound is given in Figure 1.3
along with those of other EAA antagonists.

Non-competitive NMDA antagonists acting at the channel site

Among the most potent non-competitive antagonists acting at the NMDA
channel site are MK 801 (dizocilpine), phencyclidine and dextromethorphan

(Fig. 1.3). These antagonists have potent anticonvulsant activity in many animal models of generalized convulsive seizures, with ED_{50} values in the 0.2–15 mg/kg range following systemic administration of antagonists. However, there is little or no separation of anticonvulsant and toxic doses of these non-competitive NMDA antagonists (see below), which strongly argues against chronic clinical use in epilepsy (Chapman 1991).

Recently, however, several low-affinity, non-competitive NMDA channel-site antagonists have been shown to have anticonvulsant activity against MES, seizures induced by NMDA, 4-aminopyridine and other models of generalized, convulsive epilepsy, while presenting more favorable therapeutic indices than those of MK 801 and other high-affinity antagonists (Rogawski 1993). These low-affinity antagonists include ADCI (an analogue of MK 801), the anti-Parkinsonian drug memantine, and FPL 12495, the desglycine metabolite of remacemide. The anticonvulsant action of non-competitive NMDA antagonists in human epilepsy will be discussed below.

Non-competitive NMDA antagonists acting at the glycine site

The NMDA receptor requires the binding of 2 coagonists, glutamate and glycine, for optimal activity. Antagonists acting at the glycine site reverse the glycine potentiation of the NMDA responses in in vivo and in vitro systems, and have anticonvulsant activity. However, the first generation of glycine-site antagonists (mainly chloroderivatives of kynurenic acid) did not cross the blood–brain barrier and had a very short time-course of action (Chapman 1991). Systemically active antagonists acting at the glycine/NMDA site have only recently become available. These include L 687414, ACEA-1021, and MDL 104653 (Fig. 1.3) and the partial glycine agonist, ACPC, and they have been shown to be active against MES, against NMDA-induced seizures, and against reflex-induced seizures in rodents and baboons, with ED_{50} values around 2–20 mg/kg following systemic (i.p. or i.v.) administration (Skolnick et al 1989, Saywell et al 1991, Smith & Meldrum 1992, Weber 1993, Chapman et al 1995b).

Some kynurenic acid derivatives and indole derivatives which have antagonist activity at the glycine site have been shown to have systemic activity against MES seizures in the 30–300 mg/kg range (Nichols & Yielding 1993). The systemically available glycine/NMDA antagonists have TI values around 2–6, and at least MDL 104653 has oral activity (Chapman et al 1995b).

Felbamate is active against refractory complex partial epilepsy and other forms of epilepsy in humans. Among its suggested mechanisms of action are reports of D-serine-reversible antagonism at the glycine/NMDA site. Felbamate has anticonvulsant activity against MES and other animal models of generalized convulsant seizures (Swinyard et al 1986, White et al 1992).

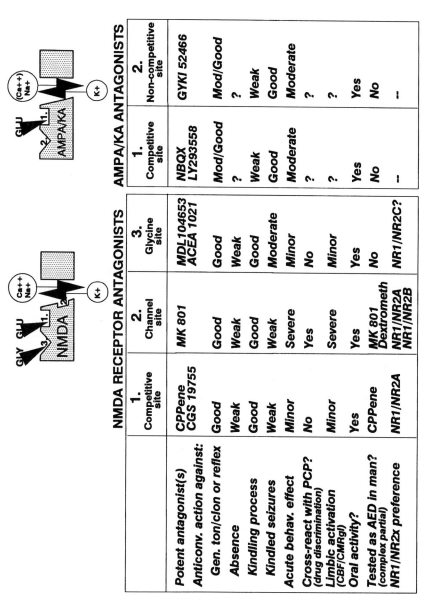

	NMDA RECEPTOR ANTAGONISTS			AMPA/KA ANTAGONISTS	
	1. Competitive site	2. Channel site	3. Glycine site	1. Competitive site	2. Non-competitive site
Potent antagonist(s)	CPPene CGS 19755	MK 801	MDL104653 ACEA 1021	NBQX LY293558	GYKI 52466
Anticonv. action against:					
Gen. ton/clon or reflex	Good	Good	Good	Mod/Good	Mod/Good
Absence	Weak	Weak	Weak	?	?
Kindling process	Good	Good	Good	Weak	Weak
Kindled seizures	Weak	Weak	Moderate	Good	Good
Acute behav. effect	Minor	Severe	Minor	Moderate	Moderate
Cross-react with PCP? (drug discrimination)	No	Yes	No	?	?
Limbic activation (CBF/CMRgl)	Minor	Severe	Minor	?	?
Oral activity?	Yes	Yes	Yes	Yes	Yes
Tested as AED in man? (complex partial)	CPPene	MK 801 Dextrometh	No	No	No
NR1/NR2x preference	NR1/NR2A	NR1/NR2A NR1/NR2B	NR1/NR2C?	--	--

Fig. 1.4   Summary of anticonvulsant and behavioural effects of *N*-methyl-D-aspartate (NMDA) and α-amino-3-hydroxy-5-methyl-4-isoxazdepropionate (AMPA)/kainate (KA) antagonists. AED = antiepileptic drug; CBF = cerebral blood flow; CMRgl = cerebral metabolic rate of glucose utilization; NR1 = NMDA receptor, subunit 1; PCP = phencyclidine.

The main properties of the different classes of NMDA antagonists have been summarized in Figure 1.4 and compared to those of the AMPA/kainate antagonists.

Antisense oligodeoxynucleotide probes of NMDA receptors

Although some classes of NMDA antagonists display a modest selectivity for specific subunit recombinants (e.g. AP5: NR1/NR2A; MK 801: NR1/NR2A = NR1/NR2B; ifenprodil: NR1/NR2B; glycine antagonist selectivity is variously reported as NR1/NR2C-preferring, NR1 preferring, or no selectivity) (Williams 1993, Yamakura et al 1993, Buller et al 1994, Hollmann & Heinemann 1994, Laurie & Seeburg 1994), it is not possible, at the present, to block pharmacologically selected NMDA or AMPA/kainate subunit recombinations. Gene manipulation is an alternative technique with which to manipulate the in vivo levels of specific subunits of EAA receptors. Receptors can be overexpressed by focally introducing the corresponding gene using, for example, a viral vector, and conversely, the expression of a receptor subunit can be reduced by focal or i.c.v. administration of an antisense oligonucleotide probe (a short piece of synthesized DNA that is complementary to, and can hybridize with, part of the messenger RNA coding for the receptor subunit, thus preventing the synthesis of the receptor protein). Though this approach is still very much in its infancy, there have been preliminary reports of prolonged (>2 weeks) enhanced seizure activity in rats following a single focal hippocampal administration of a gene expressing one of the calcium-conducting kainate subunits, GluR6 (During et al 1993). Repeated i.c.v. administration over a 30-h period before anticonvulsant testing of an antisense probe to the NMDA receptor subunit, NR1, offers complete protection against sound-induced seizures in DBA/2 mice, whereas the corresponding nonsense (scrambled nucleotide sequence) NR1 probe has no effect on the seizure activity (Chapman et al 1994b).

It may be premature to speculate on the potential clinical value of such a receptor-targeted approach to antiepileptic therapy. Each receptor family consists of many subunits with diverse properties, and it is becoming apparent that subunits respond differently to cerebral trauma in animals, e.g. in vitro hypoxia induces the NR2C subunit in cortical and hippocampal tissue, and transient or prolonged NMDA receptor changes have been reported following amygdala-kindling: there was a prolonged threefold increase in the hippocampal CA3 level of a novel population of NMDA receptors (binding CPP, but not CGS 19755) (Kraus et al 1994), as well as a reduction in NR1 and an increase in NR2A in dentate gyrus 4 h after the last kindled seizure in rats; Pratt et al 1993, Pratt & Kokaia 1994, Perez-Velazquez & Zhang 1994). It is therefore possible that some EAA receptor subunits may be critically involved in generating epileptogenic activity and would be logical targets for a gene manipulation approach to antiepileptic therapy.

AMPA/kainate antagonists

Antagonists acting at the AMPA/kainate receptor (formerly known as the quisqualate receptor) fall into two classes: competitive antagonists such as NBQX or LY293558, or non-competitive antagonists such as GYKI 52466 (Figs 1.3 and 1.4). A further level of complexity of the AMPA/kainate receptors is suggested by their interaction with the nootropic drugs aniracetam and cyclothiazide. These drugs inhibit the rapid desensitization of the AMPA-activated receptor (Vyklicky et al 1991), and it has been shown that aniracetam reverses the anticonvulsant protection provided by GYKI 52466 (Chapman et al 1993). Both classes of antagonists have reasonably good protective action against reflex induced seizures in rodents, seizures induced by AMPA and MES, with ED_{50} values around 5–10 mg/kg, TI values around 1–6 mg/kg and oral activity (Chapman et al 1991, Smith et al 1991, Bisaga et al 1993, Yamaguchi et al 1993, Chapman et al 1994a). NBQX and GYKI 52466 have relatively short time-courses of action and cause initial pronounced ataxia, while the recently described competitive antagonist, LY293558, has fewer side-effects and a longer time-course (>2 h) of action (Chapman et al 1994a).

Interestingly, both NBQX and GYKI 52466 appear to be two- to threefold more potent in a reflex primate seizure model (photically induced seizures in baboon) than in reflex rodent seizure models (Smith et al 1991), which is contrary to what has been observed with NMDA antagonists.

AMPA/kainate receptors are composed of a homomeric or heteromeric combination of four subunits (Fig. 1.1) with an unequal developmental profile, anatomical distribution and the ability to conduct calcium. The GluR1, GluR3 or GluR4 subunits permit calcium conductance through the ionophore, while the presence of GluR2 in homomeric or heteromeric recombinant receptors blocks calcium currents (Monyer et al 1992, Seeburg 1993). Subunit-selective antagonists for the AMPA/kainate receptor would therefore be expected to have differing abilities in inhibiting neuronal excitation. A GluR1/GluR2-selective antagonism by the compound Evans blue has been reported (Keller et al 1993); however, this dye has both proconvulsant and anticonvulsant effects (Dürmüller et al 1993). The currently available anticonvulsant AMPA/kainate antagonists show no selectivity for any specific subunit recombination (Hollmann & Heinemann 1994). Transient, as well as more long-lasting changes in subunit composition of the AMPA/kainate receptor have been reported following ischemia, or kindling and experimental seizures (Pollard et al 1993, Wong et al 1993, Kamphuis et al 1994, Lee et al 1994, Pellegrini-Giampietro et al 1994). However, the pattern of changes reported is not easily reconciled with enhanced excitability of neuronal tissue.

Metabotropic receptors

The metabotropic glutamate receptor family consists of seven known members (mGluR1-mGluR7 and subtypes) with very diverse properties, including both glutamate-induced excitatory and indirect inhibitory activity. The metabotropic receptors exhibit complex, reciprocal interactions with the ionotropic glutamate receptors (Schoepp & Conn 1993). Metabotropic agonists and antagonists with improved selectivity for the different receptor forms are gradually becoming available and should aid in characterizing the involvement of this class of receptors in epilepsy. Focal hippocampal injection of a metabotropic agonist [1S,3R]-ACPD, causes limbic seizures in rats (Sacaan & Schoepp 1992); there appears to be a long-lasting enhancement of amygdalar metabotropic-mediated phosphoinositide hydrolysis in kindled rats (Akiyama et al 1992); and it has recently been reported that 4-carboxy-3-hydroxyphenylglycine, an antagonist of mGluR1a (and agonist of mGluR2) protects against sound-induced seizures in DBA/2 mice (Thomsen et al 1994).

Drugs affecting glutamate release

A large number of AEDs inhibit glutamate/aspartate release indirectly through an inhibitory effect on calcium influx (Skerritt & Johnston 1984, Crowder & Bradford 1987), in addition to their presumed major mechanisms of anticonvulsant actions. However, lamotrigine and related compounds (BW1003C87) acting at sodium channels are often referred to primarily as glutamate release inhibitors. Lamotrigine (2–4 mg/kg) has a broad-spectrum anticonvulsant activity and a very favorable therapeutic index (TI >35) in experimental seizure models, including generalized seizures induced by MES, convulsants or sound stimulus (Miller et al 1986, Meldrum & Leach 1994).

Absence seizures in animals

Seizures induced by threshold doses of PTZ have historically been considered a predictive animal screening model for drugs with antiabsence efficacy. During the last decade genetic rodent models of absence epilepsy have been characterized (genetic absence epilepsy rats from Strasbourg; GAERS and albino-glaxo/rijs wijk WAG/Rij rats; lethargic, tottering, stargazer mice) that not only share the antiepileptic pharmacological profile of human absences, but also many of their anatomical, behavioral and electroencephalogram features. In particular, the GAERS model has been well-characterized physiologically and pharmacologically (Marescaux et al 1990, Vergnes et al 1990) and has been shown to have an enhanced cortical response to NMDA activation (Pumain et al 1992).

EAA antagonists

Spontaneous corticothalamic 5–10 Hz spike-and-wave discharges (SWD) are suppressed in genetic rat absence models by competitive NMDA antagonists (AP5, AP7 CPP) and non-competitive NMDA antagonists, including MK 801 at doses that are around 2–10-fold higher than those required to suppress reflex-induced seizures in rodents. At these doses major behavioral side-effects and electroencephalogram abnormalities were observed (Marescaux et al 1990).

None of the selective, systemically available AMPA/kainate antagonists appears to have been tested against rodent absence seizures. However, focal administration of AMPA aggravates SWD, and 6-cyano-7-nitro-guinoxaline-2,3-dione (CNQX), glutamic acid diethyl ester (GDEE) and kynurenate inhibit SWD in genetic rat absence models, suggesting an involvement of non-NMDA receptors in the generation of SWD (Ramakers et al 1991, Peeters et al 1994).

Focal seizures in animals

Rats that receive repetitive daily subthreshold electrical stimulation of the amygdala for 1–2 weeks gradually develop prolonged afterdischarge duration and limbic seizures in response to the kindling stimulus, and they remain permanently susceptible to stimulus-evoked partial seizures (Racine 1972). Such kindled seizures share some of the developmental, morphological and pharmacological features of complex partial epilepsy in humans, and have proven refractory to many forms of experimental anticonvulsant therapy (Lösher et al 1993).

NMDA antagonists in kindled seizures

When administered directly into the amygdala, competitive NMDA antago-nists (AP5, AP7, CGP 37849 and CGP 39551) are able to raise the kindled seizure threshold in rats with the same ranking order as their respective affinities for the NMDA receptor (Croucher & Bradford 1991). However, very high systemic doses (50–150-fold those required to block generalized reflex-induced seizures in rodents) of competitive (CGP 37849 or D-CPPene) or non-competitive (MK 801) NMDA antagonists are required to inhibit fully kindled seizures (scored as motor seizures or afterdischarge duration) in rats (Löscher & Hönack 1991, Cotterell et al 1992, Dürmüller et al 1994). These doses are associated with severe behavioral side-effects (ataxia, hyperactivity and some stereotopy) in the rodents (Löscher & Hönack 1991).

The systemically available glycine site antagonist MDL 104,653 (20 mg/kg i.p. or around 10-fold higher dose than that required to block reflex-induced seizures in rodents) has recently been shown significantly to inhibit both the motor seizures and afterdischarge duration of fully-kindled seizures without causing significant acute behavioral side effects, indicating a potential efficacy of the glycine site antagonists against complex partial seizures (Chapman et al 1995b). Less potent glycine site antagonists, though incapable of reducing overt motor seizures and afterdischarge duration, have previously been shown to raise the seizure threshold of fully kindled seizures (Croucher & Bradford 1991, Rundfeldt et al 1994).

AMPA/kainate antagonists

Both the competitive AMPA/kainate antagonist NBQX and the non-competitive antagonist GYKI 52466 have potent anticonvulsant activities against fully kindled seizures (Dürmüller et al 1994, Namba et al 1994) at doses of 10–40 mg/kg i.p., which is around 1.5–2-fold higher than the doses required to inhibit reflex-induced seizures. The AMPA/kainate antagonists therefore show more promise than the NMDA antagonists (see above) as potential anticonvulsant agents against complex partial seizures.

Drugs affecting glutamate release

Lamotrigine (6–18 mg/kg) inhibits fully kindled seizures (motor seizures and after discharge duration) in rats (Miller et al 1986), in agreement with its potent efficacy in partial seizures in humans.

Epileptogenesis

Drugs have been assessed for their ability to retard the kindling process when they are given chronically during the kindling period. All the NMDA antagonists (competitive, non-competitive and glycine site antagonists) share the ability potently to inhibit epileptogenesis (the development of amygdala-kindled seizures; Chapman et al 1991, 1995b, Dürmüller et al 1994). A behaviorally tolerated example of any of these groups of NMDA antagonists may therefore have a therapeutic prophylactic potential for posttraumatic epilepsy.

In contrast, the AMPA/kainate antagonists have only a slight protective action against epileptogenesis (Dürmüller et al 1994, Namba et al 1994).

Lamotrigine has no protective action against the kindling process in rats (O'Donnell & Miller 1991).

Behavioral side-effects of NMDA and AMPA/kainate antagonists in animals

Acute systemic administration of fully anticonvulsant doses (1–10-fold ED_{50} values) of all the classes of EAA antagonists produces some degree of ataxia and sometimes other side-effects. The severity of the side-effects differs, however, between the different classes, and to a lesser extent, between the antagonists within a class.

Non-competitive, high-affinity NMDA antagonists (e.g. MK 801, dextromethorphan) have profound behavioral effects. Anticonvulsant doses cause enhanced locomotion and stereotopy, and, based on the rotarod performance test for locomotor coordination, these antagonists have very poor therapeutic indices (Chapman 1991). It is difficult to assess cognitive side-effects in animals. The MK 801 class of antagonists does, however, cross-react with phencyclidine in drug discrimination studies (implying psychotomimetic properties of the antagonists) and they cause profound activation of cerebral blood flow and metabolism in limbic areas of the brain. These effects argue strongly against chronic clinical use of this class of antagonists (Willetts et al 1990, Chapman 1991).

Competitive NMDA antagonists (e.g. D-CPPene) cause ataxia at high doses following acute i.p., i.v. or oral administration to rodents and primates. In contrast to the non-competitive NMDA antagonists MK 801 and phencyclidine, they have only minor effects on regional cerebral blood flow and glucose utilization following the administration of fully anticonvulsant doses, and they do not cross-react with phencyclidine in drug discrimination studies in rodents and primates when administered systemically (Chapman et al 1990, Willetts et al 1990).

The impairment of learning and memory caused by EAA antagonists (Willetts et al 1990) represents a major concern for their clinical use. It has also been shown that chronic administration of MK 801 or CGP 39551 to neonatal rats causes neurochemical and behavioral alterations in the adult rat, including increased spontaneous locomotor activity (Facchinetti et al 1994).

Orally administered D-CPPene is well-tolerated in rodents (12–15 mg/kg) or baboons (32 mg/kg; Patel et al 1990). However, it has been pointed out by Löscher & Hönack (1991) that the behavioral side-effects induced by competitive NMDA antagonists are more severe in fully-kindled rats than in naïve or genetically seizure-susceptible rats, which may be related to a similar discrepancy between patients with complex partial epilepsy and volunteers (see below). In order to improve the predictive value of behavioral effects of AEDs (targeted for complex partial seizures) in animals, it would be an advantage to carry out behavioral testing, including drug discrimination studies, in kindled animals.

Antagonists acting at the NMDA/glycine site resemble the competitive NMDA antagonists with respect to behavioral side-effects. They do not cross-react with phencyclidine in drug discrimination studies or cause locomotor stimulation, and appear to have few behavioral side-effects following acute administration (high doses cause sedation and loss of muscle coordination). They (L 678414, ACEA-1021 and MDL 104653) have minimal effects on cerebral metabolism (Hargreaves et al 1993, Kemp & Leeson 1993, Weber 1993).

Clinical trials in humans

Novel AEDs are introduced into clinical use as add-on drugs in clinical trials for refractory epilepsy, which normally consist of a very high proportion of cases of complex partial epilepsy. At present, we have no information about the antiepileptic efficacy of EAA antagonists against other types of epilepsy. NMDA antagonists have been tested as add-on therapy only in small groups of patients with refractory complex partial seizures, even though the closest animal model of complex partial epilepsy (fully kindled seizures) is not significantly affected by competitive or non-competitive NMDA antagonists.

The non-competitive NMDA antagonist dextromethorphan has been used clinically for many years at low doses (around 30 mg) as an antitussive agent. It had no significant effect on seizure frequency at 120 mg/day (a five-fold higher dose is required to block generalized seizures in rodents) in 9 patients with complex partial epilepsy (Fisher et al 1990). MK 801 (0.008–0.034 mg/kg per day) was likewise without significant effect in reducing seizure frequency in 13 patients with complex partial epilepsy (0.05–0.1 mg/kg is required to inhibit generalized seizures in rodents; Troupin et al 1986).

The competitive NMDA antagonist D-CPPene (250–500 mg/day) was recently tested in add-on trials in 8 patients with refractory complex partial epilepsy (Sveinbjornsdottir et al 1993), but the trial was prematurely halted, primarily due to severe side-effects (poor concentration, sedation, ataxia, depression, amnesia, confusion) in all the patients, and also due to complete lack of antiepileptic effect at the doses tested. Interestingly, the side-effects were considerably worse in the epileptic population than among healthy volunteers (who tolerated doses of 1000 mg/day). This parallels the observation in rats, where kindled rats are much more susceptible to the behavioral side-effects of competitive NMDA antagonists than are control rats (Löscher & Hönack 1991). There is also anecdotal evidence of nightmares/anxiety among patients receiving competitive NMDA antagonists intrathecally for chronic pain (Kristensen et al 1992) or as part of clinical trials in acute stroke (Stewart et al 1993; Steinberg et al 1994). Traumatic head injury has been shown to aggravate the amnesic effect of MK 801 in rats (Hamm et al 1994). It therefore appears that patient population with complex seizures or certain types of brain injury may be more at risk for the behavioral side-effects of NMDA antagonists than is the control population.

Felbamate (400–3600 mg daily) has antiepileptic activity in refractory partial seizures and has been particularly effective against Lennox–Gastaut syndrome (Palmer & McTavish 1993). However, felbamate has recently been withdrawn from antiepileptic clinical use due to reports of aplastic anemia (and subsequently reports of hepatic failure) among the population receiving the drug (US Food and Drug Administration, 1 August 1994).

Remacemide is active against generalized convulsant seizures (MES), but not against partial seizures (fully amygdala-kindled seizures) in animals, and is currently undergoing phase 2 clinical trials for patients with generalized tonic–clonic and complex partial seizures (Palmer et al 1992).

Lamotrigine (100–300 mg/day) has clinical efficacy and a good therapeutic safety margin in refractory partial epilepsy, and in generalized epilepsy, including photosensitive epilepsy, absence epilepsy and Lennox–Gastaut syndrome (Miller et al 1986, Goa et al 1993). Lamotrigine was approved for open clinical use in the UK in 1993.

CONCLUSION

It is too early to judge the likely role of glutamate antagonists in the future therapy of epilepsy. Cognitive side-effects are a major problem with non-competitive and competitive (glutamate site) NMDA receptor antagonists. It remains possible that glycine site NMDA antagonists or more subunit-selective competitive NMDA antagonists will have a satisfactory therapeutic/cognitive profile in focal or primary generalized epilepsy. The potential of AMPA/kainate antagonists as antiepileptic drugs remains to be evaluated in humans.

REFERENCES

Akiyama K, Daigen A, Yamada N, et al 1992 Long-lasting enhancement of metabotropic excitatory amino acid receptor-mediated polyphosphoinositide hydrolysis in the amygdala/pyriform cortex of deep prepiriform cortical kindled rats. Brain Res 569: 71–77

Amara S G, Kuhar M J 1993 Neurotransmitter transporters: recent progress. Annu Rev Neurosci 16: 73–93

Bisaga A, Krzascik P, Jankowska E et al 1993 Effect of glutamate receptor antagonists on N-methyl-D-aspartate- and (S)-α-amino-3-hydroxy-5-methyl-4-isoxazolepropionic acid-induced convulsant effects in mice and rats. Eur J Pharmacol 242: 213–220

Buller A L, Larson H C, Schneider B E, Beaton J A, Morrisett R A, Monaghan D T 1994 The molecular basis of NMDA receptor subtypes: native receptor diversity is predicted by subunit composition. J Neurosci 14: 5471–5484

Chapman A G 1991 Excitatory amino acid antagonists and therapy of epilepsy. In: Meldrum B S (ed) Excitatory amino acid antagonists. Blackwell Scientific Publications, Oxford, p 265

Chapman A G, Meldrum B S 1993 Excitatory amino acid antagonists and epilepsy. Biochem Soc Trans 21: 106–110

Chapman A G, Swan J H, Patel S, Graham J L, Meldrum B S 1990 Cerebroprotective and anticonvulsant action of competitive and non-competitive NMDA antagonists. In: Lubec G, Rosenthal G A (eds) Amino Acids. Chemistry, biology and medicine. ESCOM Scientific Publishers, Leiden, p 219

Chapman A G, Smith S E, Meldrum B S 1991 The anticonvulsant effect of the non-NMDA antagonists, NBQX and GYKI 52466, in mice. Epilepsy Res 9: 92–96

Chapman A G, Al-Zubaidy Z, Meldrum B S 1993 Aniracetam reverses the anticonvulsant action of NBQX and GYKI 52466 in DBA/2 mice. Eur J Pharmacol 231: 301–303

Chapman A G, Smith S E, Parvez N, Meldrum B S 1994a The effect of aniracetam and cyclothiazide on the anticonvulsant action of 4 AMPA antagonists in rodent seizure models. Br J Pharmacol 112:14

Chapman A G, Woodburn V L, Woodruff G N, Meldrum B S 1994b Anticonvulsant activity of NMDA-R1 antisense against sound-induced seizures in DBA/2 mice. Soc Neurosci Abstr 20: 172.17

Chapman A G, Millan M H, Kingsley C, Meldrum B S 1995a Anticonvulsant activity of a novel competitive NMDA antagonist, the S-enantiomer SDZ EAB 515. Br J Pharmacol (in press).

Chapman A G, Dürmüller N, Harrison B L, et al 1995b Anticonvulsant activity of a novel

NMDA/glycine site antagonist, MDL 104,653, against kindled and sound-induced seizures. Eur J Pharmacol (in press)

Cotterell K L, Croucher M J, Bradford H F 1992 Weak anticonvulsant activity of CGP 37849 and CGP 39551 against kindled seizures following systemic administration. Eur J Pharmacol 214: 285–287

Croucher M J, Bradford H F 1991 The influence of strychnine-insensitive glycine receptor agonists and antagonists on generalized seizure thresholds. Brain Res 543: 91–96

Croucher M J, Collins J F, Meldrum B S 1982 Anticonvulsant action of excitatory amino acid antagonists. Science 216: 899–901

Crowder J M, Bradford H F 1987 Common anticonvulsants inhibit Ca^{++} uptake and amino acid neurotransmitter release in vitro. Epilepsia 28: 378–382

Danbolt N C, Storm-Mathisen J, Kanner B I 1992 An [Na^{++} K^{+}] coupled L-glutamate transporter purified from rat brain is located in glial cell processes. Neuroscience 51: 295–310

Dingledine R, McBain C J, McNamara O 1990 Excitatory amino acid receptors in epilepsy. TIPS 11: 334–338

Do K Q, Klancnik J, Gähwiler B H, Perschak H, Wieser H G, Cuenod M 1991 Release of EAA: animal studies and epileptic foci studies in human. In: Meldrum B S, Moroni F, Simon R P, Woods J H (eds) Excitatory amino acids. Raven Press, New York, p 677

During M J, Spencer D D 1993 Extracellular hippocampal glutamate and spontaneous seizure in the conscious human brain. Lancet 341: 1607–1610

During M J, Mirchandani G R, Leone P et al 1993 Direct hippocampal injection of a HSV-1 vector expressing GLUR6 results in spontaneous seizures, hyperexcitability in CA1 cells and loss of CA1, hilar and CA3 neurons. Soc Neurosci Abstr 19: 16.4

Dürmüller N, Smith S E, Meldrum B S 1993 Proconvulsant and anticonvulsant effects of Evans blue dye in rodents. Neuroreport 4: 683–686

Dürmüller N, Craggs M, Meldrum B 1994 The effect of the non-NMDA antagonists GYKI 52466 and NBQX and the competitive NMDA receptor antagonist D-CPPene on the development of amygdala kindling and on amygdala-kindled seizures. Epilepsy Res 17: 167–174

Facchinetti F, Dall'Olio R, Ciani E et al 1994 Long-lasting effects of chronic neonatal blockade of N-methyl-D-aspartate receptor through the competitive antagonist CGP 39551 in rats. Neuroscience 60: 343–353

Fisher R S, Cysyk B J, Lesser R P et al 1990 Dextromethorphan for treatment of complex partial seizures. Neurology 40: 547–549

Goa K L, Ross S R, Chrisp P 1993 Lamotrigine: a review of its pharmacological properties and clinical efficacy in epilepsy. Drugs 46: 152–176

Hamm R J, Pike B R, O'Dell D M, Lyeth B G 1994 Traumatic brain injury enhances the amnesic effect of an NMDA antagonist in rats. J Neurosurg 81: 267–271

Hargreaves R J, Rigby M, Smith D, Hill R G 1993 Lack of effect of L-687,414 ((+)-cis-4-methyl-HA-966), an NMDA receptor antagonist acting at the glycine site, on cerebral glucose metabolism and cortical neuronal morphology. Br J Pharmacol 110: 36–42

Hollmann M, Heinemann S 1994 Cloned glutamate receptors. Annu Rev Neurosci 17: 31–108

Kamphuis W, De Rijk T C, Talamini L M, Lopes da Silva F H 1994 Rat hippocampal kindling induces changes in the glutamate receptor mRNA expression patterns in dentate granule neurons. Eur J Neurosci 6: 1119–1127

Kanai Y, Stelzner M, Nussberger S et al 1994 The neuronal and epithelial human high affinity glutamate transporter. Insights into structure and mechanism of transport. J Biol Chem 269: 20599–20606

Keller B U, Blaschke M, Rivosecchi R et al 1993 Identification of a subunit-specific antagonist of α-amino-3-hydroxy-5-methyl-4-isoxazolepropionate/kainate receptor channels. Proc Natl Acad Sci USA 90: 605–609

Kemp J A, Leeson P D 1993 The glycine site of the NMDA receptor — Five years on. TIPS 14: 20–25

Kraus J E, Yeh G-C, Bonhaus D W et al 1994 Kindling induces the long-lasting expression of a novel population of NMDA receptors in hippocampal region CA3. J Neurosci 14: 4196–4205

Kristensen J D, Svensson B, Gordh T Jr 1992 The NMDA-receptor antagonist CPP abolishes neurogenic 'wind-up pain' after intrathecal administration in humans. Pain 51: 249–253

Laurie D J, Seeburg P H 1994 Ligand affinities at recombinant N-methyl-D-aspartate receptors depend on subunit composition. Eur J Pharmacol Mol Pharmacol 268: 335–345

Lee S, Miskovsky J, Williamson J et al 1994 Changes in glutamate receptor and proenkephalin gene expression after kindled seizures. Mol Brain Res 24: 34–42

Lipton S A 1993 Prospects for clinically tolerated NMDA antagonists: open-channel blockers and alternative redox states of nitric oxide. TINS 16: 527–532

Löscher W, Hönack D 1991 Responses to NMDA receptor antagonists altered by epileptogenesis. TIPS 12: 52

Löscher W, Rundfeldt C, Hönack D 1993 Pharmacological characterization of phenytoin-resistant amygdala-kindled rats, a new model of drug-resistant partial epilepsy. Epilepsy Res 15: 207–219

Louvel J, Pumain R 1991 N-methyl-D-aspartate-mediated responses in epileptic cortex in man: an in vitro study. In: Engel J (ed) Neurotransmitters, seizures and epilepsy IV. Demos, New York, p 487

Lynch D R, Anegawa N J, Verdoorn T, Pritchett D B 1994 N-methyl-D-aspartate receptors: different subunit requirements for binding of glutamate antagonists, glycine antagonists, and channel-blocking agents. Mol Pharmacol 45: 540–545

McCabe R T, Wasterlain C G, Kucharczyk N et al 1993 Evidence for anticonvulsant and neuroprotectant action of felbamate mediated by strychnine-insensitive glycine receptors. J Pharmacol Exp Ther 264: 1248–1252

Macdonald R L 1983 Mechanisms of anticonvulsant drug action. In: Pedley T A, Meldrum B S (eds) Recent advances in epilepsy, vol. 1. Churchill Livingstone, Edinburgh, p 1

McNamara J O 1994 Cellular and molecular basis of epilepsy. J Neurosci 14: 3413–3425

Marescaux C, Vergnes M, Depaulis A, Micheletti G, Warter J M 1990 Neurotransmission in rats' spontaneous generalized nonconvulsive epilepsy. In: Avanzini G (ed) Neurotransmitters in epilepsy. Demos, New York, p 453

Meldrum B S 1994 The role of glutamate in epilepsy and other CNS disorders. Neurology 44 suppl (in press)

Meldrum B S, Chapman A G 1994 Competitive NMDA antagonists as drugs. In: Watkins J C, Collingridge G L (eds) The NMDA receptor. IRL press, Oxford, p 455

Meldrum B, Leach M 1994 The mechanisms of action of lamotrigine. Rev Contemp Pharmacother 5: 107–114

Meldrum B S, Millan M H, Obrenovitch T P 1992 Excitatory amino acid release induced by injury. In: Dietrich W D, Globus M Y-T (eds) The role of neurotransmitters in brain injury. Plenum Press, New York, p 1

Miller A A, Sawyer D A, Roth B et al 1986 Lamotrigine. In: Meldrum B S, Porter R J (eds) New anticonvulsant drugs. John Libbey, London, p 165

Minamoto Y, Itano T, Tokuda M et al 1992 In vivo microdialysis of amino acid neurotransmitters in the hippocampus in amygdaloid kindled rat. Brain Res 573: 345–348

Mody I, Heinemann U 1987 NMDA receptors of dentate gyrus granule cells participate in synaptic transmission following kindling. Nature 326: 701–704

Monyer H, Sprengel R, Schoepfer R et al 1992 Heteromeric NMDA receptors: molecular and functional distinction of subtypes. Science 256: 1217–1221

Nakanishi S 1992 Molecular diversity of glutamate receptors and implications for brain function. Science 258: 597–603

Namba T, Morimoto K, Sato K et al 1994 Antiepileptogenic and anticonvulsant effects of NBQX, a selective AMPA receptor antagonist, in the rat kindling model of epilepsy. Brain Res 638: 36–44

Nicholls D, Attwell D 1990 The release and uptake of excitatory amino acids. TIPS 11: 462–468

Nichols A C, Yielding K L 1993 Anticonvulsant activity of antagonists for the NMDA-associated glycine binding site. Mol Chem Neuropathol 19: 269–282

O'Donnell R A, Miller A A 1991 The effect of lamotrigine upon development of cortical kindled seizures in the rat. Neuropharmacology 30: 253–258

Palmer K J, McTavish D 1993 Felbamate: a review of its pharmacodynamic and pharmacokinetic properties, and therapeutic efficacy in epilepsy. Drugs 45: 1041–1065

Palmer G C, Murray R J, Wilson T C M et al 1992 Biological profile of the metabolites and potential metabolites of the anticonvulsant remacemide. Epilepsy Res 12: 9–20

Patel S, Chapman A G, Graham J L et al 1990 Anticonvulsant activity of the NMDA antagonists, D(-)4-(3-phosphonopropyl)piperazine-2-carboxylic acid (D-CPP) and D(-)(E)-4-(3-phosphonoprop-2-enyl)piperazine-2-carboxylic acid (D-CPPene) in a rodent and a primate model of reflex epilepsy. Epilepsy Res 7: 3–10

Patneau D K, Mayer M L 1991 Kinetic analysis of interactions between kainate and AMPA: evidence for activation of a single receptor in mouse hippocampal neurons. Neuron 6: 785–798

Peeters B W M M, Ramakers G M J, Ellenbroek B A et al 1994 Interactions between NMDA and nonNMDA receptors in nonconvulsive epilepsy in the WAG/Rij inbred strain. Brain Res Bull 33: 715–718

Pellegrini-Giampietro D E, Pulsinelli W A, Zukin R S 1994 NMDA and non-NMDA receptor gene expression following global brain ischemia in rats: effect of NMDA and non-NMDA receptor antagonists. J Neurochem 62: 1067–1073

Perez-Velazquez J L, Zhang L 1994 In vitro hypoxia induces expression of the NR2C subunit of the NMDA receptor in rat cortex and hippocampus. J Neurochem 63: 1171–1173

Pollard H, Héron A, Moreau J et al 1993 Alterations of the GluR-B AMPA receptor subunit flip/flop expression in kainate-induced epilepsy and ischemia. Neuroscience 57: 545–554

Pratt G D, Kokaia M 1994 In situ hybridization and its application to receptor subunit mRNA regulation. TIPS 15: 131–135

Pratt G D, Kokaia M, Bengzon J et al 1993 Differential regulation of N-methyl-D-aspartate receptor subunit messenger RNAs in kindling-induced epileptogenesis. Neuroscience 57: 307–318

Pumain R, Louvel J, Gastard M et al 1992 Responses to N-methyl-D-aspartate are enhanced in rats with petit mal-like seizures. J Neural Transm 35 (suppl): 97–108

Racine R J 1972 Modification of seizure activity by electrical stimulation: II. Motor seizure. Electroencephalogr Clin Neurophysiol 32: 281–294

Ramakers G M J, Peeters B W M M, Vossen J M H, Coenen A M L 1991 CNQX, a new non-NMDA receptor antagonist, reduces spike wave discharges in the WAG/Rij rat model of absence epilepsy. Epilepsy Res 9: 127–131

Rogawski M A 1992 The NMDA receptor, NMDA antagonists and epilepsy therapy: a status report. Drugs 44: 279–292

Rogawski M A 1993 Therapeutic potential of excitatory amino acid antagonists: channel blockers and 2,3-benzodiazepines. TIPS 14: 325–331

Rogawski M A, Porter R J 1990 Antiepileptic drugs: pharmacological mechanisms and clinical efficacy with consideration of promising developmental stage compounds. Pharmacol Rev 42: 223–270

Ronne-Engström E, Hillered L, Flink R et al 1992 Intracerebral microdialysis of extracellular amino acids in the human epileptic focus. J Cereb Blood Flow Metab 12: 873–876

Rundfeldt C, Wlaz P, Löscher W 1994 Anticonvulsant activity of antagonists and partial agonists for the NMDA receptor-associated glycine site in the kindling model of epilepsy. Brain Res 653: 125–130

Sacaan A I, Schoepp D D 1992 Activation of hippocampal metabotropic excitatory amino acid receptors leads to seizures and neuronal damage. Neurosci Lett 139: 77–82

Saugstad J A, Kinzie J M, Mulvihill E R et al 1994 Cloning and expression of a new member of the L-2-amino-4-phosphonobutyric acid-sensitive class of metabotropic glutamate receptors. Mol Pharmacol 45: 367–372

Saywell K, Singh L, Oles R J et al 1991 The anticonvulsant properties in the mouse of the glycine/NMDA receptor antagonist, L-687,414. Br J Pharmacol 102: 66P

Schoepp D D, Conn P J 1993 Metabotropic glutamate receptors in brain function and pathology. TIPS 14: 13–20

Seeburg P H 1993 The TINS/TiPS lecture: The molecular biology of mammalian glutamate receptor channels. TINS 16: 359–365

Skerritt J H, Johnston G A R 1984 Modulation of excitant amino acid release by convulsant and anticonvulsant drugs. In: Fariello R, Morselli P L, Lloyd K G, Quesney L F, Engel J (eds) Neurotransmitters, seizures and epilepsy, Vol. II. Raven Press, New York, p 215

Skolnick P, Marvizón J C G, Jackson B W et al 1989 Blockade of N-methyl-D-aspartate induced convulsions by 1-aminocyclopropanecarboxylates. Life Sci 45: 1647–1655

Smith S E, Chapman A G 1993 Acute and chronic anticonvulsant effects of D(-)CPPene in genetically epilepsy-prone rats. Epilepsy Res 15: 193–199

Smith S E, Meldrum B S 1992 The glycine-site NMDA receptor antagonist, R-(+)-cis-B-methyl-3-amino-1-hydroxypyrrolid-2-one, L-687,414 is anticonvulsant in baboons. Eur J Pharmacol 211: 109–111

Smith S E, Dürmüller N, Meldrum B S 1991 The non-N-methyl-D-aspartate antagonists, GYKI 52466 and NBQX are anticonvulsant in two animal models of reflex epilepsy. Eur J Pharmacol 201: 179–183

Steinberg G K, Perez-Pinzon M A, Maier C M et al 1994 CGS-19755: Correlation of in vitro neuroprotection, protection against experimental ischemia and CSF levels in cerebrovascular surgery patients. In: Fifth International Symposium on Pharmacology of Cerebral Ischemia.

Stewart L, Bullock R, Jones M et al 1993 The cerebral haemodynamic and metabolic effects of the competitive NMDA antagonist CGS 19755 in humans with severe head injury. International Neurotrauma Symposium 1: 76

Sveinbjornsdottir S, Sander J W A S, Upton D et al 1993 The excitatory amino acid antagonist D-CPP-ene (SDZ EAA-494) in patients with epilepsy. Epilepsy Res 16: 165–174

Swinyard E A, Sofia R D, Kupferberg H J 1986 Comparative anticonvulsant activity and neurotoxicity of felbamate and four prototype antiepileptic drugs in mice and rats. Epilepsia 27: 27–34

Thomsen C, Klitgaard H, Sheardown M et al 1994 (S)-4-carboxy-3-hydroxyphenylglycine, an antagonist of metabotropic glutamate receptor (mGluR)1a and an agonist of mGluR2, protects against audiogenic seizures in DBA/2 mice. J Neurochem 62: 2492–2495

Troupin A S, Mendius J R, Cheng F, Risinger M W 1986 MK-801. In: Meldrum B S, Porter R J (eds) New anticonvulsant drugs. Current problems in epilepsy, vol. 4. John Libbey, London, p 191

Vergnes M, Marescaux C, Depaulis A, Micheletti G, Warter J M 1990 Spontaneous spike-and-wave discharges in Wistar rats: a model of genetic generalized nonconvulsive epilepsy. In: Avoli M, Gloor P, Kostopoulos G, Naquet R (eds) Generalized epilepsy: cellular, molecular, and pharmacological approaches. Birkhauser Boston, Boston, p 238

Vyklicky L Jr, Patneau D K, Mayer M L 1991 Modulation of excitatory synaptic transmission by drugs that reduce desensitization at AMPA/kainate receptors. Neuron 7: 971–984

Watkins J C, Evans R H 1981 Excitatory amino acid transmitters. Annu Rev Pharmacol Toxicol 21: 165–204

Weber E 1993 In vitro and in vivo pharmacology of a novel glycine site NMDA antagonist. In: Symposium on the glycine binding site of the NMDA receptor: molecular pharmacology and therapeutic implications

Westbrook G L 1994 Glutamate receptor update. Curr Opin Neurobiol 4: 337–346

White H S, Wolf H H, Swinyard E A et al 1992 A neuropharmacological evaluation of felbamate as a novel anticonvulsant. Epilepsia 33: 564–572

Willetts J, Balster R L, Leander J D 1990 The behavioral pharmacology of NMDA receptor antagonists. TIPS 11: 423–428

Williams K 1993 Ifenprodil discriminates subtypes of the N-methyl-D-aspartate receptor: selectivity and mechanisms at recombinant heteromeric receptors. Mol Pharmacol 44: 851–859

Wong M-L, Smith M A, Licinio J et al 1993 Differential effects of kindled and electrically induced seizures on a glutamate receptor (GluR1) gene expression. Epilepsy Res 14: 221–227

Wood P L, Rao T S, Iyengar S et al 1990 A review of the in vitro and in vivo neurochemical characterization of the NMDA/PCP/glycine/ion channel receptor macrocomplex. Neurochem Res 15: 217-230

Yamaguchi S, Donevan S D, Rogawski M A 1993 Anticonvulsant activity of AMPA/kainate antagonists: comparison of GYKI 52466 and NBQX in maximal electroshock and chemoconvulsant seizure models. Epilepsy Res 15: 179–184

Yamakura T, Mori H, Masaki H et al 1993 Different sensitivities of NMDA receptor channel subtypes to non-competitive antagonists. Neuroreport 4: 687–690

Zhang W Q, Hudson P M, Sobotka T J et al 1991 Extracellular concentrations of amino acid transmitters in ventral hippocampus during and after the development of kindling. Brain Res 540: 315–318

2

Magnetic resonance spectroscopy (MRS) in epilepsy

A. Connelly   J. S. Duncan

In the initial section we shall describe the principles, techniques, scope and limitations of in vivo magnetic resonance spectroscopy (MRS) as applied to the investigation of epilepsy. We will then review the information that may be derived regarding the neurobiology of the condition and the role of MRS in the clinical investigation and management of patients with epilepsy.

IN VIVO MRS: BACKGROUND

Nuclear magnetic resonance (NMR) began as a spectroscopic technique, and has been one of the most powerful analytical tools (particularly in the field of chemistry) over several decades. In medicine, NMR has become familiar through the more recent development of magnetic resonance imaging (MRI). The fundamental theory is the same for both techniques, since they each depend on the same nuclear properties and interactions.

Chemical shift

In NMR, the resonance frequency of a nucleus is dependent on the magnetic field strength experienced by that nucleus. In practice, this is dominated by the applied static magnetic field which, in most in vivo MRS studies in humans, will be 1.5 T or greater. The application of additional linear magnetic field gradients (i.e. magnetic fields whose strength varies with spatial position) can be used to make the total magnetic field experienced by a collection of nuclei dependent on their position within such a field. This, in turn, means that their resonance frequencies are spatially dependent. In this manner, in imaging, *frequency* is used to provide *spatial* information.

In the absence of such externally applied gradient fields, similar nuclei do not necessarily experience the same field strength, even in a homogeneous applied field. This is due to the fact that nuclei are surrounded by electrons which also experience the applied magnetic field, causing them to circulate and, in turn, to produce a second magnetic field in the opposite direction to the applied field. The magnetic field actually experienced by a nucleus is therefore a combination of the applied field and that produced by the surrounding electrons. As a result, the effective field at a nucleus (and therefore the resonance frequency of that nucleus) is different in different chemical environments. The magnitude of the frequency shift is proportional to the applied field strength. This effect is known as the chemical shift. In spectroscopy, therefore, *frequency* is used to provide *chemical* information, by means of this chemical shift. Such information is usually displayed in the form of a spectrum, which consists of a plot or graph of signal amplitude against frequency (see Fig. 2.3 below) and, in which, the area under a spectral line indicates the signal intensity at that frequency.

Signal intensity

NMR is inherently an insensitive technique, and is limited by signal-to-noise considerations. The amount of signal available is crucially dependent on the type of nucleus involved. Not all nuclei are NMR-active; for example, the most abundant isotopes of carbon and oxygen (namely ^{12}C and ^{16}O) are NMR-inactive. Only those nuclei which have non-zero nuclear spin angular momentum will give rise to an NMR signal, and these nuclei vary enormously in sensitivity. Those which have been used in a biological context include ^{1}H, ^{31}P, ^{13}C, ^{19}F, and ^{23}Na, but the most widely studied nuclei for in vivo spectroscopy are ^{1}H and ^{31}P.

The intensity of the NMR signal available from a particular type of nucleus is dependent primarily on the strength of the applied magnetic field (signal-to-noise is approximately linearly proportional to the field strength for in vivo examinations) and on a property of the nucleus known as the magnetogyric ratio. The larger this constant, the higher the signal from any individual nucleus. Each element, and each isotope of a given element, has a different magnetogyric ratio associated with the nucleus. The hydrogen nucleus, which consists of a single proton (hence the term proton NMR, commonly applied to the study of ^{1}H), has the highest magnetogyric ratio of all nuclei, with the exception of the non-naturally occurring isotope of hydrogen, tritium.

A second important factor which determines the strength of an NMR signal is the number of nuclei within the field of view of the receiver coil which contribute to the signal acquired. This is influenced primarily by three factors:

1. The concentration of the substance containing the nuclei concerned.
2. The size of the volume from which signal is acquired.
3. The natural abundance of the NMR-active isotope of the element of interest.

In studies of chemical preparations, the dependence on the first point above can frequently be dealt with by increasing the concentration of the compound of interest. In human biological studies, however, the concentrations of substances within the body are largely predefined, and, indeed, it is most likely to be this parameter which we would like to determine in disease states.

For a given concentration, the number of nuclei which can potentially contribute to the NMR signal is determined by the size of the volume from which signal is obtained (see later section on volume localization). Signal strength is therefore linearly related to volume size for a homogeneously distributed substance (with the condition that any increase in the excited volume is within the field of view of the receiver coil).

The nuclei of some elements which are potentially interesting biologically do not give sufficient signal to be studied routinely in vivo due to low natural abundance of the NMR-active isotope. For example, carbon is widely distributed throughout the body, but the main isotope of carbon (^{12}C) is NMR-inactive, while the NMR-active nucleus (^{13}C) constitutes only 1.1% of natural carbon, resulting in very low sensitivity.

Both ^{1}H and ^{31}P are of high natural abundance (99.98 and 100% respectively), relatively high sensitivity (although the sensitivity of phosphorus is only 1/15th that of hydrogen, it is still one of the more sensitive nuclei), and are present in sufficiently high concentrations in compounds that are of metabolic interest in vivo. These characteristics have resulted in the increasingly widespread use of these two nuclei for the study of in vivo metabolites, although the lower sensitivity of ^{31}P necessitates the use of larger volumes of tissue (and thus lower spatial resolution of metabolic information) than for ^{1}H MRS.

Signal-to-noise ratio

When an NMR signal is acquired, background radiofrequency noise is also acquired, even if all externally generated signals are excluded by housing the scanner in a radiofrequency-screened room. The dominant sources of noise in vivo are the radiofrequency coil and the patients themselves — the former due to coil resistance and the latter due to the fact that current flow within a conducting sample constitutes an additional resistance.

In order to detect NMR signals generated by metabolites, it is necessary to distinguish them from background noise. If the signal intensity is insufficient to allow identification of metabolite peaks, the signal-to-noise ratio can be improved by time averaging, i.e. repeatedly acquiring data under the same conditions. The NMR signal increases linearly with the number of repetitions. The noise, however, is random, and increases only as the square root of the number of scans. Thus, overall, the signal-to-noise increases as the square root of the number of signal averages.

The inefficiency of time averaging as a means of increasing signal-to-noise is a major factor in determining what is possible practically in vivo. For example, if an acquisition volume is decreased by a factor of 2 in each linear dimension (i.e. an eightfold decrease in volume) in order to increase spatial resolution, the signal amplitude will also decrease by a factor of 8. However, the noise detected by the receiver coil will be unaffected by the change in size of the selected volume, resulting in an overall decrease in signal-to-noise by a factor of 8. In order to recover the original signal-to-noise ratio by time-averaging, an increase in the experiment time by a factor of 64 would be necessary (i.e. number of averages $= 8^2$), which would be prohibitive in all but the most unusual circumstances.

In vivo MRS: detectable metabolites

The brain metabolites which are present at sufficiently high concentrations to give usable signal in vivo include the following:

For ^{31}P MRS, the metabolites used in epilepsy studies have included adenosine triphosphate (ATP), phosphomonoesters (PME), phosphodiesters (PDE), phosphocreatine (PCr), and inorganic phosphate (P_i). The last of these, P_i, has the useful NMR property of having a chemical shift which is pH-dependent. This is due to the fact that inorganic phosphate exists mainly as HPO_4 and H_2PO_4 at neutral pH. The chemical shift of these two species differs by approximately 2.4 p.p.m. In solution, however, rapid exchange between the two results in only a single resonance being detected, the resonance frequency of which is determined by the relative amounts of each species present. This equilibrium is dependent on the concentration of H^+ ions. Thus, the effective chemical shift of P_i reflects the pH of the local environment.

For ^1H MRS, the metabolites which are detectable are determined in part by the conditions used for acquisition. Some molecules, such as γ-aminobutyric acid (GABA), glutamate, glutamine and lactate, give rise to NMR signals which exhibit what is known as spin-spin coupling, which results in multiplet signals which are modulated with time. Thus, the appearance of their resonance lines is very dependent on the acquisition conditions used, in particular the echo time. Specifically, the detection of GABA in vivo has been shown to be facilitated by the use of spectral editing techniques (Rothman et al 1993). In epilepsy studies in vivo, the main signals of interest have been those from N-acetyl aspartate (NAA, 2.01 p.p.m.), creatine + phosphocreatine (Cr, 3.0 p.p.m), choline-containing compounds (Cho, 3.2 p.p.m.), and lactate (Lac, doublet signal centred at 1.35 p.p.m.). Several lines of evidence, including cell culture studies (Urenjak et al 1992, 1993), have indicated that NAA is located primarily within neurons (although it is also present in oligodendrocyte-type-2-astrocyte (O-2-A) progenitor cells, which are precursor cells). A reduction of the NAA signal is frequently interpreted, therefore, as reflecting loss or dysfunction of neurons. Such a reduction in NAA has been found in practice in many cases where neuronal loss would be expected clinically, such as in infarcts, tumours or in epilepsy. Cr and Cho are found both in neurons and in glial cells, although cell studies suggest that they are present at higher concentrations in glia (Urenjak et al 1993).

Volume localization

The acquisition of spectroscopic data in vivo is of limited use in most studies unless the spatial origin of the signals obtained is known. It is necessary, therefore, to limit the extent of the volume from which signal is acquired and to relate this volume to the anatomy of the region under investigation.

The most widely used class of localization methods is that in which amplitude and/or phase-modulated radiofrequency pulses are used in conjunction with linear magnetic field gradients. Such methods have great flexibility in terms of the positioning of a volume for signal acquisition, and are readily combined with imaging methods to provide good anatomical information for volume location. In using such methods, two distinct approaches have been used:

1. Single-voxel techniques, in which data are acquired from a single volume of interest (usually in the form of a cube of the order of 8 ml volume for ^{1}H or 60–100 ml volume for ^{31}P).
2. Chemical shift imaging (CSI) (also known as magnetic resonance spectroscopic imaging; MRSI) in which a large region is excited before spatially encoding the metabolite signals using phase-encoding gradients in a manner similar to MRI. In this way the equivalent of many single voxels can be acquired simultaneously instead of sequentially, and the increase in efficiency can be used to obtain smaller voxels (of the order of 1–2 ml for ^{1}H or 25 ml for ^{31}P) than by single-voxel methods.

Single-voxel localization

Most localized in vivo MRS to date has been done using single-voxel methods. Of these, three techniques in particular have found widespread use, all of which select cubic volumes by the use of three intersecting orthogonal slices. These are:

1. Image-related in vivo spectroscopy (ISIS).
2. Spin echo (SE; 90°–180°–180°–acquire).
3. Stimulated echo (STE; 90°–90°–90°–acquire).

ISIS (Ordidge et al 1986), works on a different principle to the other two methods above. It was designed primarily for performing phosphorus spectroscopy, in which restrictions are imposed by the short T_2 relaxation times of phosphorus metabolites, together with the effects of spin-spin coupling. Because of this, the localized magnetization is prepared in the longitudinal direction by inversion pulses (thus avoiding T_2 relaxation, other than during the rf pulses) before excitation with a single read-out pulse. A scheme of eight additions and subtractions is necessary to eliminate unwanted signals and effect localization in three dimensions. The main drawbacks of the ISIS method are the need for eight cycles to achieve localization, and the potential for subtraction errors when localizing to a small volume in the presence of a large surrounding signal. The latter problem has been reduced by the use of presaturation pulses in a later variant of the method, known as OSIRIS (outer-volume suppressed image related in-vivo spectroscopy) (Connelly et al 1988).

The two echo methods (points 2 and 3 above) have been applied extensively in the study of ^{1}H MRS. Both rely on the application of an initial shaped 90° radiofrequency pulse in the presence of a magnetic field gradient to achieve the selective excitation of a slice in a manner identical to that used in MRI. This is followed by the application of two further radiofrequency pulses in the presence of gradients in the other two spatial orientations to refocus only the spins in a cube at the intersection of all three slices. In the case of the SE method (Ordidge et al 1985), pulses 2 and 3 are 180° pulses, whereas the equivalent pulses for an STE are 90° pulses (Frahm et al 1989).

It is helpful to consider the practical consequences of the use of one or other of the echo localization methods. The STE method uses only half of the signal initially excited, whereas the SE method refocuses all of the available signal. Therefore, for the same echo time and acquisition conditions, the SE would, in theory, give twice as much signal as an STE. In the STE method, the echo time (TE) can be kept very short, with the middle time period (TM; i.e. the time between pulses 2 and 3, which does not contribute to TE) used for some of the essential switching of magnetic field gradients. All time periods contribute to TE in the case of a SE, and it is therefore more difficult to achieve such short TE values. Short TE is desirable for the detection of metabolites which have either short T_2 relaxation times or which, through spin-spin coupling, produce complex resonances which become modulated (and therefore more complex) with increasing TE. Thus, as a general rule, STE localization is best suited to achieving short TEs, while the increased signal available from an SE becomes more important at longer TE values.

Chemical shift imaging

As an alternative to the sequential excitation of (and data collection from) a series of individual voxels, it is possible to select a large region of the brain equivalent to many single voxels, and to produce spatial information within such a region by means of pulsed magnetic field gradients (Kumar et al 1975, Brown et al 1982, Maudsley et al 1983; see Fig. 2.1 for an example of the result of such a process). The volume excited can take the form of a single slab of tissue of the order of 1–2 cm thick, within which two dimensional spatial encoding is used to produce voxels of 1–2 ml volume; or the CSI volume can be a larger volume, requiring three-dimensional spatial encoding to produce similar voxel sizes, but which can provide information on metabolite distributions over a greater region of the brain.

Spatial encoding of the spectral information obtained from such large volumes is achieved by a method known as *phase encoding* (which is also used to produce one dimension of spatial information in conventional MRI). A

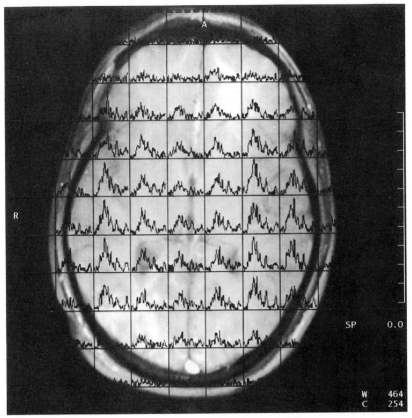

Fig. 2.1   A Example of a ^{31}P two-dimensional chemical shift imaging dataset (16 × 16 matrix), where each voxel has dimensions 25 × 25 × 40 mm. **A** shows a transverse ^{1}H anatomical image on which the 16 × 16 matrix of ^{31}P spectra has been superimposed, indicating the anatomical locations from which the ^{31}P spectra were acquired. The total acquisition time was 25 min. **B** shows an example of an individual spectrum, together with a schematic indication of its spatial location. The spectrum shows peaks corresponding to phosphomonoesters (PME), inorganic phosphate (P_i), phosphodiesters (PDE), phosphocreatine (PCR) and adenosine triphosphate (ATP). Courtesy of Dr R Sauter, Siemens, Erlangen.

pulsed magnetic field gradient is used during a time period prior to acquisition to produce a phase shift in the data whose magnitude for any given nucleus depends on the spatial location of that nucleus. The gradient has to be stepped through n different values to produce n spatial data points in any individual direction. Thus, for a slab of tissue, to divide the region into $n \times n$ voxels, n phase encoding steps are required in each of two gradient directions (i.e. a total of $n \times n$ gradient steps). To extend the spatial information into a third dimension, such that the volume is divided into $n \times n \times m$ voxels, would require a further m gradient steps in the remaining direction. Since each of these gradient steps requires $1 \times \text{TR}$ (the repetition time), where TR is of the order of 1.5–2 s, the overall time required for a CSI volume is long.

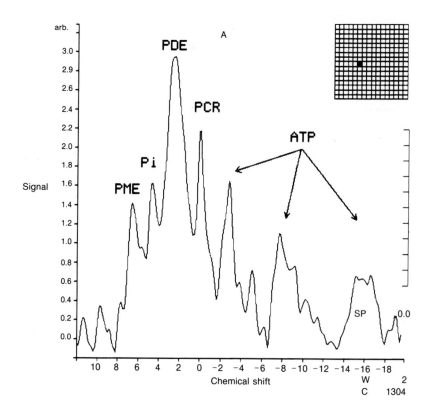

Fig. 2.1B   See previous page for caption.

However, since the whole volume is sampled each time, it is a very efficient means of data acquisition, and enables the maximum amount of metabolic information to be obtained in a given time.

MRS IN VIVO IN EPILEPSY

MRI is increasingly able to identify the anatomical abnormalities that frequently underlie partial seizure disorders, particularly hippocampal sclerosis, small discrete structural lesions such as cavernomas and areas of cortical dysplasia that have not been visualized previously (Bergen et al 1989, Brooks et al 1990, Cook et al 1992, Jackson et al 1993a, 1993b). Accurate definition of brain anatomy and the identification of regions of pathology using MRI are necessary for the adequate interpretation of functional imaging studies, such as positron emission tomography (PET) and single-photon emission computed tomography (SPECT). Such structural information is also invaluable to MRS, which has the important advantage that it can be performed with MRI in a single session. In vivo MRS investigations in epilepsy to date have focused on the use of the nuclei ^{31}P and ^{1}H, and have been largely directed at the temporal lobes of patients with intractable epilepsy in whom surgical treatment is under consideration.

^{31}P spectroscopy

PET studies have demonstrated interictal hypometabolism in the region of epileptogenic tissue in partial epilepsy (Engel et al 1982). Several studies have shown that in animal models induced epileptic seizures can produce marked changes in energy metabolism and tissue pH (Siesjö 1978, Chapman 1985). ^{31}P MRS provides the potential to measure non-invasively the levels within the brain of compounds related to high-energy phosphate metabolism and phospholipid metabolism such as ATP, PCr, PME, PDE, and P_i. It also provides a non-invasive indicator of tissue pH via the chemical shift of P_i (see earlier section). For these reasons, ^{31}P MRS has been used in several recent clinical studies to investigate the possibility of detecting metabolic abnormalities associated with seizure foci, with a view to providing lateralizing information.

Laxer et al (1992) obtained ^{31}P spectra from 84–105 ml volumes in the anterior temporal lobes of 8 patients with hippocampal sclerosis and complex partial seizures using a 2 T system. Spatial localization of the phophorus signals was achieved using the ISIS technique. The results showed no significant asymmetries between ipsilateral and contralateral temporal lobes of the concentrations of ATP, PCr or PDE. In 7 of the 8 patients, the temporal lobe ipsilateral to the focus had increased pH (mean in all 8 patients of 7.25 versus 7.08) and, in all 8, increased P_i (mean 1.9 versus 1.1 mmol/l). There was a trend towards decreased PME, although this was not statistically significant. No significant side-to-side asymmetries were noted in 8 normal subjects. There was no apparent relationship between the pH and P_i levels and severity of abnormality shown by MRI.

Since the spatial resolution of the above study was very limited and tissue heterogeneity could be a complicating factor in interpretation of the results, the same group later studied 8 epilepsy patients (7 temporal, 1 frontal) using ^{31}P CSI, with an effective voxel size of 25 cm^3, enabling more precise identification of regions of interest (Hugg et al 1992). The same lateralizing abnormalities were found; namely increased P_i, decreased PME and increased pH (7.17 ipsilateral versus 7.06 contralateral, $P<0.01$). Using the same methods, the side-to-side asymmetry of all metabolites intensities in a normal population was less than 10%. In a later study of 8 patients with frontal lobe epilepsy, increased pH in all 8 and decreased PME in 7 patients were found in the epileptogenic frontal lobes, but no alterations in P_i levels were detected (Garcia et al 1994).

Kuzniecky et al (1992) used a 1.5 T MR system to obtain ^{31}P spectra from single voxels of 72–100 cm^3 in 7 patients with temporal lobe epilepsy and 5 control subjects. In contrast to the above investigations, this study found no statistically significant difference in the pH measured in the ipsilateral and contralateral temporal lobes. However, the pH values measured were 7.11 (ipsilateral) and 7.05 (contralateral), which are similar in direction if not significance to those described above, although it should be noted that it is the *ipsilateral* value which is closer to that measured in controls (control pH 7.12). (Of the work mentioned above, only the frontal lobe study (Garcia et al 1994) quoted a control value for pH, and this was similar to the contralateral value.) No changes in the levels of PME were reported by Kuzniecky et al. The PCr/P_i ratios were found to be lower in the ipsilateral than the contralateral temporal lobe of the patients, and both sides were lower than the control data. This appears consistent with the above studies of Laxer et al and Hugg et al in that each of these two studies reported an increase in P_i with no change in PCr (giving a decrease in PCr/P_i). However, it should be noted that Kuzniecky et al interpreted this change differently in terms of a decrease in PCr, although they did not report intensity levels for individual metabolites.

The pathophysiological significance of the above results is unclear at present, although some attempts have been made to explain the findings. It has been suggested (Hugg et al 1992) that a decrease in PME may reflect altered metabolism associated with neuronal cell loss and glial proliferation, both of which are associated with hippocampal sclerosis and cortical lesions, although the data provide no direct evidence of this.

All of the above studies found a higher pH on the ipsilateral side compared to the contralateral side. In the case of Kuzniecky et al this difference was not found to be statistically significant, while the other three studies reported a higher ipsilateral pH that was statistically significant. However, all of these studies involved very small numbers of patients, and neither Laxer et al nor Hugg et al reported control pH values. Kuzniecky et al found that the higher ipsilateral pH values were close to control measurements (with the contralateral pH values lower), while Garcia et al reported that, in the frontal lobe, the contralateral pH corresponded with their control values. It would appear, therefore, that the evidence for a focal increase in pH in the location of a seizure focus is equivocal at present, and that more work in this area is necessary on larger groups of both patients and controls.

If verified, the neurobiological significance of an increase in pH associated with an epileptic focus is uncertain, particularly since seizure activity has been shown to produce acidosis. Hugg et al (1992) have suggested that an increase in pH might be explained in terms of an adaptation in brain buffering in response to repeated acidotic episodes associated with seizures, but there is no direct evidence for this.

In several of the studies quoted above, ^{31}P MRS appeared to be superior to MRI in determining the laterality of the epileptic focus. However, the specific MRI methods and analysis used were not described, and MRI methods that reliably detect mesial temporal abnormalities in epilepsy (which had previously proved difficult to visualize) have been reported recently (Jack et al 1990, 1992, Cook et al 1992, Jackson et al 1993a, 1993b). Therefore, such comparative findings should be treated with caution at present. Nevertheless, the ^{31}P MRS technique yields potentially very useful data which will be enhanced by technological developments such as the use of improved radiofrequency coils, particularly double-tuned coils which would allow ^{1}H imaging and ^{31}P spectroscopy to be carried out in the same examination without changing coils. This would be both more convenient practically and also enable simpler anatomical localization of the spectra. Future studies will need to compare ^{31}P MRS data with optimal MRI and address the question of whether CSI can make a useful contribution to the precise localization of epileptic foci in addition to lateralization.

Proton (^{1}H) spectroscopy

Accumulation of cerebral lactate has been shown by ^{1}H MRS in rabbits after bicuculline-induced status epilepticus (Petroff et al 1986). Matthews et al (1990) reported reduced NAA in the temporal lobes of 2 patients with Rasmussen's encephalitis, and focally increased lactate in 1 of the patients, who had epilepsia partialis continua. As described earlier, several lines of evidence suggest that reduced signal from NAA reflects neuronal loss or dysfunction. Proton spectroscopy has a greater signal-to-noise ratio and better spatial resolution than ^{31}P MRS and is more easily integrated with MRI in a single examination. Taken together, these data suggest a role for ^{1}H spectroscopy in the clinical investigation of epilepsy.

In a series of 82 paediatric and adult patients with a variety of seizure disorders, localized water-suppressed spectra were obtained, on a 1.5 T system, from $2 \times 2 \times 2$ cm voxels placed individually in the left and right medial temporal lobes, including part of the hippocampus, together with temporal white matter and neocortical grey matter (Fig. 2.2; Gadian et al 1994). Localization was achieved using an SE sequence, with an echo time of 135 ms. Signal intensities at 2.0 p.p.m. (NAA), 3.0 p.p.m. (Cr) and 3.2 p.p.m. (Cho) were identified on spectra and the areas under the peaks were measured by integration (Fig. 2.3). Multiplication of the signal intensity by the 90° pulse voltage compensated for differences in radiofrequency coil loading between individual patients, and enabled corrected signal intensities to be compared between subjects. As a group, the patients with epilepsy showed a reduction in the signal intensity of NAA and increases in signal intensities of Cho and Cr, with a consequent decrease in the NAA/Cho + Cr ratio, compared with a population of normal subjects.

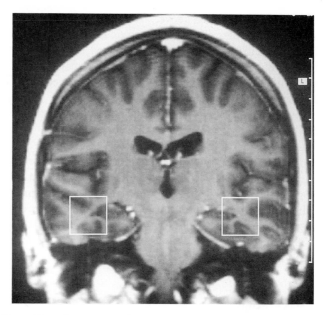

Fig. 2.2   Coronal inversion recovery T_1-weighted image showing the mesial temporal location of the two cubic volumes ($2 \times 2 \times 2$ cm) from which proton spectra were obtained by single-voxel localization. Such volumes include part of the hippocampus, but consist mainly of tissue within the temporal lobe itself and, as such, would be expected to provide information from a relatively diffuse area.

NAA in the brain is primarily located within neurons, whereas Cho- and Cr-containing compounds are also found in other cell types (see earlier section). The implication of these results is loss or dysfunction of neurons in the medial temporal lobe in patients with epilepsy. Further, the concentrations of Cr-, PCr- and Cho-containing compounds have been suggested to be higher in oligodendrocytes and astrocytes than in neurons (Urenjak et al 1993) and the increased signal from these compounds may indicate gliosis.

A subsequent investigation focused on 25 adults with well-characterized intractable temporal lobe epilepsy, on the basis of clinical, electro-encephalogram (EEG), MRI and neuropsychological data, and on 13 age-matched control subjects (Connelly et al 1994). Nineteen of the patients had hippocampal sclerosis, 3 had foreign-tissue lesions, 1 had widespread signal change suggestive of gliosis and 2 had no abnormality on MRI. Compared to normal subjects, the group data from the temporal lobes of the patients with epilepsy showed a 22% reduction in NAA, 15% increase in Cr and 25% increase in Cho ipsilateral to the epileptic focus. The mean NAA/Cho + Cr ratios were significantly less in the epilepsy patients than in the control subjects, both ipsilateral and contralateral to the focus, with the ipsilateral side being more affected (Fig. 2.4).

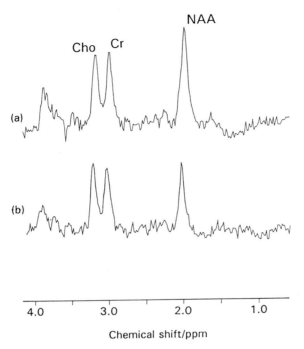

Fig. 2.3 Proton spectra obtained from 2 × 2 × 2 cm volumes located in **A** the right temporal lobe and **B** the left temporal lobe (as shown in Fig. 2.2) of a patient with left temporal lobe epilepsy. The spectra show peaks corresponding to choline-containing compounds (Cho), creatine + phosphocreatine (Cr), and *N*-acetyl aspartate (NAA). The lower spectrum shows significantly reduced NAA signal with respect both to the upper spectrum and to controls, indicating neuronal loss or dysfunction in the left temporal lobe in this patient. Each spectrum was obtained using repetition time = 1600 ms, echo time = 135 ms, and 512 averages.

On comparison of individual patients with the normative data, ^{1}H MRS showed abnormalities in the form of a reduced NAA/Cho + Cr ratio in 22 of 25 patients (88%), with 10 (40%) having bilateral abnormalities. In 6 of the 10 patients with bilateral abnormalities one temporal lobe was judged to be significantly more abnormal than the other. When lateralization was possible with MRS, this concurred with MRI findings in all but 1 case. Two patients with no abnormality shown on MRI had abnormal MRS and 3 patients with bilaterally normal MRS had hippocampal sclerosis. All 15 of these patients who have been followed for more than 1 year after temporal lobectomy have had a good seizure outcome. Seven of 8 with unilateral abnormalities were seizure-free or had auras only and 1 had >90% seizure reduction. Four of the 6 with bilateral abnormalities were seizure-free or had auras only and 2 had had single seizures.

The neurobiological implication from these data is that there is neuronal loss or dysfunction and astrocytosis in the temporal lobes of patients with

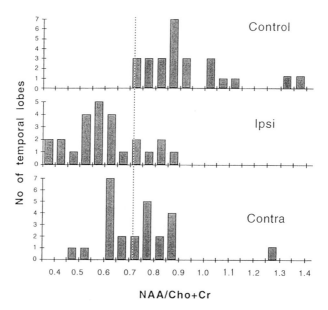

Fig. 2.4   Histogram showing the *N*-acetyl aspartate (NAA)/choline + creatine (Cho + Cr) ratio versus number of temporal lobes for 13 control subjects and 25 temporal lobe epilepsy patients. The patient data are divided into ipsi- and contralateral to the seizure focus (see text). The vertical dotted line at NAA/(Cho + Cr) equal to 0.72 corresponds to the lower limit of the 95% confidence interval for the control data. Ratios below 0.72 are therefore considered to be abnormal.

temporal lobe epilepsy. The magnitude of the reduction of NAA is such that the abnormality could not be confined to the hippocampus, as that structure occupies only a small proportion of the 8 ml voxel used. This finding is consistent with PET data on cerebral glucose metabolism in which there is commonly an area of hypometabolism that is larger than the anatomically defined focus (Sackellares et al 1990). The basis of the regional area of hypometabolism and, by inference, NAA reduction, is not certain. Comparative PET studies with ^{11}C-flumazenil and ^{18}F-deoxyglucose suggest that neuronal loss is less likely than diaschisis (Henry et al 1993). The cellular mechanisms underlying reduction of NAA, elevation of choline and creatine need to be clarified with correlative neuropathological studies, and dynamic changes in the levels of metabolites in relation to seizure activity need further evaluation.

   CSI has the advantages of being able to determine the regional distribution of metabolites and to identify areas of maximal abnormality. In a study of 10 patients with temporal lobe epilepsy and 5 controls examined on a 1.5 T system using ^{1}H CSI, the left–right asymmetry of NAA/Cr ratios was found to be significantly different from controls in all cases (Cendes et al 1994). This ratio was low in the mid temporal lobe in 5 cases and in the posterior temporal lobe in 8 patients. The asymmetry was found to be greater in the mid temporal region in 3 patients and in the posterior temporal region in 6. All patients showed a smaller focal region of asymmetry within the regions defined as mid- or posterior–temporal.

The use of such an asymmetry index alone precludes the detection of bilateral abnormalities. However, comparison of NAA/Cr ratios in patients and controls indicated that 2 patients had bilateral reduction in the NAA/Cr ratio in the posterior temporal region, and the greatest reduction was ipsilateral to the maximum EEG disturbance. One of the 10 patients had no MRI evidence of hippocampal atrophy but had a decrease of the NAA/Cr ratio in the mid posterior temporal lobe and at surgery had evidence of mild mesial temporal sclerosis.

A further CSI study, using a 2 T MR system with a 4 ml effective voxel size, was performed on 8 patients with unilateral complex partial seizures and 8 controls (Hugg et al 1994). Significant asymmetry in the intensity of the NAA signal was found in all patients. In each case the lower NAA corresponded to the side of seizure focus, as determined by EEG. No significant changes in Cho or Cr were observed.

It is apparent that CSI has distinct advantages over single-voxel techniques in terms of coverage of the brain, and it is becoming the method of choice in a number of centres for the study of epilepsy. However, it is technically more demanding than single-voxel MRS, particularly in respect to magnetic field homogeneity (shimming), water suppression and infiltration of subcutaneous fat signal into voxels other than just those adjacent to the scalp. Cendes et al (1994) noted that anterior temporal lobe structures were more accessible to single-voxel methods, and reported only posterior and mid temporal results from their CSI study. Xue et al (1993) have reported problems with suboptimal shimming when performing CSI in a large region, including both temporal lobes, and have therefore adopted the strategy of acquiring CSI volumes from each temporal lobe separately. Sauter et al (1991) have shown in a comparative study between CSI and single-voxel localization that the CSI data must be interpreted with some caution at present. Nevertheless, in the longer term, it seems likely that CSI will provide information that cannot be obtained in any other fashion.

Further work needs to be done to validate the clinical utility of temporal lobe ^{1}H-MRS, including examination of patients with epilepsy of ipsilateral and contralateral extratemporal onset, before the data can be employed with confidence in the assessment of patients with partial epilepsy of uncertain lateralization and localization. Other important questions include:

1. What is the significance and reliability of MRS data that is discordant to other information, and when other investigations are equivocal?
2. Is a bilateral abnormality of MRS an adverse prognostic factor for a good outcome from surgical treatment?

At present ^{1}H MRS appears to be a sensitive method for detecting regional cerebral metabolic disturbance, contributes to the lateralization of the epileptic focus and the identification of bilateral abnormalities and offers promise for reducing dependence on expensive and time-consuming invasive EEG studies. Firmly establishing this role will be difficult to achieve as presurgical evaluation depends on establishing a consensus between different strands of data. Examination of a larger number of patients is needed to determine the strength of the associations between MRS and other investigatory data and the clinical significance of discrepancies.

Single-voxel ^{1}H MRS applied to extratemporal epilepsy, without structural abnormalities on MRI to guide voxel placement, was not helpful in one study (Cook et al 1991). A ^{1}H CSI study has shown reduced NAA in frontal lobes ipsilateral to frontal lobe epileptic foci in 8 patients (Garcia et al 1993). This finding needs to be replicated and it is necessary to determine the extent of the area of NAA reduction in patients with seizures of frontal, temporal and posterior hemisphere onset. It is anticipated that technical advances in MR hardware and software technology, CSI and automated MRS examinations will allow further clinical applications, such as the ability to localize focal abnormalities that underly seizure disorders, in the temporal and extratemporal neocortex, when MRI does not reveal a structural abnormality.

The demonstration using proton MRS of the rise in cerebral GABA (Rothman et al 1993) consequent to the administration of vigabatrin to control subjects and to patients with epilepsy promises the possibility of non-invasive determination of cerebral neurometabolic profiles of patients prior to the initiation of drug therapy. Such information could aid considerably in the selection of the therapy that is most likely to be helpful in any individual patient and in monitoring the effects of treatment.

CONCLUSIONS

Over recent years it has become apparent that MRS offers a non-invasive method for obtaining information on cerebral metabolism. Implementation of the rapid advances now being made in MR hardware and software development over the next 5 years may enable the determination of the concentration and distribution of important metabolites in vivo, which is likely to have significant consequences for the medical and surgical management of patients with epilepsy.

REFERENCES

Bergen D, Bleck T, Ramsay R et al. 1989 Magnetic resonance imaging as a sensitive and specific predictor of neoplasms removed for intractable epilepsy. Epilepsia 30: 318–331.
Brooks B S, King D W, El Gammal T et al. 1990 MR imaging in patients with intractable complex partial epileptic seizures. Am J Neuroradiol 11: 93–99.
Brown T R, Kincaid B M, Ugurbil K. 1982 NMR chemical shift imaging in three dimensions. Proc Natl Acad Sci USA 79: 3523–3526.
Cendes F, Andermann F, Preul M C, Arnold D L. 1994 Lateralization of temporal lobe epilepsy based on regional metabolic abnormalities in proton magnetic resonance spectroscopic images. Ann Neurol 35: 211–216.

Chapman A G. 1985 Cerebral energy metabolism and seizures. In: Pedley TA, Meldrum BS (eds) Recent advances in epilepsy 2. Churchill Livingstone, Edinburgh, pp 19–63

Connelly A, Counsell C, Lohman J A B, Ordidge R J. 1988 Outer-volume supressed image related in-vivo spectroscopy (OSIRIS): a high sensitivity localization technique. J Magn Reson 78: 519–525

Connelly A, Jackson G D, Duncan J S, King M D, Gadian D G. 1994 Magnetic resonance spectroscopy in temporal lobe epilepsy. Neurology 44: 1411–1417.

Cook M J, Manford M, Gadian D G, Connelly A, Shorvon S D, Fish D R. 1991 Proton magnetic resonance spectroscopy in supplementary motor area seizures. Epilepsia 32 (suppl 3): 78

Cook M J, Fish D R, Shorvon S D, Straughan K, Stevens J M. 1992 Hippocampal volumetric and morphometric studies in frontal and temporal lobe epilepsy. Brain 115: 1001–1016.

Engel J, Kuhl D E, Phelps M E, Mazziotta J C. 1982 Interictal cerebral glucose metabolism in partial epilepsy and its relation to EEG changes. Ann Neurol 12: 510–517.

Frahm J, Gyngell M L, Merboldt K D, Hanicke W, Sauter R. 1989 High resolution proton NMR spectroscopy using stimulated echoes: initial applications to human brain in-vivo. Mag Reson Med 9: 79–93

Gadian D G, Connelly A, Duncan J S et al. 1994 ^{1}H Magnetic resonance spectroscopy in the investigation of intractable epilepsy. Acta Neurol Scand 89 (suppl 152): 116–122

Garcia P A, Laxer K D, van der Grond J, Hugg J W, Matson G B, Weiner M W. 1993 ^{1}H magnetic resonance spectroscopic imaging in patients with frontal lobe epilepsy. Epilepsia 34: 122

Garcia P A, Laxer K D, van der Grond J, Hugg J W, Matson G B, Weiner M W. 1994 Phosphorus magnetic resonance spectroscopic imaging in patients with frontal lobe epilepsy. Ann Neurol 35: 217–221

Henry T R, Frey K A, Sackellares J C et al. 1993 In vivo cerebral metabolism and central benzodiazepine-receptor binding in temporal lobe epilepsy. Neurology 43: 1998–2006

Hugg J W, Laxer K D, Matson G B, Maudsley A A, Husted C A, Weiner M W. 1992 Lateralization of human focal epilepsy by ^{31}P magnetic resonance imaging spectroscopy. Neurology 42: 2011–2018

Hugg J W, Laxer K D, Matson G B, Maudsley A A, Weiner M W. 1994 Neuron loss localises human temporal lobe epilepsy by in-vivo proton MR spectroscopic imaging. Ann Neurol 34: 788–794

Jack C R, Sharbrough F W, Twomey C K et al 1990 Temporal lobe seizures: lateralization with M R volume measurements of the hippocampal volume formation. Radiology; 175: 423–429

Jack C R, Sharbrough F W, Cascino G D et al 1992 Magnetic resonance imaging-based hippocampal volumetry: correlation with outcome after temporal lobectomy. Ann Neurol; 31: 138–146

Jackson G D, Berkovic S F, Duncan J S, Connelly A. 1993a Optimising the diagnosis of hippocampal sclerosis using MRI. Am. J Neuroradiol 14: 753–762

Jackson G D, Connelly A, Duncan J S, Grunewald R A, Gadian G D. 1993b Detection of hippocampal pathology in intractable partial epilepsy: Increased sensitivity with quantitative magnetic resonance T_2 relaxometry. Neurology 43: 1793–1799

Kumar A, Welti D, Ernst R R. 1975 NMR Fourier zeugmatography. J Magn Reson 18: 69–83

Kuzniecky R, Elgavish G A, Hetherington H P, Evanochko W T, Pohost G M. 1992 In vivo ^{31}P nuclear magnetic resonance spectroscopy of human temporal lobe epilepsy. Neurology 42: 1586–1590

Laxer K D, Hubesch B, Sappey-Marinier D, Weiner M W. 1992 Increased pH and inorganic phosphate in temporal seizure foci demonstrated by [^{31}P] MRS. Epilepsia 33: 618–623

Matthews P M, Andermann F, Arnold D L. 1990 A proton magnetic resonance spectroscopy study of focal epilepsy in humans. Neurology 40: 985–989

Maudsley A A, Hilal S K, Perman W H, Simon H E. 1983 Spatially resolved high resolution spectroscopy by "four-dimensional" NMR. J Magn Reson 51: 147–152

Ordidge R J, Bendall M R, Gordon R G, Connelly A. 1985 Volume selection for in-vivo biological spectroscopy. In: Govil, Khetrapal, Jaran (eds) Magnetic resonance in biology and medicine. Tata-McGraw-Hill, pp 387–397

Ordidge R J, Connelly A, Lohman J A B. 1986 Image selected in-vivo spectroscopy (ISIS): a new technique for spatially selective NMR spectroscopy. J Magn Reson 66: 283–294

Petroff O A C, Prichard J W, Ogino T, Avison M J, Alger J R, Shulman R G. 1986 Combined ^{1}H and ^{31}P NMR studies of bicuculline-induced seizures in vivo. Ann Neurol 20: 185–193

Rothman D L, Petroff O A C, Behar K L, Mattson R H. 1993 Localized ^{1}H NMR measurements of γ-aminobutyric acid in human brain *in vivo*. Proc Natl Acad Sci USA 90: 5662–5666

Sackellares J C, Siegel G J, Abou-Khalil B W et al. 1990 Differences between lateral and mesial temporal metabolism interictally in epilepsy of mesial temporal origin. Neurology 40: 1420–1426

Sauter R, Schneider M, Wiclow K, Kolem H. 1991 Localized ^{1}H MRS of the human brain: single-voxel versus CSI techniques. J Magn Res Imag 1: 241

Siesjö B K. 1978 Brain energy metabolism. Rochester, New York, Wiley Interscience pp 345–379

Urenjak J, Williams S R, Gadian D G, Noble M. 1992 Specific expression of N-acetylaspartate in neurons, oligodendrocyte-type-2-astrocyte progenitors, and immature oligodendrocytes in vitro. J Neurochem 59: 55–61

Urenjak J, Williams S R, Gadian D G, Noble M. 1993 Proton nuclear magnetic resonance spectroscopy unambiguously identifies different neural cell types. J Neurosci 13, 981–989

Xue M, Ng T C, Modic M, Comair Y, Kolem H. 1993 Oblique angle proton chemical shift imaging for the localization of hippocampal epilepsy. Proc Soc Magn Reson Medl, 435

3

Ictal SPECT

M. R. Newton   S. F. Berkovic

CEREBRAL BLOOD FLOW STUDIES

The current revolution in functional brain imaging is related to physiological phenomena described over a century ago when Sir Victor Horsley (1892) observed local increases in blood flow during induced seizures. This was corroborated by Penfield in 1938, and by Dymond & Crandall in 1976 using intracranial thermistors.

The techniques used by these pioneering investigators required invasive procedures, however, and gave information only on the regional perfusion changes; blood flow in other regions could not be simultaneously recorded.

Nuclide imaging

Nuclide imaging was the first major step in assessing whole-brain perfusion changes with seizures. Initially, xenon[133] was inhaled or injected whilst data were measured by scintillation counters next to the patient's head (Ingvar & Lassen 1961). Besides having limited resolution, the method did not enable seizures to be captured whenever they happened to occur, so ictal study was a rare chance event when the patient happened to have a seizure during elective study (Hougaard et al 1976, Ingvar 1973, 1975). Interictal study of patients with partial seizures sometimes revealed areas of focal hypoperfusion corresponding to the epileptic focus (Ingvar 1973, Lavy et al 1976, Touchon et al 1983, Valmier et al 1987). Positron emission tomography (PET) using fluorodeoxyglucose[19] showed hypometabolism in the epileptic zone (Engel et al 1990) in a similar patient cohort. Although PET has been shown to be a sensitive tool for identifying the interictal hypometabolic epileptic focus in about 80% of patients with temporal lobe epilepsy, it remains an expensive and elaborate technique. In addition, PET can only be routinely applied to interictal investigation as like dynamic xenon[133] single-photon emission computed tomography (SPECT), ictal data are acquired purely by chance (Engel et al 1983, Theodore et al 1983).

The use of static SPECT in the localization of seizure foci has only become possible over the last decade by the development of radioligands that are readily fixed in cerebral tissue during first-pass circulation. This has enabled ligand injection during seizures with scanning done shortly, thereafter, to produce a 'snapshot' of cerebral blood flow very close to the time of injection. The combination of this technique with video electroencephalogram (EEG) telemetry has proved to be a powerful tool for investigating the pathophysiology of partial seizures.

SPECT ligands

Iodinated ligands

The ^{123}I-iodoamines isopropyl-iodoamphetamine (IMP) and trimethyl-(hydroxy-methyl-^{123}I-iodobenzyl)-propanediamine (HIPDM) were the first of the ligands that are taken up rapidly by cerebral tissues to reflect the distribution of blood flow close to the time of injection (Winchell et al 1980, Kung et al 1983). These compounds could also be stored near the monitoring suite, facilitating injection at the time of seizure. Once the patient had recovered from the seizure and was cooperative, scanning could be done at leisure. Hill et al (1982) reported capturing a partial seizure using IMP, and Lee et al (1986, 1987, 1988a, 1988b) followed with studies of temporal lobe seizures using HIPDM. However, the iodinated[123] compounds are cyclotron products and are therefore costly and of limited availability. In addition, the long half-life of iodine[123] precludes study on sequential days.

Technetium ligand

Exametazime or hexamethyl-propyleneamineoxime (HMPAO) is a lipophilic compound that is also rapidly fixed by cerebral tissues. It has the advantage of binding to the relatively inexpensive and widely available isotope technetium[99m] (Neirinckx et al 1987) which has a much shorter half-life than iodine[123]. It can therefore be administered on sequential days if necessary. The clinically valuable localizing data from ictal SPECT have so far been derived using single-head rotating γ cameras, yet the current generations of dual- and triple-head cameras can produce superior resolution, allowing co-registration of the physiological image with the anatomic data of magnetic resonance images.

The only disadvantage of ^{99m}Tc-HMPAO is its instability, which requires mixing the isotope with the ligand immediately before use. This limitation has been largely overcome with a rapid mixing method that enables preparation of the compound within 30 s, thus allowing most seizures to be captured in the ictal or immediate postictal period (Newton et al 1993).

Conditions necessary for ictal SPECT study

Ideally, the ligand kit (vial of freeze-dried HMPAO and syringe of technetium solution) is stored next to the monitoring suite where trained personnel can instantly mix the isotope and HMPAO once they are alerted to seizure onset and inject the patient via an in situ venous cannula. In the 5-year experience of the Austin Hospital (Melbourne), ictal injections were achieved in more than 60% of cases, and as the number of available trained personnel increases, the ictal capture rate should increase accordingly.

We stress the importance of video-EEG surveillance which provides exact timing of injection relative to seizure onset and end, and correlation of the SPECT image with clinical and EEG data. Knowledge of the evolution of specific blood flow patterns, particularly in temporal lobe seizures, is essential for correct interpretation of SPECT data (Newton et al 1992b, Duncan et al 1993). This can only be achieved confidently when the timing of ligand injection is established by video telemetry.

ICTAL SPECT IN ADULTS

Temporal lobe epilepsy

Hyperperfusion of the temporal lobe was initially reported by Hill et al (1982) and Uren et al (1983) using IMP. Confirmatory findings in a larger series of patients with temporal lobe epilepsy were reported by Lee et al (1988a) using HIPDM. The use of iodinated[123] compounds was restrictive, and in 1985 Biersack et al described ictal SPECT using ^{99m}Tc-HMPAO. Isolated reports followed from Andersen et al (1990) and Rowe et al (1991a). These studies all revealed hyperperfusion of the anterior temporal lobe during temporal lobe seizures, but the extent and time-frame of perfusion changes were not delineated until we reported the *postictal switch* of blood flow (Newton et al 1992) that elaborated on Rowe et al's novel observations of postictal SPECT patterns in temporal lobe epilepsy.

The evolution of blood flow during and after temporal lobe seizures

The increased uptake of ^{99m}Tc-HMPAO in the anterior temporal lobe as seen in SPECT reflects the local increase in blood flow during the seizure (Fig. 3.1). The appearances are striking and unmistakable and provide powerful localizing data in patients being evaluated for temporal lobectomy. Side-to-side ratio analysis has shown a mean 30% increase in counts on the epileptic side compared to the interictal state. Following the end of a seizure, this ictal hyperperfusion pattern remains for about 60 s into the immediate postictal period before switching to a postictal pattern, which is found in about 70% of cases. The typical postictal pattern comprises hypoperfusion of the lateral temporal cortex on the side of focus, often with persisting increased perfusion in the mesial temporal cortex (Fig. 3.1). This was originally described by Rowe et al (1989, 1990, 1991a, 1991b), whose injections were given at a mean 6.3 min after seizure onset (about 5 min after seizure end).

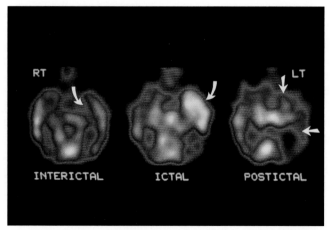

Fig. 3.1 Sequential changes in temporal lobe perfusion before, during and after complex partial seizure. **Left**: Transaxial slice through temporal lobes in the interictal condition showing reduced perfusion in the mesial temporal region (arrow). **Middle**: marked increase in perfusion in the anterior temporal lobe during seizure (arrow). **Right**: 1.5–min postictal study showing reduced lateral temporal perfusion (horizontal arrow) and with relative hyperperfusion in the mesial temporal region (vertical arrow).

Clinical value

The striking and unambiguous changes seen with ictal SPECT provide powerful lateralizing data. In a review of 119 cases of established, unilateral temporal lobe epilepsy from the Austin Hospital, Melbourne, 97% of 51 ictal SPECT studies were correctly lateralized by two blinded observers, with no incorrect lateralizations. Only 1 case was inconclusive. Second best are the postictal changes, which allowed correct lateralization in 71% of 77 studies, but were incorrect in 4%. Interictal SPECT, by contrast, allowed only 48% correct lateralizations in the 119 cases, with an unacceptable 10% being incorrectly lateralized (Newton et al 1992c, 1994a).

If is of interest that the ictal hyperperfusion during temporal lobe seizures is limited to the temporal region, in contrast to the electrical activity which frequently spreads to the contralateral hippocampus. It is not yet clear why the topography of perfusion changes does not match the electrographic spread in complex partial seizures. In partial seizures that hemigeneralize, however, hyperperfusion can be seen along the motor strip ipsilateral to the epileptic focus (Fig. 3.2), as initially reported using HIPDM SPECT by Lee et al (1987). SPECT studies of simple partial seizures that do not evolve further have rarely yielded diagnostic information in our experience.

We have seen one instance in which ictal EEG showed seizure origin in one temporal lobe which then activated the contralateral temporal lobe. Because the ligand was injected late in the seizure, the hyperperfusion was seen in the lobe contralateral to the focus. Fortunately, this has occurred in only one of more than 100 ictal SPECT studies in our experience, but it does

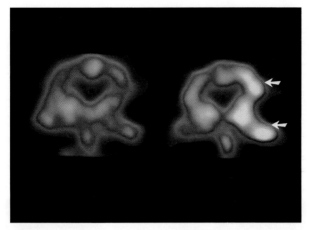

Fig. 3.2 Motor strip activation from spread of temporal lobe seizure. The central motor strip shows marked increase in perfusion (upper arrow) as seizure spreads over the left hemisphere in a patient with hemigeneralization following complex partial seizure originating from the left temporal lobe (lower arrow).

emphasize that SPECT is complementary to the clinical and electrographic data and cannot be interpreted independently.

Pathophysiological insights

Temporal perfusion subtypes.   In a study of 30 operated patients, Ho et al (1994a) found that different patterns of ictal temporal hyperperfusion were associated with different underlying pathologies. Those with hippocampal sclerosis ($n = 10$) or foreign-tissue lesions in the mesial temporal lobe ($n = 8$) had ictal SPECT patterns of ipsilateral mesial and lateral temporal hyperperfusion. Five patients with good surgical outcome but no demonstrable pathology showed ictal hyperperfusion restricted to the ipsilateral anteromesial temporal region. In contrast, patients with foreign-tissue lesions in the lateral temporal lobe ($n = 7$) had hyperperfusion bilaterally with predominant changes in the region of the lesion.

No differences were seen in the semiology of these four groups. The location of pathology may determine the spread of seizure, and the ictal SPECT patterns may reflect the connections between temporal structures.

Regional cerebral blood flow changes distant from the temporal lobe.   So far, descriptions of the rapid evolution of blood flow changes have been confined to the temporal regions. SPECT allows examination of the relative blood flow changes in all cerebral regions and therefore provides unique insights into the pathophysiology of temporal lobe seizures.

A qualitative and semiquantitative analysis of 72 ictal and postictal SPECT studies compared with the interictal condition in patients with established temporal lobe epilepsy has revealed that the peri-ictal perfusion changes

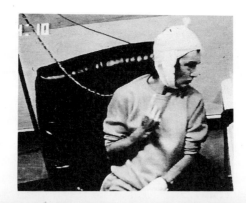

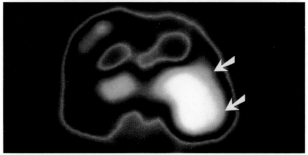

Fig. 3.3   Ictal dystonia associated with increased basal ganglia perfusion. **Top:** Dystonic posturing of patient's right arm during a complex partial seizure. **Bottom:** Coronal slice of the single-photon emission tomography (SPECT) obtained after ligand injection during the seizure. Hyperperfusion is seen in both the left temporal lobe (lower arrow) and the adjacent basal ganglia (upper arrow).

evolve at different rates in different cortical and subcortical regions (Newton et al 1994b). Whilst lateral temporal perfusion declined earlier than mesial temporal perfusion in the immediate postictal period, lateral frontal, central and parietal perfusion decreased abruptly from interictal levels at seizure end. The combination of lateral temporal hypoperfusion with these extratemporal cortical changes makes a pattern of extensive hypoperfusion throughout the hemisphere on the side of seizure origin. This appearance is useful for lateralization of the temporal lobe seizure.

Peri-ictal blood flow in subcortical grey matter structures has also been analysed. Ictal hyperperfusion of the basal ganglia ipsilateral to the epileptic temporal lobe was associated with dystonic posturing of the contralateral upper limb (Newton et al 1992a, Fig. 3.3). This observation supports the hypothesis that seizure spread from the temporal lobe to the ipsilateral basal ganglia is responsible for the dystonia (Kotagal et al 1989) rather than spread to the supplementary motor area (Bennett et al 1989).

Thalamic hyperperfusion was also seen ipsilateral to the seizure focus during the seizure but fell rapidly, like basal ganglia hyperperfusion, to interictal levels during the first 90 s of the postictal period. Perfusion in the cerebellar hemispheres, however, remained symmetrical throughout the ictal and postictal periods in complex partial seizures of temporal lobe origin (Newton et al 1994b).

Extratemporal focal epilepsies

Ictal injection of ligand has also proved of great value in localizing the onset zones of extratemporal seizures, which have long been a major diagnostic challenge. Localized hyperperfusion at the site of seizure origin has been reported by several investigators (Biersack et al 1985, Stefan et al 1990, Marks et al 1992, Harvey et al 1993b). Marks et al (1992) found that ictal SPECT was localizing in 10 of 12 studies in 11 patients with extratemporal foci. Seizures of extratemporal origin are commonly brief, shorter than temporal lobe seizures, and therefore allow little time for ^{99m}Tc-HMPAO preparation and injection, which, in our hands, takes 30 s. Examination of our postictal injections in the extratemporal cases has been of little localizing value. Postictal SPECT suggested localization in 10 of 26 patients with no other diagnostic data, in contrast to ictal SPECT, which suggested a seizure focus in 8 of 9 patients who were injected with ligand during their seizure. Furthermore, in 12 patients with established parietal, frontal or occipital foci, ictal SPECT was congruent in all 9 when ictal injection was achieved (Fig. 3.4). Postictal studies in this group, however, revealed changes in only 2 of 5 patients studied in that condition. These data make the ictal injection of ligand an even greater priority than in the case of temporal lobe seizures.

Ho et al (1994b) studied the clinical and ictal SPECT features of 14 patients with parietal lobe epilepsy. The images showed focal hyperperfusion in all cases and corresponded with structural lesions, which were present in 9. Semiquantitative analysis of side-to-side ratios in the parietal regions of interest revealed increases of 11–15% (mean 25.5) compared to interictal scans. In addition, two main clinical seizure patterns were recognized in association with the SPECT patterns: a syndrome of sensorimotor manifestations characterized by hyperperfusion in the anterior parietal area, and a syndrome of complex partial seizures of the psychoparetic type associated with hyperperfusion in the posterior parietal region. These patterns may reflect seizure propagation via association and commissural fibres that connect the anterior parietal region to the primary motor, premotor and supplementary motor areas. The posterior parietal region, however, is connected to the cingulate gyrus, insula and parahippocampal gyrus, so that seizure propagation to these structures may well imitate the psychoparetic seizures of temporal lobe epilepsy.

So far the extratemporal epilepsies have proved difficult to study with EEG and PET. Ictal SPECT in these disorders is providing valuable data which more than rewards the efforts required to achieve seizure capture with the ligand.

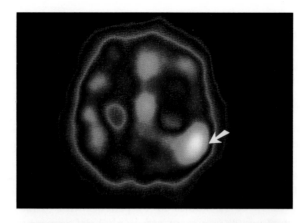

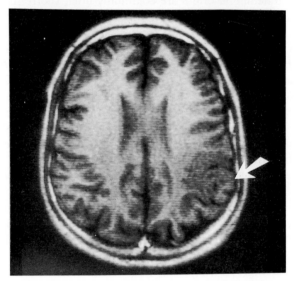

Fig. 3.4 Parietal lobe seizure. **Top:** Transverse slice of ictal single-photon emission tomography (SPECT) study showing focal hyperperfusion (arrow) in a patient with parietal lobe seizures arising from a discrete region of cortical dysgenesis, revealed by magnetic resonance scan (**bottom arrow**).

ICTAL SPECT IN CHILDREN

Physiological considerations

Brain development in the child is associated with maturational changes in regional cerebral blood flow. Knowledge of these changes is essential for accurate interpretation of pathological conditions. The most critical development occurs in the first years of life, where cerebral blood flow values exceed those of adults and the regional patterns of blood flow differ (Kennedy &

Sokoloff 1957, Kennedy et al 1970, Chugani & Phelps 1986, Chugani et al 1987, 1990).

At birth, the mean regional cerebral blood flow is the same as adults (50 mg/100 g per min) but increases rapidly to 60 mg/100 g per min by 1 year and to 70 mg 1100/g per min by 3 years. The mean cerebral blood flow gradually decreases after the age of 10 to reach adult values by age 20. These changes parallel most markers of synaptic activity (Huttenlocher 1979, Farkas-Bargeton et al 1984, Seeman et al 1987, McDonald & Johnston 1990), which is most prolific in the first few years of life, stabilizing after the first decade.

The regional changes in cerebral blood flow are characterized by intermittent increases that mirror an anteroposterior gradient of cortical maturation. Increased cerebral blood flow in the sensorimotor and posterior cortex is found at birth and followed by increased flow in the primary visual cortex by 3 months and posterior associative cortex by 6 months (Rubinstein et al 1989, Chiron et al 1992, Denays et al 1992). Frontal cortex regional cerebral blood flow gradually increases after the first year of life (Chiron et al 1992), in contrast to the specific spurts of increased regional cerebral blood flow seen in the posterior cortex which have stabilized by that age. This evolution corresponds with the sequence of cognitive development whereby visual and auditory faculties develop in the first year of life and are followed by the development of frontal lobe functions in succeeding years.

Changing cerebral blood flow in childhood and epilepsy

The fact that more than 50% of epilepsies begins in childhood years (particularly in infancy; Hauser & Kurland 1975) provides support for the suggested relationship between synaptogenesis and epileptogenicity (Sutula et al 1989). Plasticity is also related to synaptogenesis and is important in learning, as well as in 'after-damage recovery'. Childhood therefore seems to be the most favourable time for rehabilitation after surgery.

Clinical observations of childhood epilepsy parallel the age-related changes in regional cerebral blood flow. Rolandic and occipital epilepsy are relatively common in young children, whereas frontal lobe epilepsy rarely occurs. Pre-existing epileptogenic areas may become symptomatic at different ages, depending on their location. In tuberous sclerosis, for example, tubers at different sites may produce seizures at different times of life. West syndrome, which has a peak onset at 6 months of age can be associated with lesions in the occipital and associated posterior areas (Dulac et al 1987, Chugani et al 1990) the age at which regional cerebral blood flow normally increases in those regions.

Temporal lobe epilepsy

The regional cerebral blood flow patterns associated with temporal lobe epilepsy in children as shown by SPECT are similar to those seen in adults in the interictal, ictal and postictal conditions. Lateralization rates up to 80% or more (Hwang et al 1987, Harvey et al 1993a) have been found with ictal studies compared with the interictal SPECT perfusion defects which are seen in 40–60% of cases (Denays et al 1988, Chiron et al 1989, Uvebrant et al 1991, Hwang et al 1990). The high proportion of correct localizations has been supported by congruence with other investigative data and pathological findings following surgery. This makes ictal SPECT a useful tool in the presurgical work-up of children with temporal lobe epilepsy.

Extratemporal focal epilepsies

Seizures arising in sites other than the temporal lobe have often been difficult to localize in children as in adults. When localizing, data from clinical and EEG study are sparse, there remain few options for further investigation. Ictal SPECT, however, can demonstrate the epileptic region in frontal lobe epilepsy as reported by Harvey et al (1993b; Fig. 3.5), who studied 22 children with this condition. Focal frontal hyperperfusion was seen in 20 of 22 (91%) cases, the distribution being lobar in 1 child and restricted to focal frontal regions in the remainder. Semiquantitative measurement using side-to-side ratios of counts revealed a mean 20% increase in flow at the epileptic focus

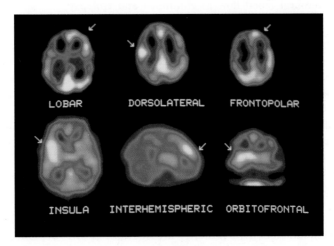

Fig. 3.5   Single-photon emission tomography (SPECT) patterns of frontal lobe seizures in children. Ictal SPECT study in 6 children with frontal lobe epilepsy shows regional hyperperfusion in the left lobar distribution (**top left**), focal hyperperfusion in the right dorsolateral region (**top middle**) and frontopolar hyperperfusion (**top right**). A seizure arising from right insula is associated with regional hyperperfusion (**bottom left**), and an interhemispheric focus is shown on the sagittal slice (**bottom middle**), whilst orbitofrontal hyperperfusion is demonstrated on the coronal slice (**bottom right**).

compared to the interictal state. The ictal studies frequently showed ipsilateral basal ganglia hyperperfusion and contralateral cerebellar hyperperfusion, presumably reflecting regions of subcortical activation via corticostriatoponto-cerebellar connections. Occipital and parietal seizure foci have been localized using ictal SPECT by the same authors (personal communication).

LIMITATIONS OF ICTAL SPECT

Seizures of very brief duration (e.g. less than 30 s) are likely to be associated with short-lived hyperperfusion of small magnitude. These factors militate against capturing the seizure using ^{99m}Tc-HMPAO SPECT due to the 30 s required to prepare the ligand. In addition, the prolonged postictal hypoperfusion that is often present in the temporal SPECT studies is not found in postictal SPECT of the extratemporal seizures that we have studied so far. Furthermore, hyperperfusion confined to a very small cortical area, as in epilepsia partialis continua or simple partial seizures, may elude detection by SPECT. Seizures that spread rapidly to a distant cortical focus or secondarily generalize may not show a single area of increased perfusion with ictal ligand injection. Fortunately, these circumstances are relatively uncommon in the spectrum of refractory partial seizures. In our experience of over 100 ictal SPECT studies in patients being investigated for prospective temporal lobectomy, only 1 has shown rapid contralateral spread of seizure, thereby giving false lateralization on the SPECT.

CONCLUSIONS

Ictal SPECT is a reliable and highly accurate method of lateralizing temporal lobe seizures. Injection of ligand during the seizure or immediately after produces striking and obvious changes that are readily and precisely interpretable. Such studies can be securely undertaken only in the context of video-EEG monitoring which enables the precise timing of injection relative to seizure end. Knowledge of the postictal switch in blood flow is essential to the proper interpretation of SPECT images, whether ictal or postictal studies.

Initial experience with ictal SPECT in extratemporal seizures promises that this method will also be valuable in localizing the epileptic focus. This has been the case in children with frontal lobe epilepsies where ictal SPECT has demonstrated frontal foci in more than 90% of cases in one series (Harvey et al 1993b). Although ictal SPECT data have not been as rigorously validated in children as in adults, it appears to provide almost identical lateralizing data.

Ictal SPECT has developed into a powerful tool for the localization of refractory partial seizures in both adults and children. In addition, SPECT also provides unique scientific insights into the pathophysiology of epilepsy. The widespread availability of ^{99m}Tc-HMPAO SPECT, its ease of use and relative economy make it a desirable diagnostic test for the evaluation of partial seizures.

KEY POINTS FOR CLINICAL PARCTICE

- Ictal injection of radioligand is the method of choice for the SPECT localization of seizures. It is imperative that radioligand injection is made under video-EEG surveillance to determine the nature of the seizure being studied and the precise time of injection relative to seizure onset and end.

- Interpretation of SPECT images in temporal lobe epilepsy requires a knowledge of the rapidly changing perfusion patterns that characterize temporal lobe seizures. Hyperperfusion of the epileptic temporal lobe persists for up to 1 min into the immediate postictal period, whereafter the lateral temporal cortex becomes rapidly hypoperfused compared to the mesial temporal region which often remains relatively hyperperfused throughout the postictal epoch.

- Ictal SPECT study of temporal lobe seizures yeild more than 90% lateralization rates because of the striking and unmistakable increase in anterior temporal blood flow. Postictal studies are lateralizing in 70% of temporal lobe seizures whereas interictal SPECT has a lower yeild of true positives and an unacceptable false positive rate.

- Increasing experience of SPECT in extra-temporal epilepsies, both in children and adults, indicates that ictal injection of isotope is achievable in many cases and provides powerful localizing data. Brief seizures remain difficult to capture with ictal injection of ^{99m}Tc-HMPAO but the development of stabilized forms will undoubtedly improve the capture rate.

- Ictal SPECT study is establishing a secure place in the investigation of refractory focal epilepsy. The widespread availability of SPECT and the relative simplicity of rapid isotope injection provide accurate and powerful localizing data in addition to unique scientific insights into the pathophysiology of epilepsy.

REFERENCES

Anderson A R, Waldemar G, Dam M, Fuglsang-Frederiksen A, Herning M, Kruse-Larsen C. 1990 SPECT in the presurgical evaluation of patients with temporal lobe epilepsy — a preliminary report. Acta Neurochir (Wien) 50: 80–83

Bennett D A, Ristanovic R K, Morrell F, Goetz C G. 1989 Dystonic posturing in temporal lobe seizures (letter). Neurology 39: 1270–1271

Biersack H J, Reichmann K, Winkler C et al 1985 ^{99m}Tc-labelled hexamethylpropyleneamine oxime photon emission scans in epilepsy. Lancet 2: 1436–1437

Chiron C, Raynaud C, Dulac O, Tzourio N, Plouin P, Tran-Dinh S. 1989 Study of the cerebral blood flow in partial epilepsy of childhood using the SPECT method. J Neuroradiol 16: 317–324

Chiron C, Raynaud C, Mazière B et al. 1992 Changes in regional cerebral blood flow during brain maturation in children and adolescents. J Nucl Med 33: 696–670

Chugani H T, Phelps M E. 1986 Maturation in cerebral function in infants determined by (18)FDG positron emission tomography. Science 231: 840–843

Chugani H T, Phelps M E, Mazziotta J C. 1987 Positron emission tomography study of human brain functional development. Ann Neurol 22: 487–497

Chugani H T, Shields W D, Shewdon D A et al 1990 Infantile spasms: PET identifies focal cortical dysgenesis in cryptogenic cases for surgical treatment. Ann Neurol 27: 406–413

Denays R, Rubinstein M, Ham H, Piepsz A, Noël P. 1988 Single photon emission computed tomography in seizure disorders. Arch Dis Child 63: 1184–1188

Denays R, Ham H R, Tondeur M, Piepsz A, Noël P. 1992 Detection of bilateral and symmetrical anomalies in Tc-99m HMPAO brain SPECT studies. J Nucl Med 33: 485–490

Dulac O, Chiron C, Jambaqué I, Plouin P, Raynaud C. 1987 Infantile spasms. Prog Clin Neurosci 2: 97–109

Duncan R, Patterson J, Roberts R, Hadley D, Bone I. 1993 Ictal/postictal SPECT in the presurgical localization of complex partial seizures. temporal lobe epilepsy. J Neurol Neurosurg Psychiatry 56: 141–148

Dymond A M, Crandall PH. 1976 Oxygen availability and blood flow in the temporal lobes during spontaneous seizures in man. Brain Res 102: 191–196

Engel J Jr, Kuhl D E, Phelps M E et al 1983 Patterns of human local cerebral glucose metabolism during epileptic seizures. Science 218: 64–66

Engel J Jr, Henry T, Risinger M W et al. 1990 Presurgical evaluation for partial epilepsy: relative contributions of chronic depth-electrode recordings versus FDG-PET and scalp-sphenoidal ictal EEG. Neurology 40: 1670–1677

Farkas-Bargeton E, Deibleer M F, Rosenberg B, Wehrle R. 1984 Histochemical changes of the developing human cerebral neocortex. Neuropediatrics 15: 82–91

Harvey A S, Bowe J M, Hopkins I J, Shield L K, Cook D J, Berkovic S F. 1993a Ictal ^{99m}Tc-HMPAO single photon computed tomography in children with temporal lobe epilepsy. Epilepsia 34: 869–877

Harvey AS, Hopkins IJ, Bowe JM, Cook DJ, Shield LK, Berkovic SF. 1993b Frontal lobe epilepsy: clinical seizure characteristics and localization with ictal ^{99m}Tc-HMPAO SPECT. Neurology 43: 1966–1980

Hauser A, Kurland LT. 1975 The epidemiology of epilepsy in Rochester Minnesota, 1935 through 1969. Epilepsia 16: 1–66

Hill TC, Holman L, Lovett R et al 1982 Initial experience with SPECT of the brain using N-isopropyl I-123 p-iodoamphetamine: concise communication. J Nucl Med 23: 191–195

Ho SS, Berkovic SF, McKay WJ et al. 1994a Temporal lobe epilepsy subtypes: differential patterns of cerebral perfusion on ictal SPECT. (Submitted)

Ho SS, Berkovic SF, McKay WJ et al. 1994b Parietal lobe epilepsy: clinical features and localization by ictal SPECT. Neurology (in press)

Horsley V. 1892 An address on the origin and seat of epileptic disturbance. Br Med J 1: 693–696

Hougaard K, Oikawa T, Sveinsdottir E et al. 1976 Regional cerebral blood flow in focal cortical epilepsy. Arch Neurol 33: 527–535

Huttenlocher P. 1979 Synaptic density in human frontal cortex: developmental changes and effects of aging. Brain Res 163: 195–205

Hwang P, Gilday DL, Ash JM et al. 1987 Perturbations in regional cerebral blood flow detected by SPECT scanning with ^{99}Tc HMPAO correlate with EEG abnormalities in children with epilepsy. J Cereb Blood Flow Metab 7 (suppl 1): S573

Hwang P, Adams C, Gilday D L et al. 1990 SPECT studies in epilepsy: applications to epilepsy surgery in children. J Epilepsy (Suppl): 83–92

Ingvar D H, Lassen N A. 1961 Quantitative determination of regional cerebral blood flow in man (letter). Lancet ii: 806–807

Ingvar D H. 1973 Regional cerebral blood flow in focal cortical epilepsy. Stroke 4: 359–360

Ingvar D H. 1975 CBF in focal cortical epilepsy. In: Langfitt T W, McHenry L C Jr, Reivich M, Wollman H, eds. Cerebral circulation and metabolism. New York: Springer-Verlag.

Kennedy C, Sokoloff L. 1957 An adaptation of the nitrous oxide method to the study of the cerebral circulation in children: normal values for cerebral blood flow and cerebral metabolic rate in childhood. J Clin Invest 36: 1130–1137

Kennedy C, Grave G D, Jehie J W, Sokoloff L. 1970 Blood flow to white matter during maturation of the brain. Neurology 20: 613–618

Kotagal P, Lüders H, Morris H H et al. 1989 Dystonic posturing in complex partial seizures of temporal lobe onset: a new lateralizing sign. Neurology 39: 196–201

Kung H F, Trampsch K M, Blau M. 1983 A new brain perfusion imaging agent: (I-123) HIPDM: N,N,N'-trimethyl-N'-(2-hydroxy-3-methyl-5-iodobenzyl)-1,3-propaneamine. J Necl Med 24: 66–72

Lavy S, Melamed E, Portnoy Z et al. 1976 Interictal regional cerebral blood flow in patients with partial seizures. Neurology 26: 418–422

Lee B I, Markand O N, Siddiqui A R et al. 1986 Single photon emission computed tomography (SPECT) brain imaging using HIDPM: intractable complex partial seizures. Neurology 36: 1471–1477

Lee B I, Markand O N, Wellman H N et al. 1987 HIPDM single photon emission computed tomography brain imaging in partial onset secondarily generalized tonic-clonic seizures. Epilepsia 28: 305–311

Lee B I, Markand O N, Wellman H N et al. 1988a HIPDM-SPECT in patients with medically intractable complex partial seizures: ictal study. Arch Neurol 46: 397–412

Lee B I, Park, H M, Siddiqui A R et al. 1988b Interictal HIPDM-SPECT in patients with complex partial seizures. Neurology 38 (suppl 1): 406

McDonald J W, Johnston M V. 1990 Physiological pathophysiological roles of excitatory aminoacids during central nervous system development. Brain Res Rev 15: 41–70

Marks D A, Katz A, Hoffer P, Spencer S S. 1992 Localization of extratemporal epileptic foci during ictal single photon emission computed tomography. Ann Neurol 31: 250–255

Neirinckx R D, Canning L R, Piper I M et al. 1987 Technetium-99m HM-PAO: a new radiopharmaceutical for SPECT imaging of regional cerebral blood perfusion. J Nucl Med 28: 191–202

Newton M R, Berkovic S F, Austin M C, Reutens D C, McKay W J, Bladin P F. 1992a Dystonia, clinical lateralization and regional cerebral blood flow in temporal lobe seizures. Neurology 42: 371–377

Newton M R, Berkovic S F, Austin M C, Rowe C C, McKay W J, Bladin P F. 1992b A postictal switch in blood flow distribution characterizes human temporal lobe seizures. J Neurol Neurosurg Psychiatry 55: 891–894

Newton M R, Berkovic S F, Austin M C, Rowe C C, McKay W J, Bladin P F. 1992c The lateralizing power of ictal ^{99m}Tc-HMPAO SPECT in the presurgical evaluation of temporal lobe epilepsy. J Nucl Med 33: 929

Newton M R, Austin M C, Chan J G, McKay W J, Rowe C C, Berkovic S F. 1993 Ictal SPECT using technetium-99m-HMPAO: methods for rapid preparation and optimal deployment of tracer during spontaneous seizures. J Nucl Med 34: 666–670

Newton M R, Berkovic S F, Austin M C et al. 1994a Ictal, postical and interictal SPECT in the lateralization of temporal lobe seizures. Eur J Nucl Med 21: 1067–1071

Newton M R, Berkovic S F, Austin M C et al. 1994b A SPECT study of the distribution and time course of cerebral blood flow during and after temporal lobe seizures. (Submitted)

Penfield W. 1938 The circulation of the epileptic brain. Assoc Res Nerv Dis Proc 18: 605–637

Rowe CC, Berkovic SF, Sia STB et al. 1989 Localization of epileptic foci with postical single photon emission computed tomography. Ann Neurol 26: 660–668

Rowe C C, Berkovic S F, Austin M C, Bladin P F, McKay W J. 1990 Interictal and postical blood flow in temporal lobe epilepsy. In: Focal epilepsy: clinical use of emission tomography. eds. Baldy-Moulinier M, Lassen NA, Engel J Jr, Askienazy S, John Libbey, London, pp 143–150

Rowe C C, Berkovic S F, Austin M, McKay W J, Bladin P F. 1991a Patterns of postical cerebral blood flow in temporal lobe epilepsy: qualitative and quantitative analysis. Neurology 41: 1096–1103

Rowe CC, Berkovic SF, Austin MC et al. 1991b Visual and quantitative analysis of interictal SPECT with Tc-99m HMPAO in temporal lobe epilepsy. J Nucl Med 32: 1688–1694

Rubinstein M, Denays R, Ham HR et al. 1989 Functional imaging of brain maturation in humans using iodine-123 iodoamphetamine and SPECT. J Nucl Med 30: 1982–1985

Seeman P, Bzowej N, Guan II et al. 1987 Human brain dopamine receptors in children and aging adults. Synapse 1: 399–404

Stefan H, Bauer J, Feistel H et al. 1990 Regional cerebral blood flow during focal seizures of temporal and frontocentral onset. Ann Neurol 27: 162–166

Sutula T, Cascino G, Cavazos J, Parada I, Ramirez L. 1989 Mossy fiber synaptic reorganization in the epileptic human temporal lobe. Ann Neurol 26: 321–330

Theodore WH, Newmark ME, Sato S et al 1983 [^{18}F] Fluorodeoxyglucose positron emission tomography in refractory complex partial seizures. Ann Neurol 14: 429–437

Touchon J, Valmier J, Baldy-Mouinier M. 1983 Regional cerebral blood flow in temporal lobe epilepsy: interictal studies. In: Baldy-Moulinier B, Ingvar DH, Meldrum BE, eds. Current problems in epilepsy: cerebral blood flow, metabolism and epilepsy. London: Libbey

Uren RF, Magistretti PL, Royal HD et al. 1983 Single-photon emission computed tomography: a method of measuring cerebral blood flow in three dimensions (preliminary results of studies in patients with epilepsy and stroke). Med J Aust 1: 411–413

Uvebrant P, Bjure J, Hedstrom A, Ekholm S. 1991 Brain single photon emission computed tomography (SPECT) in neuropediatrics. Neuropediatrics 22: 3–9

Valmier J, Touchon J, Daures P et al. 1987 Correlations between cerebral blood flow variations and clinical parameters in temporal lobe epilepsy: an interictal study. J Neurol Neurosurg Psychiatry 50: 1306–1311

Winchell HS, Bladwin RM, Lin TH. 1980 Development of I-123-labelled amines for brain studies: localization of I-123 iodophenylalkyl amines in rat brain. J Nucl Med 21: 940–946

4

The Wada test: a critical review

M. J. Hamberger   T. S. Walczak

Unlike most psychometric tests that are administered, scored and interpreted in a uniform fashion, intracarotid amobarbital testing has remained unstandardized. The Wada test (Wada 1949), therefore, refers not to a particular protocol but to a class of procedures that assess aspects of cognitive function during temporary anaesthesia of one cerebral hemisphere induced by injection of sodium amobarbital into the internal carotid artery. Because surgical treatment for medically intractable epilepsy frequently entails resection of brain regions that support important cognitive functions, surgical candidates are at risk for postoperative cognitive decline. The Wada test provides an opportunity to identify these patients, in that temporary anesthesia of brain regions perfused by the internal carotid artery can be viewed as a crude reversible analog of resective surgery. The test was originally developed to determine hemispheric language dominance (Wada 1949), but it was subsequently modified to include assessment of hemispheric memory competence (Milner et al 1962) after several patients developed amnesia and severe memory impairment following bilateral (Scoville & Milner 1957) and unilateral (Penfield & Milner 1958) temporal lobectomy. More recent clinical experience and investigation have further defined the utility of the Wada test (Rausch et al 1993) and also identified many limitations that complicate interpretation of test results (Loring et al 1992a). In this review, we summarize current data regarding traditional uses as well as recent applications of the Wada test; methodological variations and their associated implications; issues of validity and reliability; and alternative procedures for acquiring similar information. We also propose guidelines for clinical practice.

THE PROCEDURE

Patients with medically intractable seizures arising from the temporal lobe constitute the majority of candidates for resective surgery. Because the temporal lobe is intimately involved in language and memory functions, these patients are at risk for postoperative decline in these domains, especially when the resection involves the language-dominant hemisphere (Ivnik et al

1987, Jones-Gotman 1987, Jones-Gotman et al 1993). The Wada test, therefore, primarily involves evaluation of language and memory functions during the period of hemispheric anesthesia. Protocols vary widely in almost every detail, including amobarbital dose, speed and volume of the injection, language and memory assessment techniques, pass/fail criteria, and interpretation of test performance (Rausch et al 1993). An exhaustive review of the techniques used by different epilepsy centers to perform the Wada test is beyond the scope of this chapter and can be found elsewhere (e.g. Loring et al 1992c). The following pretest and test procedures are reasonably routine.

A comprehensive neuropsychological evaluation administered within a few weeks of the actual Wada test provides the examiner with an assessment of the patient's baseline level of cognitive functioning. On the day of the procedure, a practice Wada test is performed to familiarize the patient with the anticipated protocol; to ensure that the patient is functioning at a normal level; and to provide a baseline performance with which to compare that demonstrated following amobarbital injection. Usually before, but sometimes after amobarbital is administered, carotid angiography is carried out to determine if there is cross-flow into the contralateral hemisphere (typically by the anterior communicating artery), perfusion of the posterior cerebral artery, or anomalous, potentially hazardous, neurovascular patterns. Angiography also serves to confirm catheter placement. Patients receive only local anesthesia for the femoral artery puncture, as the effects of even a mild sedative or anxiolytic drug would interfere with cognitive testing.

Just before injecting the amobarbital, the patient, who is lying supine, is asked to hold the arms straight up, with the fingers either wiggling or fisted around the physician's fingers to provide a baseline measure of grip strength. The patient is then instructed to count aloud, at which time 100–200 mg of sodium amobarbital is injected into either the left or right internal carotid artery. Within several seconds after the injection, the patient develops contralateral weakness which ranges from mild paresis to profound plegia. Counting typically stops following injection of the speech-dominant hemisphere. Occasionally, perfusion of the non-dominant hemisphere interrupts counting but this pause is brief and is quickly succeeded by resumption of counting and normal language ability. Language assessment typically includes object naming, repetition, and execution of verbal commands. Memory evaluation consists of either a discrete item presentation or continuous recognition memory format, with the majority of centers employing the former (Loring et al 1992c). With discrete item presentation, acquisition of new information (anterograde memory) is measured by presenting items such as pictures, objects, words or shapes, during the period of drug effect (determined differently at different centres — see below) and recall or recognition of these items is assessed upon return of normal functioning (Milner 1972). Alternatively, a continuous recognition memory task affords assessment of both acquisition and retrieval of information during the drug effect (Fedio & Weinberg 1971, Rausch et al 1984). Presentation of a stimulus (e.g. a picture of an object) is followed by a distractor task (e.g. reading a sentence), after which the patient is required to recall or recognize the previously presented item. Throughout these procedures, physiological measures such as grip strength and electroencephalogram (EEG) activity are obtained to monitor the degree of hemispheric anesthesia during the postinjection period. The contralateral injection is typically performed 30–60 minutes later, although some centres conduct the contralateral injection on the following day to ensure the absence of any residual amobarbital effects.

GOALS

Determination of cerebral language dominance

Most centers concur that one of the principal objectives of the Wada test is to determine hemispheric language dominance. This information potentially affects the decision to pursue surgery and may influence the extent of the resection. Although better seizure relief is generally associated with larger surgical resections, the risk of postoperative cognitive decline may increase as more brain tissue is removed. Consequently, resections within the language-dominant hemisphere tend to be more conservative compared to resections within the non-dominant hemisphere. Additionally, knowledge of hemispheric language dominance can clarify atypical seizure-related language behavior, assist in the interpretation of an unusual neuropsychological profile, and provide confirmatory evidence of early left hemisphere seizure involvement by demonstrating pathological shifting of language to the right hemisphere (Rausch et al 1991).

Validity of the Wada test in determining language lateralization

Although it was previously assumed that hemispheric language dominance could be reliably inferred from handedness, several investigators have demonstrated inconsistencies in the relationship between these two variables (Gloning et al 1969, Rasmussen & Milner 1975, Rausch & Walsh 1984, Strauss & Wada 1988). Although most right-handed individuals are left hemisphere language-dominant, the relation between handedness and language dominance is particularly precarious among epilepsy patients, because early functional or structural lesions can cause intra- or interhemispheric shifting of cortical language areas (Snyder et al 1990, Rausch et al 1991). For instance, Rausch & Walsh (1984) reported that 15% of their right-handed patients with left temporal lobe seizures were right hemisphere language-dominant. Reports of right-handed seizure patients with right temporal lobe epileptogenic foci and right hemisphere language dominance (Rosenbaum et al 1989, Loring et al 1992c) underscore the need for amobarbital testing of all surgical candidates, as knowledge of handedness and seizure laterality are not reliable indicators of language laterality. Although such cases are relatively uncommon, the potentially devastating effects of postoperative aphasia require that all surgical candidates undergo amobarbital testing for more definitive determination of hemispheric language representation.

Comparing data derived from amobarbital studies of language lateralization, cases of postsurgical aphasia (Branch et al 1964) and results of functional cortical mapping (Rosenbaum et al 1989, Loring et al 1990b), the Wada test can currently be considered the gold standard for determining hemispheric language dominance. Nonetheless, despite the strong correspondence between Wada test results and other measures of language laterality, discrepancies have occasionally been reported (Stanulis et al 1989, Loring et al 1992a). Wyllie et al (1990a) found that, whereas Wada test results demonstrating left hemisphere language dominance were highly reliable, findings indicating right hemisphere language did not necessarily indicate exclusive right hemisphere language representation. They described 2 patients who were right hemisphere language-dominant by amobarbital testing but who demonstrated significant left hemisphere language representation when language was mapped extraoperatively using cortical electrical stimulation. Snyder et al (1990) reported similar findings and argued that exclusive right hemisphere language dominance is extremely rare. Rather, they proposed that language dominance, like handedness, is a continuous rather than dichotomous variable.

Several investigators have cautioned that failure to disrupt language functioning with intracarotid amobarbital injection is insufficient evidence to conclude that the injected hemisphere does not support language function (Loring et al 1992a). The absence of language impairment following internal carotid amobarbital injection could be attributable to a number of factors. For instance, the type of task administered may not be suitably demanding. Overlearned phrases such as counting sequences or nursery rhymes are not equivalent to, and are therefore probably not a sound measure of, voluntary productive speech. Additionally, there are currently no standard criteria regarding the nature of vocalizations that constitute language nor the error types that signify language impairment (Snyder et al 1990). Thus, some centers infer language representation based on a period of muteness immediately following injection (Jones-Gotman et al 1993), whereas others disregard the mute phase, which frequently occurs following non-dominant hemisphere injection as well (Oxbury & Oxbury 1984), instead requiring the production of paraphasic errors (Gershenghorn et al 1992).

Although it is generally accepted that the Wada test is a powerful tool for assessing expressive language skills, its adequacy in accurately lateralizing receptive language abilities has been questioned. During the period of expressive aphasia, many patients successfully execute simple commands and show adequate knowledge of semantic relationships such as word–picture matching (Hart et al 1991). McGlone (1984), however, reported impaired execution of complex verbal commands when contextual cues were unavailable. Hart et al (1991) proposed that posterior language regions are probably not sufficiently perfused to test adequately hemispheric receptive language function. However, Loring and colleagues (1992a) have contended that complete anesthesia of all intrahemispheric language areas is not a necessary condition for accurate inference of hemispheric language dominance.

Assessment of hemispheric memory competence

Another goal of amobarbital testing is to identify patients at risk for postsurgical amnesia. Although relatively rare, unilateral temporal lobectomy can result in a global amnesic syndrome if the contralateral temporal lobe cannot support new learning (Penfield & Milner 1958).

Variability among centers in how memory is tested is even greater than that for language testing. There is no uniformity with respect to the type of procedure employed (i.e. continuous or discrete), characteristics of the memory test stimuli, timing of item presentation, criteria for passing, or even how the memory performance should affect surgical decisions. Depending upon the philosophy of the particular center, if a patient 'fails' the Wada memory test with injection ipsilateral to the epileptogenic temporal lobe, any of the following may ensue:

1. The results may be disregarded and the patient will proceed to surgery.
2. The procedure may be repeated using a lower dosage of amobarbital.
3. Other measures assessing the epileptogenic temporal lobe's memory may be implemented (see below).
4. A selective posterior cerebral artery amobarbital test may be performed (Jack et al 1988; see below).
5. Surgery may be cancelled.
6. The resection may be modified to spare the hippocampus and parahippocampal gyrus (Milner, 1972).

Features of Wada memory testing

Memory assessment techniques.   Little is known about the predictive power of the various Wada memory protocols or the extent to which they yield compatible findings. Most centers employing discrete item presentation protocols have reported poorer memory performances following injection of the side contralateral to the seizure focus (Engel et al 1981). Fedio & Weinberg (1971) found that performance using a continuous recall memory format was sensitive to language lateralization but not seizure laterality. Rausch et al (1984) used a modification of this task and reported effects of both language and seizure lateralization as well as an interaction between these two variables, although this appeared to be attributable to a performance asymmetry observed only in the right hemisphere seizure group.

Dodrill (1993) has made the only systematic comparison among Wada memory tasks. He combined three assessment techniques into one Wada protocol to compare performances on the following:

1. continuous recall memory during drug effect (Seattle procedure);
2. post-drug recognition for discrete items presented during the drug effect (Montreal procedure);
3. post-drug recall for events experienced during the procedure (e.g. memory of aphasia, hemiplegia; Interview procedure).

Concordance rates for pass/fail results following injection ipsilateral to the proposed surgery were 70% for the Montreal and Seattle procedures; 71% for the Montreal and interview procedures, and 51% for the Seattle and Interview procedures. All three methods elicited consistent findings in only 18% of their patient sample ($n = 126$). As most centers employ only a single technique, these discordances imply that the same patient may undergo surgery without hesitation at one institution but be denied surgery at another. Such discrepant findings generated by different assessment procedures should be investigated further.

Item characteristics.   There is considerable variation among centers regarding the characteristics of the to-be-remembered stimuli. Rausch et al (1989) asserted the importance of using items that are easily processed by the hemisphere undergoing evaluation (i.e. verbal items should not be critical for memory performance of the non-dominant hemisphere). Perrine et al (1993c) reported that material-specificity is reduced on the epileptogenic side, and therefore these stimuli are most sensitive to hemispheric dysfunction. For dually encodable items, both groups found that right temporal lobe epilepsy patients showed the expected pattern of better memory performance following injection ipsilateral compared to contralateral to the seizure focus, whereas left temporal lobe epilepsy patients demonstrated intact memory following both right and left injections. At odds with these findings are those reported by Christianson et al (1990), in which dually encodable items elicited the expected pattern in both right and left temporal lobe epilepsy groups. Similar findings were reported by Loring et al (1993) who deliberately selected items that were encodable by multiple strategies in order to minimize the effects of aphasia. The underlying cause for these discrepant findings is unclear, but may involve methodological variations or differences in patient populations.

Timing of item presentation.   The optimal time to present stimuli after the injection is controversial (Rausch et al 1993). Although it has been argued that stimuli should be presented immediately post injection when memory-sensitive structures are maximally dysfunctional, anesthetic effects on other cognitive functions that interact with learning (e.g. attention, language processing) are likely to be maximal as well. To minimize the non-specific effects of these other impairments on new learning, Jones-Gotman (1987) recommended presenting items when at least minimal language abilities had recovered. Unfortunately, this typically results in later presentation of items following injection of the language-dominant hemisphere which confounds hemispheric comparison of memory performances. Additionally, several investigators have demonstrated that, although patients may appear inattentive during the early postinjection period, even with the dominant hemisphere injection, there are no significant differences in recognition performances between items presented early versus late after injection (Aasly & Silfvenius 1990, Lesser et al 1986, Loring et al 1990a). In fact, there is some evidence that the hemispheric asymmetry score for early items is a more sensitive measure than for items presented later after injection (Loring et al 1992a. Loring et al in press).

Pass/fail criteria. Over time and among centers, pass/fail criteria have been arbitrarily determined. Early on, Milner et al (1962), considered a single error on postinjection recognition testing as a failure for that injection. As this excluded many patients from surgery, failure was subsequently redefined as greater than two recognition errors (Milner 1972). Current criteria vary widely, with some centers using a postdrug recognition criterion of >67% of items to define pass (Blume et al 1973, Lesser et al 1986, Rausch & Risinger 1990), but other centers use less stringent criteria (e.g. >33% of items recognized, Sass et al 1991). More recently, instead of absolute scores, comparison scores (e.g. fail defined as ≥20% difference between number of items recognized following right and left injections) have been used to identify relatively dysfunctional performances (Loring et al 1993, Wyllie et al 1990). However, <50% correct following each injection was considered a failure for both sides (Wyllie et al 1991a).

Another source of variability in amobarbital memory testing involves the approach to false-positive recognition responses (i.e. guessing). Whereas Powell et al (1987) considered that presence of false positives invalidated memory performance, Loring et al (1992a) employed a calculation to control response biases and guessing. Most reports of Wada memory testing do not address this issue.

Recent applications of Wada memory testing

Predicting material-specific memory decline. Whereas global postoperative amnesia occurs infrequently, detectable postoperative material-specific memory declines are not uncommon, especially following dominant hemisphere resective surgery (Ivnik et al 1987). The Wada memory test was initially developed to predict global postoperative amnesia, and it has been claimed that the technique lacks the sensitivity to predict more subtle postoperative abnormalities (Jones-Gotman 1987). However, given the relative frequency of subtle memory deficits and their potentially significant effect on daily functioning and quality of life, recent efforts have been made to extend the sensitivity of the Wada memory test paradigms. Wyllie et al (1991a) examined 6-month postoperative material-specific memory performances of patients with right and left temporal lobe resections. A significant decline was defined as greater than 10% reduction of their modality-specific index which was comprised of subtest scores from the Wechsler memory scale—Revised (Wechsler 1987). As expected, left temporal lobectomy patients performed worse relative to right temporal lobectomy patients. More importantly, they found that although absolute ipsilateral Wada memory scores were not predictive of postoperative memory performance, the relationship between postoperative memory performance and a comparison score between right and left injection performances approached significance. Rausch & Langfitt (1991) reported that, among a small sample of patients, all of whom has passed the ipsilateral memory test, poorer postoperative performance on a measure of verbal learning correlated with failure to recall a printed word. These findings suggest that the ability to predict postoperative material-specific decline probably requires inclusion of material-specific memory items during Wada testing. Failure to include such items may account for the absence of statistically significant findings reported by Wyllie et al (1991a). A multicenter trial employing identical, sensibly designed Wada tests could probably determine the procedure's ability to predict mild material-specific postoperative memory deficits.

Lateralization of a seizure focus. There is an accumulating body of evidence that the discrepancy between memory of performance following right and left carotid artery injections is a fairly powerful indicator of the laterality of a seizure focus (Wyllie et al 1991b, Loring et al 1993, Perrine et al 1993b). At some centers, a patient may be spared intracranial grid or depth recordings and allowed to proceed directly to surgery if Wada memory comparison data are consistent with other localizing information acquired during the presurgical evaluation (Rausch & Langfitt 1991).

Defining failure as a >20% difference between sides, Wyllie et al (1991b) reported that significantly more patients (80%) failed the injection contralateral than ipsilateral (20%) to the side of the seizure focus. To investigate the ability of performance asymmetries to predict seizure lateralization, we calculated memory lateralization scores by subtracting percentage items recognized following left hemisphere anesthesia from percentage items recognized following right hemisphere anesthesia. Memory lateralization scores accurately predicted side of seizure onset in 100% of right hemisphere seizure patients and 77% of left hemisphere seizure patients. Other investigators have reported similar findings (Powell et al 1987, Rausch et al 1989, Walker & Laxer, 1989). This phenomenon has also been investigated by examining the relationship between amobarbital memory performance and the histological integrity of the contralateral hippocampal region. Although Rausch et al (1989) reported reliably poor memory performance only for patients with severe hippocampal damage (>80% cell loss), Sass et al (1991) found a significant correlation between CA3 cell density and Wada memory scores. Using a discriminant function analysis derived from difference scores for both Wada memory performance and magnetic resonance imaging hippocampal volume asymmetries, Loring et al

(1993) accurately lateralized 75% of left and 100% of right temporal lobe seizure foci. These data provide evidence that Wada memory performance is related to the structural integrity of the contralateral temporal region.

Predicting postsurgery seizure outcome. A recent application of the Wada memory test has been to predict postsurgical seizure outcome. Loring et al (1994) reported that 89% of their patient sample ($n = 55$) with memory asymmetry scores of at least 3 (memory items were 8 dually encodable stimuli) were seizure-free 1 year postsurgery, whereas only 63% of patients with asymmetry scores less than 3 were seizure-free. Similar findings were reported by Sperling et al (1993). Based on the memory asymmetry scores, patients were classified as either lateralized (i.e. ipsilateral minus contralateral injection score >0) or not correctly lateralized (score ≤0). Correctly lateralized patients were more likely to be seizure-free 1 year postoperatively. Loring and colleagues proposed that Wada memory testing, therefore, provides an additional measure with which to counsel patients regarding surgical outcome.

Validity of Wada memory testing

Predicting postoperative global amnesia. Several factors preclude statistically rigorous validation studies of amobarbital memory testing. Assessment of the test's ability to identify patients at risk for postoperative amnesia or significant memory decline requires knowledge of the natural occurrence (i.e. base rate) of the phenomenon. This information has remained elusive for several reasons: because the decision to recommend surgery takes into account the results of the Wada tests, the outcome variable (i.e. postoperative memory functioning) is confounded with the predictor variable (i.e. Wada memory performance; Loring et al 1992a). Consequently, the base rate of postoperative amnesia cannot be determined. Proper assessment of the adequacy of the Wada test to identify patients at risk for postoperative amnesia would require that a series of patients undergo temporal lobectomy without regard to Wada findings.[1] Clearly, this is unrealistic due to ethical and legal concerns. Some measure other than postoperative amnesia is needed with which to compare results of memory testing. However, as no gold standard currently exists, the true base rate of postoperative amnesia cannot be determined. As a result, the validity of the Wada memory test cannot be empirically tested (Rausch & Langfitt 1991).

Another limitation in assessing the validity of the Wada test is that the base rate of postoperative amnesia is probably quite low. Although previously estimated to be 10–20% (Walker 1957), the natural occurrence of postoperative amnesia is probably as low as 1% (Loring et al 1992c). Of the 7766

---

[1] For a detailed discussion on base rates and validity, see Loring et al (1992c). For a detailed discussion on relevant issues of sensitivity and specificity, see Rausch & Langfitt (1991).

temporal lobe resections[2] since 1925 (Engel 1993), to date, there have been 12 reported cases of postoperative amnesia (Perrine 1993). Six of these failed the Wada test and 6 apparently passed. Different protocols were used and technical adequacy of these was not always clear. Nonetheless, at least 50% of patients with postoperative amnesia failed the Wada tests. Patients failing Wada tests do undergo temporal lobectomy without developing global amnesia (Loring et al 1990a). Although the numbers are unknown, the situation is not rare. If we assume for purposes of illustration that 1% of patients undergoing temporal lobectomy fail the Wada test without developing global amnesia (Table 4.1), it is clear that most patients failing the Wada

Table 4.1 Incidence of postoperative global amnesia as a function of Wada memory performance

Wada performance	Global amnesia	No global amnesia
Fail	6	77
Pass	6	7623
Total	12	7700

test do not develop global amnesia after surgery. However, a far greater percentage of the small group who develop postoperative amnesia fail the Wada test than of the much larger group that do not develop postoperative amnesia.

Despite these constraints, several investigators have explored the relationship between memory performance on the Wada test and postoperative memory function. There is substantial evidence that failing the Wada memory test does not always, or even usually, result in a postoperative amnesic syndrome. Loring et al (1990a) reported that 10 of 13 patients who failed the Wada memory test but performed satisfactorily on memory tests during hippocampal stimulation or intraoperative thermal cooling did not develop postoperative amnesia. In fact, most patients either showed no change or improved on selected memory tests administered 1 year postoperatively.[3] Girvin et al (1987) and Novelly & Williamson (1989) have also described patients who failed Wada memory tests but showed no evidence of postoperative amnesia. In contrast, Jones-Gotman et al (1993) demonstrated that patients who failed the ipsilateral amobarbital memory tests and underwent resective surgery sparing the hippocampus performed significantly worse on several delayed Wechsler memory scale — Revised measures (Wechsler 1987) than patients who had passed the amobarbital memory test, even though the

---

[2] This figure includes anterior temporal lobectomy and amygdalohippocampectomy.
[3] Due to poor performance on these ancillary tests, 3 patients underwent surgery with sparing of the hippocampus.

hippocampus had been spared. This suggests that patients who fail amobarbital memory testing have poorer memory abilities preoperatively and decline proportionally after surgery. In addition to comparing the compatibility of findings among different Wada protocols (see above), Dodrill (1993) compared the three procedures regarding the ability of each to predict postoperative memory decline (defined as >40% reduction on two of three measures of verbal memory from the Wechsler memory scale 1 year postsurgery). Six patients exhibiting significant memory decrements were compared with 6 patients who showed no postoperative memory reduction. The Seattle, Montreal and Interview procedures correctly classified 92, 50 and 42% of these patients, respectively. These findings, if confirmed, carry important implications for Wada test protocols, as most centers utilize Montreal-like procedures.

It has been proposed that the high success rate of patients passing the memory test with injection contralateral to the epileptogenic side poses a significant threat to the validity of the Wada test (Loring et al 1992a). Using absolute or percentage recognition scores, Rausch et al (1989) and Jones-Gotman (1987) reported a substantial number of patients who passed the Wada memory test following injection contralateral to the seizure focus. They claimed that the Wada test failed to demonstrate dysfunction of the epileptogenic temporal lobe. However, this conclusion does not take into account possible explanations for the intact performance (e.g. inadequate drug effect, variable perfusion patterns, insufficiently sensitive test paradigms). Additionally, there is an underlying assumption that brain tissue involved in seizure activity is completely and continuously dysfunctional — a hypothesis that has not been empirically verified.

Alternative approaches to assessing the validity of Wada memory testing. Another way of assessing the validity of the Wada test to measure memory function is to compare Wada memory performances with other measures of cognitive functioning. We reasoned that results of hemispheric memory testing should correlate with performances on corresponding material-specific memory functioning (convergent validity). Similarly, non-memory functioning should be unrelated to outcomes of Wada memory (tests divergent validity). We correlated performance on the Wada test following both dominant and non-dominant injections for both right and left hemisphere seizure patients with performance on several measures of attention obtained during the presurgical neuropsychological evaluation (trail making A and B 1944, digit span forward and backward, Wechsler 1981). None of these correlations approached significance, indicating that Wada memory performance is not highly related to, or contingent upon, baseline attentional levels.

Collapsed across right and left temporal lobe epilepsy, Wada performance following left or right internal carotid artery injections did not correlate with any verbal memory measures (Wechsler memory scale — Revised immediate and delayed logical memory, immediate paired associate learning, Buschke Selective Reminding Test). In contrast, following dominant hemisphere anesthesia, the relationship between Wada memory performance and scores on immediate ($r = 0.44$, $P < 0.05$) and delayed ($r = 0.62$, $P < 0.05$) visual reproduction subtests of the Wechsler memory scale — Revised were significant. (Separate correlations for right and left hemisphere seizure groups revealed a similar but not statistically significant pattern for the ipsilateral injection in the left hemisphere seizure group.) This correlation between Wada memory performance and measures of visual memory is reasonable given that most of the Wada memory stimuli are presented visually.

Reliability of Wada memory testing

Because failing the Wada memory test following injection of the epileptogenic hemisphere may exclude a patient from surgery, it is common practice at many centers to repeat the procedure when these circumstances arise (Rausch et al 1993). Reports of patients passing the repeat test (Dinner et al 1987, Novelly 1987) have called into question the reliability of the Wada test. At issue is the reason for the improved performance: was it because of changes in patient characteristics (psychological state, time since most recent seizure, type/dosage of antiepileptic drug), changes in technical aspects of the procedure (amobarbital dose, stimulus characteristics, rate and volume of injection) or changes due to practice effects? McGlone & MacDonald (1989) investigated same-hemisphere retesting (alternate forms reliability, $n = 18$) as well as the effects of practice by comparing performance between the first injection and second (opposite hemisphere) injection ($n = 71$). Of 8 within-hemisphere repeated injections that resulted in changes in pass/fail status, 6 were attributable to external factors that had made initial tests technically unsatisfactory. Additionally, of 8 other cases that were repeated to reinvestigate unexpected language or memory findings, pass/fail status remained the same in 7. Comparison of performances across hemispheres revealed no significant practice effects or relation to which hemisphere was injected first (dominant versus non–dominant, ipsilateral versus contralateral to the seizure focus). Our protocol also demonstrated adequate test–retest reliability in that neither right nor left hemisphere seizure patients showed significant performance differences following same-hemisphere repeated injections. These findings support the conclusion that the Wada test is a reliable procedure if properly executed.

TECHNICAL FACTORS

Methodological variability in Wada test procedures persists, in part due to the paucity of data indicating which variables yield the most reliable and valid results. As the medical community has become aware of the wide inconsistency in test performance and interpretation, systematic investigations of the technical aspects of amobarbital testing have begun to appear in the literature. Critical factors include amobarbital dose and administration, criteria employed as evidence that an appropriate drug effect has been attained (e.g. grip strength, EEG characteristics), cerebral perfusion patterns, and effects of antiepileptic drugs.

Amobarbital dose

Currently, amobarbital dosages among centers range from 60 to 200 mg per injection (Rausch et al 1993). Although 200 mg may have been necessary to elicit a sufficient effect when amobarbital was injected into the common carotid artery (Wade & Rasmussen 1960), lower doses (e.g. 100–125 mg) are adequate when the drug is injected directly into the internal carotid artery. Loring et at (1992b) reported significantly poorer memory performance following injection ipsilateral to the seizure focus with higher doses (up to 250 mg); they subsequently standardized their procedure using 100 mg. It is also important to remember that speed of injection and amobarbital volume and concentration significantly influence the nature, intensity and duration of the drug effect (Rausch et al 1993).

Criteria used to monitor effects of anesthesia

Criteria used to infer adequate hemispheric anesthetization also vary among centers. According to a recent survey (Rausch et al 1993), most centers (79%) regard contralateral hemiparesis as evidence of a sufficient drug effect and 26% reported using loss of antigravity tone. When grip strength was utilized (55% of respondents), some centers required stringent criteria of 0/5, whereas others accepted a grip strength of 4/5 as evidence of continuing drug effect. Loring et al (1992b) reported considerable variability both within and across individuals regarding the amount of amobarbital necessary to produce contralateral hemiplegia. However, their effort to match all patients according to degree of weakness resulted in systematic unmatching on memory performance, the critical variable, because increased doses of amobarbital resulted in poorer memory performance. Several investigators have reported uncoupling of cognitive and sensory/motor dysfunction; that is, dysphasia often outlasts hemiparesis (Rausch et al 1984, Aasly & Silfvenius 1990). Thirty-seven per cent of survey respondents monitored drug-induced EEG slow activity. However, the proportion of delta activity considered as evidence of continued drug effect was arbitrarily determined and varied markedly (Rausch et al 1993). To our knowledge, the relationship between EEG characteristics and memory performance has not been systematically investigated. Rausch et al (1984) reported that, similar to the recovery of language and memory abilities, unilateral EEG slowing lasted longer following injection of the hemisphere contralateral to the seizure focus.[4] It is possible

---

[4] The particular EEG characteristics (e.g. δ–θ transition versus return to baseline) were not specified.

that the time course of EEG recovery may more closely parallel the recovery of cognitive functioning, yet this requires further study.

Perfusion patterns

The significance of arterial perfusion patterns in assessing memory competence is controversial, especially with regard to filling of the posterior cerebral artery (PCA). Although the internal carotid artery typically perfuses the anterior one-third of the hippocampus via the anterior choroidal artery, the posterior portion of the hippocampus is irrigated principally by the vertebrobasilar system through the PCA. In approximately 9% of patients, the PCA originates from the internal carotid artery (Osborne 1980) which enables perfusion of the PCA following carotid artery injection. In another small proportion of patients, the PCA fills from the internal carotid artery by way of the posterior communicating artery (Osborne 1980). Thus, during the majority of Wada tests, some memory-sensitive temporal lobe structures are not perfused with amobarbital. Gotman et al (1992), using depth electrode recording during amobarbital injection, reported slow activity developing throughout the hippocampus, despite perfusion of only the anterior regions. They hypothesized that carotid injection produces complete hippocampal dysfunction because of functional deafferentation of the hippocampus from anesthetized surrounding cortical areas. However, this reasoning is potentially problematic. Although increased EEG δ activity was also recorded from contralateral structures, it is unlikely that these regions had been rendered dysfunctional because of deafferentation. Furthermore, as the relationship between EEG changes and memory function, is not well-characterized, the finding of hippocampal EEG δ activity is difficult to interpret. Other measures of brain function during carotid amobarbital injection have produced discrepant findings. At odds with Gotman et al's EEG findings are single-photon emission tomography (SPECT) studies (Jeffrey et al 1991) showing decreased cerebral blood flow *only* in regions supplied by the anterior and middle cerebral arteries. Although a few centers have experimented with selective PCA injections to ensure amobarbital perfusion of critical mesial temporal lobe structures, this procedure carries a high risk of stroke and is therefore not widely utilized.

Although some case reports have suggested that perfusion of the PCA is critical for interpretation of performance on the Wada test, there is also evidence that PCA filling does not significantly influence the findings (Rausch et al 1989, Perrine 1993). There has also been concern that filling of the contralateral anterior cerebral artery (ACA) via the anterior communicating artery would have potential effects on attention. However, Perrine et al (1993a) could not find any consistent relations between contrateral ACA filling and attentiveness; they observed that obtundation was associated with higher dosages and baseline mental retardation.

Effects of sedative/hypnotics

It is conceivable that patients treated with barbiturates may respond differently to amobarbital than barbiturate-naïve subjects. Although investigators have acknowledged that antiepileptic drugs may influence test performance (Rausch et al 1993), we know of no published reports that have specifically addressed this issue. In our sample, 4 of 9 patients (44.4%) taking sedative hypnotics had an ineffective first injection, compared to 5 of 43 (11.6%) patients not on sedative hypnotic medication. This difference approached, but did not reach statistical significance, probably because of the relatively small sample size.

SELECTIVE AMOBARBITAL TESTS

As previously noted, injection of amobarbital into the internal carotid artery does not affect much of the medial temporal lobe regions. Accordingly, several selective amobarbital tests, have been developed that aim to anesthetize medial temporal regions while leaving other areas relatively unaffected. Two major methods have been described. In one, a catheter is advanced just distal to the anterior choroidal artery and the artery is temporarily occluded at this location. In this situation amobarbital injections selectively perfuse the anterior choroidal territories. Arterial flow carries sufficient amounts of the drug through the posterior communicating artery to the PCA and its branches to allow some anesthesia of the majority of the medial temporal lobe (Wieser 1991). In the other technique, the catheter is advanced through the vertebral and basilar arteries to the peduncular segment of the PCA where amobarbital is injected. This allows more direct administration of amobarbital to the arterial branches perfusing the majority of the medial temporal lobe structures (Jack et al 1989).

These techniques offer several advantages. In contrast to the standard internal carotid injection, aphasia is not produced. Because less amobarbital is necessary, global inattention rarely occurs. Therefore, poor memory performance cannot be attributed either to aphasia or inattentiveness. Most importantly, the structures anesthetized by the procedure correspond more closely to areas resected during radical hippocampectomy and to regions directly involved in learning and memory.

However, both procedures are technically difficult and carry substantially higher risks than intracarotid injections. Vessel tortuosity or other factors prevent adequate catheter placement in 16% of cases, even in expert hands (Jack et al 1989). Major complications (stroke) occur in 2% and minor complications in another 2% (Jack et al 1989). Reflux of amobarbital into the basilar artery with anesthesia of the respiratory center is possible but very rare. These procedure are not used routinely, although they may be used in special cases. Because selective injections are only performed unilaterally, hemispheric memory differences cannot be assessed. Finally, selective amobarbital tests do not allow assessment of language dominance.

Validity issues related to selective injections are even more difficult to evaluate than with standard internal carotid injections. Far fewer selective amobarbital tests have been performed, and the failure rate appears to be low (Jack et al 1988). Jack et al (1989) found a correlation between results of the procedure and change in a post hoc measure of learning after surgery. This was one of seven analyses of a single test performed on 13 selected patients. Reliability of selective amobarbital tests has not been examined.

While selective amobarbital tests have much theoretical appeal, they should be reserved for patients who repeatedly fail standard intracarotid amobarbital injection, especially when failure may be related to aphasia or inattention, or when high drug doses are necessary to achieve hemispheric anesthesia. They are contraindicated in uncooperative patients or when severe arterial tortuosity is present. They should only be performed by interventional neuroradiologists experienced with the technique.

OTHER METHODS OF EXAMINING LANGUAGE DOMINANCE AND HEMISPHERIC MEMORY COMPETENCE

Direct electrical stimulation of cortex can be used to examine language and memory either intraoperatively or extraoperatively using implanted intracranial electrodes. Experience is more extensive with language evaluation. Stimulating current is increased until either disruption of language or electrical afterdischarge occurs. Language is tested by confrontation naming, reading, repetition, and occasionally more complex tasks. Speech arrest is the most common disruption of language observed during stimulation studies. Motor inhibition must be excluded before concluding that speech arrest indicates language cortex.

Electrical stimulation allows detailed mapping of multiple aspects of language, especially during the more lesiurely extraoperative studies. Language disturbances are often evoked outside the traditional Wernicke's and Broca's areas and sites vary widely among patients. Resection of anterior temporal regions where language disruption is induced results in subtle speech defects (Ojeman & Dodrill 1985). However, stimulating medial and lateral superior frontal gyrus and basal temporal areas often disrupts speech as well, and these regions can usually be resected without permanent language deficits (Lüders et al 1991, Ojemann et al 1993). Wyllie et al (1990) found that stimulation studies always confirmed left hemispheric language dominance demonstrated by the Wada test. However, substantial left hemispheric language function was occasionally detected in patients found to be right hemisphere language-dominant by the Wada test. Electrical stimulation may therefore be more accurate than the Wada test in patients with right hemispheric language dominance.

It is less clear that direct electrical stimulation can identify cortical areas critical for memory. One group has reported that memory deficits are commonly induced with stimulation of lateral temporal cortex, and that resection of these regions worsens memory (Ojemann & Dodrill 1987). Others however, have not found memory deficits during stimulation of lateral temporal cortex, even though detailed testing was performed extraoperatively (Ojemann et al 1993). The validity and reliability of direct electrical stimulation in assessing hemispheric memory competence require further study.

Two studies have reported using *transcranial magnetic stimulation* to lateralize language (Pascual-Leone et al 1991, Jennum et al 1994). Magnetic stimulation delivered by a coil placed over the anterior temporal scalp region was used to inactivate the underlying cerebral cortex. Frequency and intensity of the magnetic stimuli were increased until speech arrest occurred in 20 of 27 patients in the two studies. Slowing of speech occurred in the others. Language dominance determined in this manner corresponded to language dominance determined by the Wada test in 26 of 27 cases.

Unlike the Wada test, magnetic coil stimulation does not require hospitalization, is easily repeated, and appears to pose little risk. It also appears to inactivate more discrete areas than amobarbital infusion. However, stimulation of the anterior temporal region often results in contraction of facial and laryngeal muscles which may make the distinctions between anarthria and aphasia difficult. Most importantly, coils allowing sufficient rates of stimulation to inactivate language cortex are not widely available. Though the technique remains experimental, it deserves further study.

Functional positron emission tomography and, more recently, *dynamic magnetic resonance imaging* provide other non-invasive means of evaluating brain function. These techniques measure local changes in cerebral glucose utilization, cerebral blood flow, and blood oxygenation due to local neuronal activity. They will almost certainly demonstrate language dominance with sufficient resolution to be clinically useful and may eventually provide useful information regarding structures critical for memory in individual patients. The validity of both procedures will have to be established as with the Wada test.

KEY POINTS FOR CLINICAL PRACTICE

Although many of the procedural issues discussed in this chapter remain controversial, a number of questions have been addressed systematically within the past several years. As a result of these efforts, many of the arbitrary decisions regarding Wada procedures are no longer justified. In actuality, several investigations now form the basis for systematizing components of the procedure. The protocol currently used at the Neurological Institute of New York is given in Table 4.2.

Table 4.2   Current Wada protocol in use at the Neurological Institute of New York, Columbia Presbyterian Medical Center

†Time	Record patient response	Memory performance (multiple choice)	Confidence rating: 1 = guess 3 = sure
Preinjection	Patient begins counting aloud		
Inject	Patient reaches '5'		
Assess grip strength			
Execution of verbal commands			
Point to ceiling			
Stick out tongue			
Assess grip strength			
Name pictured objects:			
Tie*			
Rabbit			
Assess grip strength			
Name real objects			
One-dollar bill			
Comb			
Assess grip strength			
Name pictured object			
Lamp			
Drum			
Assess grip strength			
Name Sounds			
Telephone touch-tone			
Cat meow			
Assess grip strength			
Language testing			
Name body parts			
Nose, thumb			
Repeat words:			
Gingerbread			
Snowman			
Repeat phrases:			
Down to earth			
No ifs, ands, or buts			
The spy fled to Greece			
Answer questions:			
What is the colour of an apple?			
Are 2 lbs of flour heavier than one?			
Assess neurological functioning and mental status. If normal, proceed to memory assessment (approximately 15 min postinjection)			

*Items shown are examples. Different items are used for right and left internal carotid artery injections.
†Include in memory assessment only items presented during full hemiplegia and electroencephalogram slowing. Passing performance ≥67% correct on recognition testing.

- Given the unreliability of handedness and seizure laterality in determining cerebral language dominance, all surgical candidates should undergo a Wada test to ascertain this information. Right hemisphere language dominance determined by the Wada test is not necessarily indicative of exclusive right hemisphere language dominance.

- Amobarbital 100–125 mg produces an adequate drug effect in adults, smaller dosages are insufficient, and larger dosages impair performance.

- Despite the immediate postinjection effects of aphasia or inattention, there is substantial evidence that patients can recognize items presented during this early postinjection period. Testing based on items presented early seems to be more sensitive to contralateral dysfunction than testing using items presented later after injection.

- Hemispheric asymmetry scores may be more useful than absolute pass/fail criteria in evaluating hemispheric memory competence and in predicting lateralization of the epileptogenic zone.

- Selective Wada tests should be attempted only when standard testing has failed to generate the necessary information, and only by neuroradiologists with extensive experience in these techniques.

- Given the potentially high rate of false-positive results, failure to pass the ipsilateral Wada memory test is not an absolute contraindication to resective surgery and should be considered within the context of other data. Further evaluation (repeat standard Wada, selective Wada, intra- or extraoperative stimulation, intraoperative cooling) may be necessary.

REFERENCES

Aasly J, Silfvenius H. 1990 Evaluation of early and late presented tasks in the intracarotid amytal test for epileptic patients. Epilepsy Res 7: 155–164

Army Individual Test Battery 1944 Manual of directions and scoring. Washington DC: War Department, Adjutant General's Office

Blume W T, Grabow J D, Darley F L et al. 1973 Intracarotid amobarbital test of language and memory before temporal lobectomy for seizure control. Neurology 23: 812–819

Branch C, Milner B, Rasmussen T. 1964 Intracarotid sodium amytal for the lateralization of cerebral speech dominance: observations in 123 patients. J Neurosurg 21: 399–405

Buschke H, Fuld P A. 1974 Evaluating storage, retention and retrieval in disordered memory and learning. Neurology 24: 1019–1025

Christianson S A, Saisa J, Silfvenius H. 1990 Hemispheric memory differences in sodium amytal testing of epileptic patients. J Clin Exp Neuropsychol 12: 681–694

Dinner D S, Lüders H Morris H H III, Wyllie E, Kramer R E. 1987 Validity of intracarotid sodium amobarbital (Wada test) for evaluation of memory function. Neurology 37 (S): 142

Dodrill C B. 1993 Preoperative criteria for identifying eloquent brain: intracarotid amytal for language and memory testing. Neurosurg Clin North Am 4: 211–216

Engel J Jr. 1993 Overview: Who should be considered a surgical candidate? In: Engle J Jr, ed. Surgical treatment of the epilepsies, 2nd edn New York: Raven Press, pp 341–357

Engel J, Rausch R, Lieg J P et al. 1981 Correlation of criteria used for localizing epileptic foci in patients considered for surgical therapy of epilepsy. Ann Neurol 9: 215–224

Fedio P, Weinberg L K. 1971 Dysnomia and impairment of verbal memory following internal carotid injection of sodium amytal. Brain Res 31: 159–168

Gershenghorn J, Brown E, Haywood et al. 1992 Criteria for assessing bilateral language dominance in the IAP. Neurology 42: 148

Girvin J P, McGlone J, McLachlan R S et al. 1987 Validity of the sodium amobarbital test for memory in selected patients. Epilepsia 26: 636

Gloning K. 1977 Handedness and aphasia. Neuropsychologia 15: 355–358

Gloning I, Gloning K, Harb G, Quatember R. 1969 Comparison of verbal behavior in right-handed and nonright-handed patients with anatomically verified lesions of one hemisphere. Cortex 5: 43–52

Gotman J, Bouwer M S, Jones-Gotman M. 1992 Intracranial EEG study of brain structures affected by internal carotid injection of amobarbital. Neurology 42: 2136–2143

Hart J, Lesser R P, Fisher R S et al. 1991 Dominant-side intracarotid amobarbital spares comprehension of word meaning. Arch Neurol 48: 55–58

Ivnik R J, Sharbrough F W, Laws E R. 1987 Effects of anterior temporal lobectomy on cognitive function. J Clin Psychol 43: 128–137

Jack C R, Nichols D A, Sharbrough F W et al 1988 Selective posterior cerebral artery amytal test for evaluating memory function before surgery for temporal lobe seizure. Radiology 168: 787–793

Jack C R, Nichols D A, Sharbrough F W et al. 1989 Selective posterior cerebral artery injection of amytal: new method of preoperative memory testing. Mayo Clin Proc 64: 965–975

Jeffrey P J, Monsein L H, Szabo A et al. 1991 Mapping the distribution of amobarbital sodium in the intracarotid Wada test by use of Tc-99m HMPAO with SPECT. Radiology 178: 847–850

Jennum P, Friburg L, Fuglsang-Frederiksen A, Dam M. 1994 Speech localization using repetitive transcranial magnetic stimulation. Neurology 44: 269–273

Jones-Gotman M. 1987 Commentary: Psychological evaluation–testing hippocampal function. In: Engel J, ed. Surgical treatment of the epilepsies. New York: Raven Press, pp 203–211

Jones-Gotman M, Barr W B, Dodrill C B et al. 1993 Postscript: controversies concerning the use of the intraarterial amobarbital procedures. In: Engel J Jr, ed. Surgical treatment of the epilepsies, 2nd edn. New York: Raven Press, pp 445–449

Lesser R P, Dinner D S, Lüders H et al, 1986 Memory for objects presented soon after intracarotid amobarbital sodium injections in patients with medically intractable complex partial seizures. Neurology 36: 895–899

Loring D W, Lee P L, Meador K J et al. 1990a The intracarotid amobarbital procedures as a predictor of memory failure following unilateral temporal lobectomy. Neurology 40: 605–610

Loring D W, Meador K J, Lee P L et al. 1990b Crossed aphasia in a patient with complex partial seizures: evidence from intracarotid sodium amytal testing, functional cortical mapping and neuropsychological assessment. J Clin Exp Neuropsychol 12: 340–354

Loring D W, Meador K J, Lee P L. 1992a Criteria and validity issues in Wada assessment. In: The neuropsychology of epilepsy. New York: Plenum Press, pp 233–245

Loring D W, Meador K J, Lee P L. 1992b Amobarbital dose effects on Wada memory testing. J Epilepsy 5: 171–174

Loring D W, Meador K J, Lee P L et al. 1992c Amobarbital effects and lateralized brain function: the Wada test. New York: Springer Verlag

Loring D W, Murro A M Meador K J. 1993 Wada memory testing and hippocampal volume measurements in the evaluation for temporal lobectomy. Neurology 43: 1789–1793

Loring D W, Meador K J, Lee P L et al. 1994 Stimulus timing effects on Wada memory testing. Arch Neurol 51: 806–810

Lüders H, Lesser R P, Hahn J et al. 1991. Basal temporal language area. Brain 114: 743–754

McGlone J. 1984 Speech comprehension after unilateral injection of sodium amytal. Brain Lang 22: 150–157

McGlone J, MacDonald B H. 1989 Reliability of the sodium amobarbital test for memory. J Epilepsy 2: 31–39

Milner B. 1972 Disorders of learning and memory after temporal lobe lesions in man. Clin Neurosurg 19: 421–446

Milner B, Branch C, Rasmussen T. 1962 Study of short-term memory after intracarotid injection of sodium amytal. Trans Am Neurol Assoc 87: 224–226

Novelly, R A. 1987 Relationship of intracarotid sodium amytal procedure to clinical and neurosurgical procedures to clinical and neurological variables in epilepsy surgery. J Clin Exp Neuropsychol 9: 33

Novelly R A, Williamson P D. 1989 Incidence of false positive memory impairment in the intracarotid amytal procedure, Epilepsia 30: 711

Ojemann G A, Dodrill C B. 1985 Verbal memory deficits after left temporal lobectomy for epilepsy. J Neurosurg 62: 101–107

Ojemann G A, Dodrill C B. 1987 Intraoperative techniques for reducing language and memory deficits with left temporal lobectomy. In: Wolf P, Dam M, Janz F, Dreifuss F E, eds. Advances in epileptology, vol 16. New York: Raven Press, pp 327–330

Ojemann G A, Sutherling W W, Lesser R P, Dinner D S, Jayakar P, Saint-Hilaire J M. 1993 Cortical stimulation In: Engel J Jr, ed. Surgical treatment of the epilepsies, 2nd edn. New York: Raven Press, pp. 399–414

Oxbury S M, Oxbury J M. 1984 Intracarotid amytal test in the assessment of language dominance. In: Rose F C, ed. Advances in neurology, vol 42. Progress in aphasiology. New York: Raven Press, 115–123

Pascual-Leone A, Gates J R, Dhuna A. 1991 Induction of speech arrest and counting errors with rapid-rate transcranial magnetic stimulation. Neurology 41: 697–702

Penfield W, Milner B. 1958 Memory deficits produced by bilateral lesions in the hippocampal zone. Arch Neurol Psychiatry 79: 475–497

Perrine K. 1993 Future directions for functional mapping. Miami, FL: American Epilepsy Society

Perrine K, Devinsky O, Luciano D et al. 1993a Behavioral correlates of arterial filling in the intracarotid amobarbital procedure. Epilepsia 34: 85

Perrine K, Sass K J, Choi I S et al. 1993b Interhemispheric difference scores in IAP memory testing. J Clin Exp Neuropsychol 15: 24

Perrine K, Gershengorn J, Brown E R et al. 1993c Material-specific memory in the intracarotid amobarbital procedure. Neurology 43: 706–711

Powell G E, Polkey C E, Canavan A G M. 1987 Lateralization of memory functions in epileptic patients by use of the sodiumamytal (Wada) technique. J Neurol Neurosurg Psychiatry 50: 665–672

Rasmussen T, Milner B. 1975 Clinical and surgical studies of the cerebral speech areas in man. In: Zulch K J Creutzfelft O, Galbraith G C, eds. Cerebral localization: an Otrfid Foerster symposium. New York: Springer Verlag, pp 238–257

Rausch R, Langfitt J T. 1991 Memory evaluation during the intracarotid sodium amobarbital procedure. In: Lüders H, eds. Epilepsy surgery: pp 507–514

Rausch R, Risinger M. 1990 Intracarotid sodium amobarbital procedure. In: Boulton A A, Baker G B, Hiscick M, eds. Neuromethods 17: Clifton, NJ: Humana Press

Rausch R, Walsh G. 1984 Right-hemisphere language dominance in right-handed epileptic patients. Arch Neurol 41: 1077–1080

Rausch R, Fedio P, Ary C et al. 1984 Resumption of behavior following intracarotid sodium amytal injection. Arch Neurol 15: 31–35

Rausch R, Babb T L, Engel J, Crandall P H. 1989 Memory following intracarotid sodium amobarbital injection contralateral to hippocampal damage. Ann Neurol 46: 783–788

Rausch R, Boone K, Ary C M. 1991 Right-hemisphere language dominance in temporal lobe epilepsy: clinical and neuropsychological correlates. J Clin Exp Neuropsychol 13: 217–231

Rausch R, Silfvenius H, Weiser H et al. 1993 Intraarterial amobarbial procedures. In: Engle J Jr, ed. Surgical treatment of the epilepsies, 2nd edn. New York: Raven Press, pp 341–357

Rosenbaum T, DeToledo J, Smith D B et al. 1989 Preoperative assessment of language laterality is necessary in all epilepsy surgery candidates: a case report. Epilepsia 30: 712

Sass K J, Lencz T, Westerveld M et al. 1991 The neural substrate of memory impairment demonstrated by the intracarotid amobarbital procedure. Arch Neurol 48: 48–52

Scoville W B, Milner B. 1957 Loss of recent memory after bilateral hippocampal lesions. J Neurol Neurosurg Psychiatry 20: 11–21

Snyder P H, Novelly R A, Harris L J. 1990 Mixed speech dominance in the intracarotid sodium amytal procedure: validity and criteria issues. J Clin Exp Neuropsychol 12: 629–643

Sperling M R, Glosser G, Saykin A J et al. 1993 Intracarotid amobarbital test predicts seizure relief after temporal lobectomy. Epilepsia 34: 70–71

Stanuli R G, Valentine R V, Kramer R E et al. 1989 ISA and grid mapping of language: a case of divergent findings? Epilepsia 30: 712

Strauss E, Wada J. 1988 Hand preference and proficiency and cerebral speech dominance determined by the carotid amytal test. J Clin Exp Neuropsychol 10: 169–174

Wada J 1949 [A new method of determining the side of cerebral speech dominance: a preliminary report on the intracarotid injection of sodium amytal in man.] Igaku to Seibutsugaki 14: 221–222 (in Japanese)

Wada J, Rasmussen T. 1960 Intracarotid injection of sodium amytal for the lateralization of cerebral speech dominance: experimental and clinical observations. J Neurosurg 17: 266–282

Walker J A. 1957 Recent memory impairment in unilateral temporal lesions. Arch Neurol Psychiatry 78: 543–552

Walker J A, Laxer K D. 1989 Comparison of recall and recognition memory in the Wada test. Epilepsia 30: 712–713

Wechsler D. 1981 Wechsler adult intelligence scale–revised. New York: Psychological Corporation

Wechsler D. 1987 Wechsler memory scale–revised: manual. New York: Psychological Corporation

Wieser H G. 1991 Anterior cerebral artery amobarbital test. In: Lüders H, ed. Epilepsy surgery. New York: Raven Press, pp 515–523

Wyllie E, Naugle R, Awad I et al. 1991a Intracarotid amobarbital procedure. I. Prediction of decreased modality-specific scores after temporal lobectomy. Epilepsia 32: 857–864

Wyllie E, Naugle R, Chelune G et al. 1991b Intracarotid amobarbital procedure: II. Lateralizing value in evaluation for temporal lobectomy. Epilepsia 32: 865–869

5

Cortical localization of cognitive functions

C. E. Elger   Th. Grunwald   C. Helmstaedter   M. Kurthen

The cortical localization of mental processes has been a major topic of scientific research in neurology since the latter half of the 19th century, when Broca, Lichtheim and Wernicke developed their theories on aphasias and the cerebral language system. Their hypotheses made them the pioneers of a conception later apostrophized as connectionism. According to this view, which was further elaborated by researchers like Norman Geschwind, higher cortical functions are associated with distinct cortical regions and the pathways between them. This concept was vehemently opposed by followers of the so-called holistic view of brain function, held by investigators such as Lashley, Head and Goldstein, although the analyses of individual patients by followers of both schools are much less incompatible than it might seem at first sight.

The only method available to early neuropsychologists was to explore single cases thoroughly and to generate hypotheses based on the location of underlying brain lesions which were fully characterized by postmortem neuropathological analysis. Clinical neuropsychology became independent of brain pathology with the introduction of *structural imaging* methods (brain computed tomography (CT) and magnetic resonance imaging (MRI), which today can visualize location and extent of lesions in the living brain with great accuracy. Valuable knowledge has been accumulated by these kinds of studies, but they are nevertheless subject to some important restrictions. In patients with lesions, one can only test those functions that the injured brain can still perform and describe how these performances deviate from normal cognitive processes. Thus, Hughlings Jackson's criticism that the location of the brain lesion of an aphasic patient shows only in which cortical area language can be disturbed, not in which it resides, is still valid (Head 1915). Furthermore, the brain can exhibit considerable neuronal plasticity which can affect strategies of cognitive processing as well as their cortical localization. Therefore, lesional studies may reflect the adaptation of the injured brain to a lesion rather than 'normal' cortical localizations and processing. This is especially true for patients with focal epilepsies as a result of early childhood brain damage which can result in considerable shifts of the cortical representation of cognitive functions. As has been shown by intracarotid amobarbital studies (see below), there are considerably more cases of atypical patterns of language dominance than previously expected. Neuronal plasticity is the basis by which the brain copes with early acquired damage, this plasticity results in a variability in the localization of brain functions that must be taken into account in lesional studies.

Physicians interested in epilepsy surgery were aware early of the need to determine the localization of cognitive functions in individual patients because of the necessity to perform operations in cortical areas that are macroscopically normal. There is a risk of producing additional neuro-psychological deficits when operations are performed within eloquent brain regions. Efforts to minimize this risk led to the technique of electrical stimulation mapping, which made it possible to activate or disturb cortical functions by the application of an electrical current to the intrasurgically exposed brain. The epoch-making work of Penfield and colleagues (Penfield & Jasper 1954, Penfield & Roberts 1959) gave new impetus to the search for the cortical localization of cognitive functions. However, applicable test paradigms as well as the performance of the patient in these kind of studies are certainly restricted by the operating-room setting and open craniotomy. Modern electrocorticography, using chronically implanted intracranial elec-trodes that can remain in situ for a longer time and can be used for electrical stimulation mapping as well, is the response to this criticism. It must again be kept in mind that patients undergoing presurgical evaluation have morpho-logical or functional lesions, and the implantation of grid electrodes, for example, is usually designed to cover lesional areas. So the objection still holds that the location of a lesion that correlates with impaired cognitive functions cannot be taken immediately as proof for the normal localization of these functions. The issue of plasticity can also be addressed using the intracarotid amobarbital procedure (IAP or Wada test), which was designed to identify hemispheric dominance for language and, later memory abilities in the individual patient. The selective narcosis of one hemisphere permits testing the abilities of the isolated remaining hemisphere, but of course, this method is a dramatic interference with normal brain function − and of course, normal controls are not available for Wada tests for ethical reasons. (For further discussion of the Wada test, see Chapter 4.)

The search for a *physiological* localization of cognitive processes within the cortex thus makes it necessary to compare results between lesional studies with examinations of healthy subjects. This calls for non-invasive physiologi-cal studies of cognitive processes, a demand that is met by *functional imaging techniques* which do not depend on analysing suppressed or impaired cognitive functions. A breakthrough in this field was a method for studying regional cerebral blood flow (rCBF) using isotope clearance (Ingvar & Lassen 1965). Higher spatial resolution is obtained using the newer techniques of single-photon emission computed tomography (SPECT), positron emission tomography (PET), and most recently functional MRI. While the spatial resolution of functional imaging techniques has been considerably improved, their temporal resolution is still a problematic issue for the analysis of cognitive processes. In this domain, however, *electrophysiological studies* using event-related electrical potential and magnetic fields are helping to clarify the time-course of cognitive processes. Combining functional imaging with electro-encephalograms (EEG), electrocorticography and magnetoencephalography (MEG)-studies seems, therefore, to be a promising new approach in modern psychophysiology. Last but not least, it was the introduction of standardized *neuropsychological tests* that made methodologically sound intra- and inter-individual comparisons possible.

Results of lesional as well as physiological studies have clearly demon-strated that the view of there being a few unvaryingly delimited cortical centres, each completely representing one special function, is oversimplistic. While certain cortical areas do participate in special neuropsychological processes, the concept of *single* functional centres has been replaced by a theory of distributed neuronal assemblies participating preferably (though not exclusively) in the processing of special external or internal stimuli. Thus, it seems likely that a certain cortical area may be of importance for different aspects of cognitive functions, like the dominant perisylvian area for language processing as well as for declarative verbal memory. Converging evidence of studies using different methodologies has made it possible to identify cortical areas associated with neuropsychological functions in this way. Figure 5.1 summarizes the current discussion of these areas in the form of a tentative map with an attribution to the hemispheres that should be understood given all the above mentioned limitations.

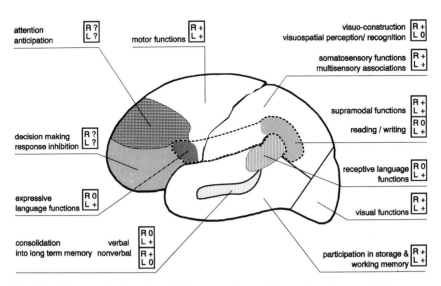

Fig. 5.1 Schematic drawing of cortical areas associated with cognitive functions. The function is attributed to a certain brain region by a line. L = left; R = right; + = function; 0 = no function; ? = possible function.

Cortical functions are affected by epilepsy in several ways. Ictal and interictal activity cause functional disturbances, and underlying brain lesions may produce permanent deficits. Additionally, medical and surgical treatment can interfere with cortical abilities. Most studies of patients with epilepsy involve language and memory. Therefore we will concentrate in the following two sections on these two cognitive functions which are both central to human neuropsychology and of utmost importance in the diagnosis and therapy of epileptic patients. Both may be affected by the pathological process itself, and the protection of both must be an essential goal of epilepsy surgery which is most often performed on temporal lobe structures.

LANGUAGE

Cortical localization of language functions was the major issue separating the connectionist and holistic conceptions mentioned above. While early research was methodologically confined to the postmortem analysis of lesions in aphasic patients and focused on rather circumscribed cortical areas such as Broca's area in the gyrus opercularis of the lower frontal gyrus and Wernicke's area in the posterior part of the superior temporal gyrus of the left hemisphere, current research using CT or MRI has shown a higher than expected variability in the topography of the classical speech centres. Basso et al (1985) reported unexpected lesions in 17% of a large group (n = 207) of right-handed fluent or non-fluent aphasics studied with CT. They even found cases of clinically defined Broca's or Wernicke's aphasia in which the classical speech regions were unaffected. Damasio (1989) found that Broca's and Wernicke's area varied interindividually in site and extension. Hence, these areas seem to be related to cortical areas which are larger than was assumed in earlier studies.

Most *functional imaging* studies of language function have involved PET. Wise et al (1991) found that comprehension and retrieval of single words were accompanied by the activation of variable cortical areas in addition to the constant involvement of Wernicke's area. Other studies support the involvement of the left inferior frontal cortex in the syntactic processing of sentences (Rumsey et al 1994) and the major role of the left superior temporal and left dorsolateral prefrontal regions in intrinsic word generation assessed by a word fluency task (Friston et al 1991). These results support earlier hypotheses concerning language-associated areas, but are, at the present, frequently discussed within the framework of a distributed-network view of cortical language representation (see below).

Electrophysiological studies of language using electrical stimulation of awake patients undergoing brain surgery or of patients with implanted grids or subdural electrodes permit functional cortical mapping with a spatial resolution of about 10 mm. Recent work confirms the major contribution of the left perisylvian cortex to language, although other widespread cortical areas are also involved in linguistic processing (Ojemann 1991). However, stimulation mapping also demonstrates a great variability in language-associated areas, especially for the most thoroughly investigated subfunctions of naming and reading (Ojemann et al 1989). More innovatively, stimulation mapping has led to the assumption that in some patients there is a hitherto unrecognized third language area in the left fusiform gyrus (Lüders et al 1991). The specific role of this basal temporal language area remains unknown, because resection of the basal temporal cortex does not produce aphasic symptoms. When interpreting these results, it must be kept in mind that this method maps areas in which language processes can be disturbed by the application of an electric current. This does not necessarily mean that the underlying cortex processes language.

Neuropsychological tests for memory processes can also contribute to understanding the cortical basis of language functions, as demonstrated by the work of Baddeley et al (1988), Gathercole & Baddeley (1990) and Papagno et al (1991). Their studies indicate that the left perisylvian cortex is crucial for the short-term storage of verbal stimuli for phonological analysis, and thus may provide the morphological correlate of phonological working memory. However, language test batteries designed for the examination of aphasic patients prove, as a rule, to be unsuitable for testing patients with focal epilepsies, because deviations in their language performance are usually too subtle to be accounted for by common test measures. In this field there is a need for new test material tailored to the special demands of examining epileptic patients. It may well be that careful analyses of speech acts on the level of linguistic pragmatics can differentiate language performance of patients with epileptogenic foci in different cortical areas.

In the IAP or Wada test that was designed for determining the dominant hemisphere (Wada & Rasmussen 1960), barbiturate injection into the internal carotid artery contralateral to the side of language dominance leads to short-term dose-dependent aphasic syndromes, while the contralateral injection leaves linguistic functions unimpaired (see Chapter 8). Earlier IAP studies with very short language tests (mostly naming and serial speech) yielded an elementary differentiation of left, right and bilateral speech representation. On the basis of more extended language testing, the degree of asymmetries in language representation can be evaluated more precisely. Combined with clinical and neuroimaging data, results from IAP language testing will also give clues to the aetiology and intrahemispheric topography of language representation patterns.

In the Bonn IAP series (Kurthen et al 1994), candidates for epilepsy surgery underwent a total of six short language subtests in each IAP: serial speech, sentence comprehension, body commands, naming, repetition and reading. For a quantitative evaluation of dominance patterns, spontaneous speech was considered as a seventh criterion. Then, a simple score for performance in either IAP was defined as the sum of subscores in tasks 1–6 and spontaneous speech. In each task, two points were given for a faultless performance, one point for an impaired performance, and no point for a complete failure. The lateralization index L was then computed according to the formula

$$L = ((IAP_{right} - IAP_{left})/(IAP_{left} + IAP_{right})) / (n / m)$$

where the $(R - L) / (R + L)$ term yields a value between $+1$ (i.e. complete left-hemisphere dominance, CLD) and -1 (i.e. complete right-hemisphere dominance (CRD), while the right-sided quotient (n / m) serves as a correction factor for patients with a zero-score in one IAP and incomplete failure in the other (n stands for the score with incomplete failure, m for the highest possible score, that is, 14). In a group of 173 patients we found a high proportion of patients with bilateral language representation (BR; $n = 63$). The distribution of lateralization indices in these BR patients shows that in the most cases there is still a relative superiority of one hemisphere (Fig. 5.2). This presentation also reveals a partially continuous gradation of language lateralization with minor gaps, especially between strongly bilateral representation ($L = 0$) and right-hemisphere dominance ($L = -1$). These results suggest that language dominance is a continuous rather than a discrete variable (cf. Loring et al 1990), and that the extreme indices of $+1$, 0, and -1 can be seen as lateralization attractors (Kurthen et al 1994).

With respect to the aetiology and inter- and intrahemispheric topography of language representation patterns, cases with extreme bilaterality (indices around 0) are most interesting, as the following example demonstrates. An 18-year-old right-handed woman suffered from medically uncontrolled com-

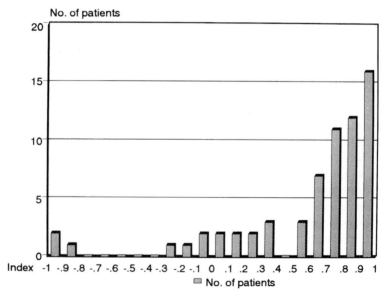

Fig. 5.2 Distribution of laterality indices (L) in 63 epileptic patients with bilateral language representation as indicated by intracarotid amobarbital procedure (IAP).

plex partial seizures since the age of 3 years. Electrocorticography revealed ictal onset in the right orbital–frontal area, with epileptic activity spreading to frontopolar and frontolateral areas. CT and MRI scans were normal, but SPECT images showed right frontal hypoperfusion postictally as well as ictal hyperperfusion in the same area. This patient showed isolated preservation of expressive language functions during right IAP, while left-sided amobarbital injection left only receptive language functions unimpaired. This suggests an interhemispheric dissociation of expressive and receptive functions, with the posterior language area located in the right hemisphere, and the anterior language area in the left. It can be assumed that in the absence of right frontal lobe dysfunction, this patient would have developed right-hemisphere language dominance. The circumscribed right frontal focus, however, led to the shift of expressive — but not of receptive — functions to the left hemisphere. After a right frontal resection, no aphasic symptoms occurred in this patient (Kurthen et al 1992).

Thus, it seems that a conception of strictly circumscribed and unvarying cortical centres processing language cannot account for the individually differing language representation patterns. On the other hand, results of the studies referred to in this section strongly argue against a distribution of language throughout the whole brain. Rather, there is emerging evidence for the association of special linguistic processes with distributed — but identifiable — neuronal assemblies within certain cortical areas, primarily the perisylvian region. Clinical, neuropsychological and neuroimaging data as well as results of intracarotid amobarbital testing contribute to the analysis of the inter- and intrahemispheric topography of language functions. Functional imaging using cognitive activation and electrophysiological studies using the techniques of cortical stimulation mapping and registration of event-related potentials are of increasing importance, as will be pointed out later. Thus, a multidisciplinary neurophysiological–neuropsychological–neuroimaging approach seems to offer promising possibilities for a better understanding of brain mechanisms related to language.

MEMORY

Even more than for language it may seem impossible to identify topological correlates for such an intricate and complex function as memory, especially in view of growing evidence for the existence of multiple memory systems. While the distinction between *short-term* and *long-term memory* emphasizes temporal aspects of memory processes, more recent findings prove that long-term memory itself is no single entity, but rather comprises different components with regard to its contents. Thus, the notion of *declarative memory* refers to the storage of events and facts that can be consciously recalled and consists of both episodic and semantic items. *Non-declarative memory*, on the other hand, includes different forms of learning and storage processes associated with skills and habits that cannot be recollected consciously but express themselves through performance (cf. Squire et al 1993). Analyses of the localization of lesions in patients with amnesic syndromes, however, revealed that certain memory processes can indeed be associated with special brain systems. It was especially shown that the declarative memory system depends on the function of medial temporal and diencephalic structures (Squire & Zola-Morgan 1991, Zola-Morgan & Squire 1993).

Since the seminal work of Milner (Milner et al 1962), *intra-arterial amobarbital procedures* have been used to determine the lateralization of material-specific memory functions. Performance in short memory tests after unilateral injection of amobarbital is thought to represent the amnestic capacities of the unaffected hemisphere. Data from IAP studies largely support the hypothesis of a left-hemisphere dominance for verbal memory functions and a right-hemisphere superiority for non-verbal memory (Silfvenius et al 1988). One disadvantage of the memory-oriented IAP is the unavoidable anesthesia of undesirably large cortical areas in combination with an inconstant and interindividually variable effect on medial temporal structures (Hart et al 1993). To minimize these undesirable features, selective techniques have been developed to allow amobarbital injection into the posterior cerebral artery (Jack et al 1988) or the anterior choroid artery (Wieser et al 1989). These selective amobarbital procedures can demonstrate more specifically the role of mesial temporal structures in material-specific memory. Although these results are definitely relevant to localizationalist approaches to memory, the clinical value of memory-oriented IAP, especially its predictive power with respect to possible postoperative memory deficits, is still a matter of controversy (Loring et al 1991).

Neuropsychological testing, on the other hand, has proved to be highly relevant for evaluating memory functions in patients with focal epilepsies, and can even contribute to the topological diagnosis. Because of data obtained in early hippocampal models of amnesia (Scoville & Milner 1957), much effort has been directed towards the functional organization of the temporolimbic system and its involvement in memory processes. Now, there is converging evidence that multiple memory systems (declarative/non-declarative) are subserved by different neuronal substrates, and that these can be affected selectively. Investigations of global amnesia show that bilateral lesions of the hippocampi and related cortical structures can lead to severe impairment of episodic and semantic declarative memory performance, while non-declarative procedural or skill-oriented learning, conditioning and priming are largely preserved. Apart from this differentiation, the medial temporal lobe system may be preferentially involved in fast and time-limited consolidation processes of memory contents, i.e. the hippocampus mediates long-term declarative memory. Short-term (or working) memory as well as the actual storage of information are believed to be provided by neocortical structures (Eichenbaum et al 1992, Squire 1992). Finally, the left and right medial temporal lobe systems and associated cortical structures are assumed to perform different forms of material-specific information processing depending on the pattern of cerebral language dominance (Milner 1972).

Examples of neuropsychological methods used to evaluate the dominant temporal lobe in terms of verbal learning and memory are tests which require word-list learning, paired associate learning or learning short stories (Jones-Gotman et al 1993). Although these tests differ with respect to the test paradigm (immediate versus delayed recall, recognition versus cued recall) as well as the test material (concrete versus abstract, semantically or phonologically related to unrelated), the most consistent and reliable finding in non-resected patients with left temporal lobe epilepsy is their difficulty in the delayed free recall of previously learned verbal information (Fig. 5.3; Lavadas et al 1979, Delaney et al 1980, Mungas et al 1985, Herman et al 1987, Helmstaedter et al 1992). Immediate recall and recognition appear to be less sensitive measures for the localization of left temporal dysfunction. As mentioned above, the performance of short-term memory depends strongly on neocortical functions and thus is significantly interrelated with and influenced by receptive and expressive language performance, as well as selective attention and speed (Helmstaedter & Elger 1992, Herman et al 1992a).

Findings regarding the relation between dysfunctions of the *non-dominant temporal lobe* and non-verbal, visuospatial memory are less clear-cut. Typical tests on visuospatial memory require learning and immediate/delayed retention of more or less complex and abstract designs, face recognition, and learning of locations (Jones-Gotman et al 1993). The inhomogeneous findings on visuospatial memory can partly be explained by interfering verbalization or dual encoding, which can be largely excluded by the choice of abstract and difficult-to-verbalize items. Parallel to the dependence of verbal learning and memory on language functions, most figural tests make demands on attention, perception and visuoconstruction, which, when impaired, may also affect learning and memory (Fig. 5.3; Helmstaedter et al 1994). However, recent findings in non-resected patients with strictly lateralized right temporal lobe epilepsy prove that immediate recall within the list learning of abstract designs is a sensitive and reliable measure for identifying right temporal lobe dysfunction (Helmstaedter et al 1991, Jones-Gotman et al 1993). The observation that with immediate recall of visuospatial information and delayed recall of verbal memory items different processes appear to be preferentially impaired in patients with right versus left temporal lobe epilepsy needs further investigation.

Verbal and non-verbal memory assessment reliably differentiates healthy controls from patients with unilateral epilepsy and those with bilateral temporal lobe epilepsy. Thus, neuropsychological tests provide valuable information about the lateralization and localization of dysfunctions associated with temporal epileptogenic foci. Results which deviate from morphological and electrophysiological findings may indicate dysfunction that extends

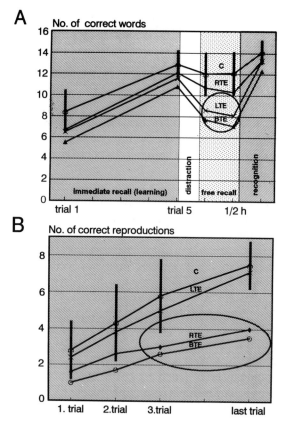

Fig. 5.3 Learning and memory in healthy controls (C, *n* = 30) and patients with left temporal (LTE, *n* = 30), right temporal (TRE, *n* = 30) and bitemporal epilepsy (BTE, *n* = 30). Bars show the confidence intervals of the group of controls. **A** Results of the adapted Rey verbal learning and memory test (15 concrete and unrelated words/five learning trials, each followed by immediate recall/distraction/free recall after distraction and a delay of 30 min/recognition. Learning, free recall and recognition phases are indicated by different headings. Significant differences (analysis of variance; ANOVA) are circled. **B** Learning of figural material (DCS = Diagnostikum für Cerebralschäden — nine abstract designs/six learning trials, each followed by immediate reproduction; cf. Helmstaedter et al 1991). Significant differences (ANOVA) are circled.

beyond the primary epileptogenic area, reduced compensatory capacities after surgery, or an atypical dominance pattern.

Until recently, *neuroimaging techniques* used in the search for morphological correlates of memory processes were confined to demonstrating brain pathology in patients with memory impairment. Volumetric MRI measurements of hippocampal asymmetries, however, offer the possibility of correlating hippocampal measurements with findings on intracarotid amobarbital testing as well as neuropsychological parameters (Loring et al 1993, Trenerry et al 1993). Likewise, *functional imaging* is beginning to contribute to the localization of memory processes (Goldman-Rakic & Friedman 1991). These methods may contribute to a still closer localization of functions within the temporolimbic system (amygdala, fornix, hippocampus, temporolateral cortex). Additional evidence comes from studies which compare hippocampal sclerosis or neuronal loss with presurgical memory deficits and postoperative memory changes (Herman et al 1992b, Sass et al 1993). The different contribution of medial temporal and lateral temporal structures to memory processes may also be elucidated by the evaluation of postoperative neuropsychological outcome, with respect to different strategies of epilepsy surgery. Wieser & Yasargil (1982), for example, stated that selective amygdalohippocampectomy (AH) did not produce additional impairment compared to en block resection of the anterior two-thirds of the temporal lobe. Goldstein & Polkey (1993) found that temporal lobectomy (TL) produced more deficits than selective AH, as evaluated by tests of paired associate learning and immediate recall of visuospatial material. However, there are reports that do not find the assumed relationship between hippocampal pathology and memory or the dependence of neuropsychological changes on the extent of medial or lateral temporal resections (McMillan et al 1987, Wolf et al 1993). Thus, postoperative findings have to be treated with care until results from controlled studies on patients with AH, TL and pure lateral resections are available. Furthermore, there is a need for further investigations of the constructive validity of the different dependent measures of memory in use.

The relevance of research described in this section for the localization of memory processes is evident. However, it should be kept in mind that most localizational conclusions are in fact inferences made from pathological conditions. Therefore, it still has to be proved that they are of value for the localization of memory processes in the healthy brain. In the following section we will briefly consider methods that may turn out to be helpful in meeting this demand.

NEW PERSPECTIVES

The recording of event-related potentials (ERPs) has been used extensively during the last two decades to identify specific stages of information processing and elucidate the time-course of neuropsychological processes. There is ample literature on the basis and principles of this method and its relevance for psychophysiological analyses (see the review by Hillyard & Kutas 1983). In short, ERPs are phasic brain potentials elicited by the processing of sensory, motor or cognitive events that can be recorded by non-invasive scalp recordings. Because of this non-invasiveness, ERP recordings are perfectly suited for psychophysiological studies in healthy subjects. Though they have contributed valuable insights into stages of cognitive processes relevant for language and memory, the technique of recording from the intact scalp implied that the main relevance of ERP studies was tied to the time domain, while it was difficult to draw upon their results for the cortical localization of cognitive processes.

A possible method for the spatial analysis of ERPs is the topographical mapping of scalp current source density. In this way, for example, Münte & Heinze (1994) were able to demonstrate that the negativity evoked by syntactical incongruities had a more frontal distribution than the negative component evoked by semantic incongruities. Friederici et al (1993) found that sentences containing a violation of syntactic phrase structure evoke a negativity with a mean latency of 180 ms and a maximum amplitude over the Broca area, while potentials evoked by violations of semantic or morphological constraints did not show this spatial distribution. A new approach to the spatial analysis of ERP voltage and current density patterns on the scalp is inverse dipole modelling. Localization of the model dipoles within the brain is used to hypothesize on the neural generators of the corresponding neuropsychological processes. If we can combine information on regional cognitive activation as demonstrated by functional imaging with careful ERP analysis of the activating process, it will be possible to obtain information on the temporospatial distribution of stages of cognitive processes.

Promising possibilities for research on the cortical localization of cognitive processes are provided by recordings of event-related — or cognitive — potentials from intracranial electrodes. As already pointed out, temporal lobe epilepsies are frequently associated with specific memory deficits. Presurgical evaluation of patients considered for epilepsy surgery often requires the implantation of subdural and hippocampal depth electrodes for invasive electrocorticographic monitoring when the localization of the primary epileptogenic focus cannot be determined by non-invasive scalp EEG. During the time-consuming process of electrocorticographic monitoring, it is possible to record ERPs without any additional risk to the patient. Several studies have found that hippocampal cognitive potentials are associated with the surface P300 component or can be evoked by the presentation of verbal as well as non-verbal visual stimuli (Halgren et al 1980; Meador et al 1987). As for recognition memory paradigms making use of verbal or non-verbal stimuli, a prominent recognition effect was found for a negative component with an average latency of 460 ms and a later positive potential with a mean latency of 620 ms (Smith et al 1986, Puce et al 1991), indicating the involvement of limbic structures in memory processes. However, the nature and localizing value of these potentials remained to be established.

In a study of 25 patients with medically intractable temporal lobe epilepsy (9 left, 16 right) and left hemisphere language dominance, we studied intrahippocampal and also lateral temporal cognitive potentials by means of a word and a picture recognition paradigm (Grunwald et al 1994). Single stimuli (words, concrete pictures or abstract) shapes were presented visually and 50% of these were repeated later. Subjects had to judge whether each stimulus was a first presentation or a repetition, and they indicated their choice by pressing one of two buttons. ERPs were averaged selectively for

correctly identified first- or second-word presentations after rejecting recordings contaminated by spikes or sharp waves. Neuropsychological evaluation of
the patients included a German version of the Rey auditory verbal learning
test, in which a list of 15 words had to be listened to and repeated in five
subsequent trials and a delayed recall of the memorized words was required
after an interval of 30 min. In both hemispheres a negative potential with a
latency comparable to the results of previous studies was found only in
anterior contacts of depth electrodes, implanted stereotactically via the
longitudinal axis of the hippocampus. Typical examples of these potentials are
shown in Figure 5.4. We were able to show that, while potentials of the right
medial temporal lobe correlated with the patients' recognition rate for visual
stimuli, amplitudes of the negative component recorded in the left anterior
hippocampus were highly significantly correlated with the number of words
patients could recall after a 30-min delay in the neuropsychological test of
verbal learning and memory. This correlation of the left anterior hippocampal
potentials with neuropsychological performance is so strong that it seems

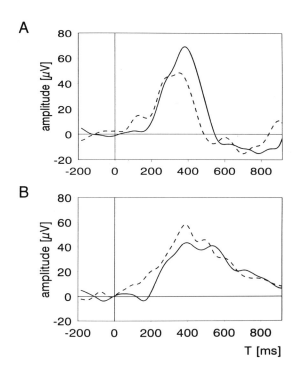

Fig. 5.4 Typical examples of cognitive potentials from the anterior hippocampus evoked by
a word recognition paradigm (patient with right temporal lobe epilepsy and left hemispheric
language dominance). **A** Left hippocampus; **B** Right hippocampus. Solid line = first
presentation; broken line = repetition.

possible to predict with high accuracy from their amplitudes how many words can be stored in verbal long-term memory.

While these kinds of studies on verbal memory can only be conducted in patients with temporal lobe epilepsy, it has to be kept in mind that 16 of the subjects had no left temporal pathology. Thus, the strong predictive value of left medial temporal potentials for the performance of verbal long-term memory processes holds, irrespective of the presence or absence of epileptogenic lesions or verbal memory deficits. Although recordings of intracranial potentials are ruled out in normal, non-epileptic subjects, it seems possible that this kind of direct evidence for the association of electrophysiological correlations of cognitive processes with neuropsychological performance, and for the effects of morphological or functional lesions on both, may be able to close the gap between lesional studies of neuropsychological deficits and neurobiological research of cognitive processes.

CONCLUSIONS

The search for the cortical localization of cognitive processes has received fresh impetus by the convergence of multidisciplinary methods that combine neuropsychological, electrophysiological and neuroimaging techniques. It has become clear that language and memory cannot be attributed to few unvaryingly delimited cortical areas, nor can they be described as amorphous properties of the brain is a whole. Rather, there is growing and converging evidence that they comprise neuropsychological processes subserved by distributed neuronal assemblies. Progress in localizing such 'networks' has been achieved, strongly stimulated not least by clinical needs of the presurgical evaluation of patients with focal epilepsies and made possible by the application and combination of improved or new methods. These advances are met by neuroscientific developments on the molecular biological level of cellular and subcellular physiology. There is increasing evidence for the involvement of N-methyl-D-aspartate-receptor mediated long-term potentiation or depression in learning and memory processes. Moreover, it has been shown that long-term potentiation is a frequent phenomenon in hippocampal neuronal assemblies and that extrahippocampal, e.g. prefrontal, long-term potentiation can be induced by high-frequency electrical stimulation of the CA1 area of the hippocampus (Doyère et al 1993). This suggests a possible neurobiological mechanism of how hippocampal activity can contribute to the long-term storage of items in declarative memory. If it can be shown that neuropsychological relevant intracranially recorded cognitive potentials are related to similar synaptic processes and the same connections between different levels of analysis hold in the presence or absence of pathological processes, a next and truly multidisciplinary approach to the neurobiology of cognitive processes may develop. Research in epileptology is challenged to contribute to this development, because the improvement of presurgical evaluation makes it necessary not only to learn about the localization of cognitive processes in the brain but also in the *individual* brain.

REFERENCES

Baddeley A D, Papagno C, Vallar G. 1988 When long-term depends on short-term storage. J Memory Lang 27: 586–595

Basso A, Lecours A R, Moraschini S, Vanier M. 1985 Anatomoclinical correlations of the aphasias as defined through computerized tomography: exceptions. Brain Lang 26: 201–229

Damasio H. 1989 Neuroimaging contributions to the understanding of aphasia. In: Goodglass H, Damasio A R, eds. Handbook of neuropsychology, vol. 2. Amsterdam: Elsevier, pp 3–46

Delaney R C, Rosen A J, Mattson R H, Novelly R A. 1980 Memory function in focal epilepsy: a comparison of nonsurgical, unilateral temporal lobe and frontal lobe samples. Cortex 16: 103–117

Doyère V, Burette F, Rédini-Del Negro C, Laroche S. 1993 Long-term potentiation of hippocampal afferents and efferents to prefrontal cortex: implications for associative learning. Neuropsychologia 31: 1031–1053.

Eichenbaum H, Cohen N J, Otto T, Wible C. 1992 Memory representation in the hippocampus: functional domain and functional organization. In: Squire L R, Lynch G, Weinberger N M et al, eds. Memory: organization and locus of change. New York: Oxford University Press, pp 163–204

Friederici A D, Pfeifer E, Hahne A. 1993 Event-related brain potentials during natural speech processing: effects of semantic, morphological and syntactic violations. Cognitive Brain Res 1: 183–192

Friston K J, Frith C D, Liddle P F, Frackowiak R S. 1991 Investigating a network model of word generation with positron emission tomography. Proc R Soc Lond B244: 101–106

Gathercole S E, Baddeley A D. 1990 The role of phonological memory in vocabulary acquisition: a study of young children learning new names. Br J Psychol 81: 439–454

Goldman-Rakic P S, Friedman C R. 1991 The circuitry of working memory revealed by anatomy and metabolic imaging. In: Levin H S, Eisenberg H M, Benton A L, eds. Frontal lobe function and dysfunction. New York: Oxford University Press, pp 72–91

Goldstein L H, Polkey C E. 1993 Short-term cognitive changes after unilateral temporal lobectomy or unilateral amygdalo-hippocampectomy for the relief of temporal lobe epilepsy. J Neurol Neurosurg Psychiatry 56: 135–140

Grunwald T, Elger C E, Lehnertz K et al. 1994 Intrakranielle Potentiale bei Gedächtnisprozessen. In: Deecke L, ed. Proceedings of the German and Austrian Congress of Neurologists (in press)

Halgren E, Squires N K, Wilson C L, Rohrbaugh J W, Babb T L, Crandall P H. 1980 Endogenous potentials generated in the human hippocampal formation and amygdala by infrequent events. Science 210: 803–805

Hart J, Lewis P J, Lesser R P et al. 1993 Anatomic correlates of memory from intracarotid amobarbital injections with technetium Tc 99m hexamethylpropyleneamine oxide SPECT. Arch Neurol 50: 745–750

Head H. 1915 Hughlings Jackson on aphasia and kindred affections of speech. Brain 38: 81

Helmstaedter C, Elger C E. 1992 Beziehungen zwischen Verbalgedächtnis und Sprachleistung am Beispiel fokaler Temporallappenepilepsien. Z Geriatrie 1: 1–5

Helmstaedter C, Pohl C, Hufnagel A, Elger C E. 1991 Visual learning deficits in non-resected patients with right temporal lobe epilepsy. Cortex 27: 547–555

Helmstaedter C, Hufnagel A, Elger C E. 1992 Preoperative memory profiles in patients with temporal lobe epilepsy are related to postoperative seizure outcome. J Epilepsy 5: 17–23

Helmstaedter C, Pohl C, Elger C E. 1994 Kognitive Teilleistungsdefizite bei Temporallappenepilepsien. In: Deecke L, ed. Proceedings of the German and Austrian Congress of Neurologists (in press)

Herman B P, Wyler A R, Richey E T, Rea J M. 1987 Memory function and verbal learning ability in patients with complex partial seizures of temporal lobe origin. Epilepsia 28: 547–554

Herman B P, Seidenberg M, Haltiner A, Wyler A R. 1992a Adequacy of language function and verbal memory performance in unilateral temporal lobe epilepsy. Cortex 28: 423–433

Herman B P, Wyler A R, Somes G, Berry A D, Dohan C. 1992b Pathological status of the mesial temporal lobe predicts memory outcome from left anterior lobectomy. Neurosurgery 31: 652–657

Hillyard S A, Kutas M. 1983 Electrophysiology of cognitive processing. Annu Rev Psychol 34: 33–61

Ingvar D H, Lassen N A. 1965 Regional cerebral blood flow. Kopenhagen Munksgard. Jack C R, Nichols D A, Sharbrough F W, Marsh W R, Petersen R C. 1988 Selective posterior cerebral artery test for evaluating memory function before surgery for temporal lobe seizures. Radiology 168: 787–793

Jones-Gotman M, Smith M L, Zatorre R J. 1993 Neuropsychological testing for localization and lateralization of the epileptogenic region. In: Engel J Jr, ed. Surgical treatment of the epilepsies. New York: Raven Press, pp 245–262

Kurthen M, Helmstaedter C, Linke D B, Solymosi L, Elger C E, Schramm J. 1992 Interhemispheric dissociation of expressive and receptive language functions in patients with complex-partial seizures. Brain Lang 43: 694–712

Kurthen M, Helmstaedter C, Linke D B, Solymosi L, Elger C E, Schramm J. 1994 Quantitative and qualitative evaluation of patterns of cerebral language dominance: an amobarbital study. Brain Lang 46: 536–564

Lavadas E, Umilta C, Provinciali L. 1979 Hemisphere-dependent cognitive performances in epileptic patients. Epilepsia 20: 493–502

Loring D W, Meador K J, Lee G P et al. 1990 Cerebral language lateralization: evidence from intracarotid amobarbital testing. Neuropsychologia 28: 831–838

Loring D W, Lee G P, Meador K J, King D W. 1991 Does memory assessment during amobarbital testing predict postsurgical amnesia? J Epilepsy 4: 19–24

Loring D W, Murro A M, Meador K J et al. 1993 Wada memory testing and hippocampal volume measurements in the evaluation of temporal lobectomy. Neurology 43: 1789–1793

Lüders H, Lesser R P, Hahn J et al. 1991 Basal temporal language area. Brain 114: 743–754

McMillan T M, Powell G E, Janota I, Polkey C E, 1987 Relationship between neuropathology and cognitive functioning in temporal lobectomy patients. J Neurol Neurosurg Psychiatry 50: 167–176

Meador K J, Loring D W, King D W et al. 1987 Limbic evoked potentials predict site of focus. Neurology 37: 494–497

Milner B. 1972 Disorders of learning and memory after temporal lobe lesions in man. Clin Neurosurg 19: 421–446

Milner B, Branch C, Rasmussen T. 1962 Study of short-term memory after intracarotid injection of sodium amytal. Trans Am Neurol Assoc 87: 224–226

Mungas D, Ehlers C, Walton N, McCutchen C B. 1985 Verbal learning differences in epileptic patients with left and right temporal foci. Epilepsia 26: 340–345

Münte T F, Heinze H J. 1994 ERP negativities during syntactic processing of written words. In: Heinze H J Plunte T F, Mangun G R, eds. Cognitive electrophysiology: basic and clinical research, Boston: Birkhäuser pp 211–239

Ojemann G A. 1991 Cortical organization of language. J Neurosci 11: 2281–2287

Ojemann G A, Ojemann J, Lettich E, Berger M. 1989 Cortical language localization in left dominant hemisphere. J Neurosurg 71: 316–326

Papagno C, Valentine T, Baddeley A D. 1991 Phonological short-term memory and foreign language vocabulary learning. J Memory Lang 30: 331–347

Penfield W J, Jasper H H 1954 Epilepsy and the functional anatomy of the human brain. Boston: Little, Brown

Penfield W J, Roberts L. 1959 Speech and brain mechanisms. Princeton: Princeton University Press

Puce A, Andrewes D G, Berkovic S F, Bladin P F. 1991 Visual recognition memory. Neurophysiological evidence for the role of white matter in man. Brain 114: 1647–1666

Rumsey J M, Zametkin A J, Andreason P et al. 1994 Normal activation of frontotemporal language cortex in dyslexia, as measured with oxygen 15 positron emission tomography. Arch Neurol 51: 27–38

Sass K J, Spencer D D, Kim J H, Westerveld M, Novelly Lencz T. 1993 Verbal memory impairment correlates with hippocampal pyramidal cell density. Neurology 40: 1694–1697

Scoville W B, Milner B. 1957 Loss of recent memory after bilateral hippocampal lesions. J Neurol Neurosurg Psychiatry 20: 11–21

Silfvenius H, Christianson SA, Nilsson L-G, Säisä J. 1988 Preoperative investigation of cerebral hemisphere speech and memory with the bilateral intracarotid amytal test. Acta Neurol Scand 78: (suppl 117) 79–83

Smith ME, Stapleton JM, Halgren E. 1986 Human medial temporal lobe potentials evoked in memory and language tasks. Electroencephalogr Clin Neurophysiol 63: 145–159

Squire LR. 1992 Memory and the hippocampus: a synthesis from findings with rats, monkeys and humans. Psychol Rev 99: 195–231

Squire LR, Zola-Morgan S. 1991 The medial temporal lobe memory system. Science 253: 1380–1386

Squire LR, Knowlton B, Musen G. 1993 The structure and organization of memory. Annu Rev Psychol 44: 453–495

Trenerry MR, Jack CR, Ivnik RJ et al. 1993 MRI hippocampal volumes and memory function before and after temporal lobectomy. Neurology 43: 1800–1805

Wada J, Rasmussen T. 1960 Intracarotid injection of sodium amytal for the lateralization of cerebral speech dominance. J Neurosurg 17: 266–282

Wieser HG, Yasargil MD. 1982 Selective amygdalohippocampectomy as a surgical treatment of mesiobasal limbic epilepsy. Surg Neurol 17: 445–457

Wieser HG, Landis T, Regard M, Schiess R. 1989 "Selective" and "superselective" temporal lobe amytal tests: II. Neuropsychological test procedure and results. In: Manelis J Bental E, Loeber J M et al, eds. Advances in epileptology, vol. 17. New York: Raven Press, pp 28–33

Wise RJ, Chollet F, Hadar U, Friston K, Hoffner E, Frackowiak R. 1991 Distribution of cortical neural networks involved in word comprehension and word retrieval. Brain 114: 1803–1817

Wolf RL, Ivnik RJ, Sharbrough FW, Cascino GD, Marsh WR. 1993 Neurocognitive efficiency following left temporal lobectomy: standard versus limited resection. J Neurosurg 79: 76–83

Zola-Morgan S, Squire LR. 1993 The neuroanatomy of memory. Annu Rev Neurosci 16: 547–563

6

Microdialysis in epilepsy

M. J. During

Recent advances in neurochemical methods, in combination with the development of intracerebral microdialysis, have enabled in situ measurements of neurotransmitters, metabolites and drugs in defined regions of the brain. A large number of experimental animal studies using microdialysis have focused on amino acids associated with seizures. Although pioneering studies by Bradford and colleagues reported a rise in glutamate with seizures using a push–pull method, many early microdialysis studies in a variety of seizure models did not demonstrate an ictal rise in glutamate, presumably due to limitations in the technique, including tissue injury, probe size with an inability to sample synaptic fluid and high-affinity uptake of excitatory amino acids preventing the synaptically released transmitter from spilling out into the extrasynaptic space. More recently, the microdialysis technique has been coupled with intracranial electrode recording in patients with medically intractable seizures to monitor neurochemical changes associated with epilepsy, specifically transmitter release during the generation and arrest of spontaneous and electrically stimulated hippocampal seizures. These studies have consistently observed an increase in the excitatory amino acids aspartate and glutamate during epileptiform activity. Morever, in patients with established unilateral-onset hippocampal seizures, interictal levels of glutamate are elevated and γ-aminobutyric acid (GABA) levels are diminished in the epileptogenic hippocampus compared to the contralateral, 'control' hippocampus. Immediately prior to the onset of spontaneous hippocampal seizures, levels of glutamate rise and increase further during the ictal period. In secondarily generalized seizures, levels of glutamate remain elevated postictally in the epileptogenic hippocampus, whereas levels in the contralateral hippocampus fall immediately following seizure arrest. This imbalance in excitatory transmission is further enhanced by an attenuated ictal increase in extracellular levels of the brain's major inhibitory neurotransmitter, GABA, in the epileptogenic compared to the contralateral hippocampus. In addition to changes in these amino acid transmitters, adenosine increases markedly during seizures to levels which in vitro suppress epileptiform discharges. Lactate also increases significantly during seizures and similarly to adenosine remains elevated in the postictal period. These data suggest that there is an underlying abnormality in the regulation of extracellular glutamate and GABA in human epileptogenic hippocampus favoring excitation; moreover, a preictal rise in glutamate release may trigger spontaneous seizures and the extracellular generation of adenosine and lactate may be in part responsible for seizure arrest and postictal refractoriness.

There have been a great number of studies investigating the neurochemistry of the epilepsies (for review, see Snead 1983, Jobe 1984; Wasterlain et al 1985, Delgado-Escueta et al 1986). Despite such an enormous research effort, there are few definitive, consistent neurochemical changes associated with epilepsy. In animal studies, each model appears to have individual features and specific artefacts associated with its generation. Human epilepsies are a heterogeneous group of disorders with multiple etiologies and pathologies so it would perhaps be naïve to assume that a single animal model would reflect this complexity and, as a corollary, it is highly probable that there are different neurochemical signatures for each of the different epilepsies. Ideally, of course, the neurochemistry of the human disease itself should be investigated in well-controlled studies. However, this has not been generally possible except for postmortem or excised tissue studies, which reveal little about dynamic, in vivo function. In addition, there have been major problems in clinical studies with respect both to the selection of patients and the area of brain excised and studied. Such dramatic differences underlie several of the problems associated with the study of excised foci, in that the changes observed may either be primary and reflect the original injury with perhaps etiological significance or alternatively may be secondarily adaptive changes in the brain's attempt to limit seizure generation and spread. These studies must therefore be done in conjunction with experimental animal studies using a variety of developmental, electrophysiological and neuroanatomical techniques to ensure that an appropriate interpretation is made. Over the past decade, methods have been developed to investigate dynamic changes in neurochemicals in the brain of experimental animals in vivo. Most recently, these techniques have been applied in the clinical setting and have begun to contribute to our knowledge of the in vivo neurochemistry of human epilepsy.

MICRODIALYSIS

Several invasive intracerebral monitoring techniques are becoming established as methods to measure extracellular levels of neurochemicals in defined brain regions in vivo in experimental animals. These techniques include cortical cup perfusion (MacIntosh & Oborin 1953), push–pull perfusion (Gaddum 1961), in vivo voltametry (Adams & Marsden 1982) and, most recently, intracerebral microdialysis. Although Bito et al first described a brain dialysis technique in 1966, it was not until Delgado et al (1972) and particularly Ungerstedt and his colleagues (Ungerstedt & Pycock 1974, Ungerstedt et al 1982) refined the technique that the method became established as a valid technique to monitor dynamic changes in the extracellular fluid (ECF). The major limitation in the development of the technique as a rapid sampling method was the low sensitivity of the majority of neurochemical assays. With the development of high-performance liquid chromatography (HPLC) systems coupled to highly sensitive electrochemical and fluorescent detectors in the 1970s and 1980s, precise quantification of neurotransmitters could be determined in the small microliter volumes obtained by microdialysis. This development in trace analytical chemistry has led to microdialysis becoming the most widely used and preferred method for the in vivo neurochemical investigation of experimental animals.

The basic principle of microdialysis is simple and has been discussed in detail in several recently published review articles (Ungerstedt 1984, Westerink et al 1987, Benveniste 1989; Di Chiara 1990, During 1992). In brief, fluid is perfused using a syringe pump, via inlet and outlet tubing, through a hollow dialysis fiber (implanted within the brain) to a collecting vial. It is essentially similar to push–pull perfusion, apart from a dialysis membrane which links the inlet and outlet tubes and thus only requiring the 'push'. The inlet and outlet tubing generally run side by side with the membrane, either forming a loop between them or alternatively in concentrically designed probes; the distal end of the hollow dialysis fiber is sealed and forms the tip of the probe. The end of the inlet tube is flush with the distal, plugged end of the membrane and the outlet is at a variable distance proximally. The distance between the inlet and outlet determines the membrane area exposed for diffusion of neurochemicals. A simpler and less commonly used probe is the transcranial or linear probe in which the inlet tube enters one side of the brain and the outlet exits directly out the other side with the hollow dialysis fiber lying in between with an impermeable surface coating of the membrane applied to restrict dialysis to defined regions.

The rate of flow through dialysis probes is slow, generally ranging from 0.2 to 5 μl/min. As the perfusing fluid passes through the dialysis fiber, the concentration gradient generated between the regional brain ECF and the intraluminal fluid drives molecules either into the probe or alternatively may be used to deliver compounds from the dialysate into the brain ECF. The amount of brain chemical recovered therefore represents some percentage of its actual ECF concentration. This recovery efficiency depends on many factors, including the molecular weight, charge and stickiness of the compound, diffusion and tortuosity factors in the extracellular microenvironment, uptake and metabolism, as well as dialysis membrane length and composition (Benveniste 1989, Hsiao et al 1990, Morrison et al 1991).

There are several major limitations of the dialysis method. Most notably, the time resolution of the technique is several orders of magnitude above that of events at the neuronal membrane. Even with the most sensitive assays and on-line recording in the case of lactography (direct, on-line monitoring of dialysis fluid lactate; see below), the response time of a dialysis probe to changes in the extracellular environment is in the order of 40 s (Kuhr & Korf

1988b,c). As events at the synaptic membrane occur in the millisecond time frame, it is evident that the microdialysis probe is a rather crude index of neurotransmission. Moreover, the dimensions of even.the smallest concentric probes are orders of magnitude greater than the size of synapses. The question of what intracerebral microdialysis actually measures and of its relevance when it is so removed from the actual scale of synaptic transmission is critical. Perhaps an appropriate way to look at the technique is that, although it clearly is not measuring release or even levels of transmitters within the synaptic cleft, it is a pooled, integrated measure of ECF levels in the immediate vicinity of the probe over a defined time interval. Dialysate measurements are clearly most influenced by the ECF concentration directly adjacent to the probe membrane surface, and although most estimates and models of in vivo probe recovery assume that the probe has not significantly disturbed the neuronal microenvironment and also that at any one moment there is a relatively fixed absolute ECF concentration, it is likely that both these assumptions are false for the majority of neurotransmitters (Benveniste 1989, Morrison et al 1991).

There are likely to be local variations in the ECF concentrations of most neurotransmitters, clearly an extremely high concentration within synaptic vesicles and at the release site of the presynaptic cell membrane, with complex gradients of the concentration of the transmitter as one approaches the ECF immediately adjacent to the probe membrane. For most transmitters, the absolute ECF concentration, which many investigators have pursued with a variety of modeling kinetics, may be a rather futile search for a concentration which bears little resemblance to the concentration at the active site, be it the pre- or postsynaptic receptor. For extrasynaptic receptors it may have more relevance, and certainly for drugs or metabolites, whose ECF production is non-synaptic, the concentrations may also be more relevant. The transmitter molecules found outside the synapse, sampled by the dialysis probe, have either escaped uptake or degradation from within the synapse or are extrasynaptically released transmitters. Dialysis measurements represent therefore a balance between several dynamic processes which include release, uptake, bulk flow or egress, capillary exchange, transmembrane diffusion, synthesis and degradation as well as extracellular volume and tortuosity. In addition, measurements are clearly influenced by membrane recovery, which may change both chronically with the tissue reaction surrounding the probe (Benveniste & Diemer 1987), as well as more rapid changes in membrane efficiency perhaps relating to temperature, neuronal activity, pH and changes in the blood–brain barrier.

In summary then, dialysis might best be considered as a method which does not monitor synaptic transmission (wiring transmission) but is an index of volume transmission in the brain (Fuxe & Agnati 1991), i.e. the diffusional or paracrine, extrasynaptic chemical communication between cells in the brain.

Although originally used as a passive probe to monitor extracellular levels of neurotransmitters and metabolites in the ECF, microdialysis has evolved rapidly over the past 5 years. In addition to determining dynamic changes in extracellular levels of neurotransmitters, microdialysis has become an established tool in defining brain metabolism and glucose utilization (Kuhr & Korf 1988), enzymatic activity (Westerink et al 1990) and receptor function both presynaptically (Bean et al 1990) and postsynaptically (Egawa et al 1988).

Microdialysis has not only been used to measure endogenous compounds but is also useful for pharmacological studies. As the blood–brain barrier (in those few animal studies in which it has been tested) is intact within 30–60 min following probe implantation (Benveniste 1989), microdialysis is an important technique in defining drug and metabolite entry into the brain as well as comparing brain pharmacokinetics with peripheral (plasma) pharmacokinetics (Scheyer et al 1994b).

In addition to the measurement of chemicals, ion concentrations in the ECF have also been determined by microdialysis. Extracellular changes in calcium, potassium as well as sodium have all been followed with the technique (Vezzani et al 1985, Lazarewicz et al 1986a 1986b, Chastain et al 1989). Fluxes in the concentration of these ions coupled to the use of specific channel agonists and/or antagonists may extend the method to be able to determine ion channel function in vivo.

It is clear from the above discussion that the development of microdialysis represents a significant advance in the investigation of in vivo neurochemistry. The biological questions which have been investigated using this technique in studies of experimental animals include defining the neurochemical changes associated with: cerebral ischemia, hypoxia and anoxia; hypoglycemia; meningitis; cerebral trauma; excitotoxins; seizures; hepatic encephalopathy; eating; sleeping; stress and cerebral transplantation. In addition, a major research effort has used microdialysis to determine neurotransmitter and metabolite effects of centrally acting drugs, and the characterization of interactions between various transmitter systems.

In contrast to this enormous research effort in experimental animal studies, there have been few investigations of the human brain using microdialysis.

However, recently several investigators have been using invasive methods to study the neurochemistry of the human brain and specifically epilepsy in vivo (During et al 1989, 1994, During, 1991, Do et al 1991, Carlson et al 1992, During & Spencer 1992, 1993, Ronne-Engstrom et al 1992).

MICRODIALYSIS STUDIES OF EPILEPSY

Glutamate and GABA

Perhaps the most established neurochemical hypothesis of epilepsy is the imbalance theory — a chemical imbalance favoring excitation underlies the development of spontaneous seizures (Dichter & Ayala 1987) and epilepsy-related neuropathology (Meldrum 1983). Specifically, epilepsy may result from an increase in glutamate-mediated excitation and/or a reduction in GABA-mediated inhibition. Local infusion of glutamate can result in seizures (Hayashi 1952, Biscoe & Straughan 1966) and neuroanatomical injury similar to that found in epilepsy (Meldrum & Corsellis 1984), while glutamate receptor antagonists have anticonvulsant and neuroprotective properties (Croucher et al 1982, Choi 1988). Further evidence of glutamate involvement in epilepsy has come from the study of animal models of focal epilepsy, including intracerebral cobalt (Dodd & Bradford 1976, Dodd et al 1980), folate (Lehmann 1987) and kainate (Jacobson & Hamberger 1985, Wade et al 1987) application as well as in the electrically kindled amygdala (Peterson et al 1983), in which seizure activity is associated with an increase in the release of glutamate. However, investigators were unable to find a significant increase in glutamate during seizures induced by systemic kainate, bicuculline (Lehmann et al 1985), picrotoxin, locally applied bicuculline (Millan et al 1991) or quinolinic acid (Vezzani et al 1985).

Recently, several investigators have performed invasive recording in humans. Do et al (1991), using push–pull cannulation, reported increases in excitatory amino acids during brief intraoperative recordings in anesthetized humans undergoing electrical stimulation. Similarly, Carlson and colleagues (Carlson et al 1992, Ronne-Engstrom et al 1992), using microdialysis, reported marked increases in the amino acids aspartate, glutamate, glycine and serine with smaller increases in other animo acids, including taurine, during intraoperative recording. These studies however were limited in their duration, had no control regions for comparison and were not able to investigate spontaneous seizures in awake, conscious humans. Moreover, these studies did not investigate the release of the brain's major inhibitory neurotransmitter, GABA.

At Yale, we have now had extensive experience with microdialysis in humans and have begun characterizing the epileptogenic hippocampus (During et al 1989, 1994, During & Spencer 1990, 1992, 1993, During 1991). Patients with an established epileptogenic hippocampus as determined by intracranial electroencephalogram (EEG) monitoring and subsequent surgical resection and confirmation of mesial temporal sclerosis on histological examination were studied. In this group of patients, basal (interictal) levels of glutamate were approximately 10% higher in the epileptogenic hippocampus compared to the contralateral side. In contrast, basal concentrations of GABA in dialysates were approximately 25% lower in the epileptogenic hippocampus compared to the non-epileptogenic hippocampus. Both glutamate and GABA increased during spontaneous hippocampal seizures with secondary generalization. Of particular interest was the increase in glutamate in the epileptogenic hippocampus which preceded the seizure onset. Moreover, the increase in glutamate in this hippocampus was greater and more sustained than the contralateral side. Furthermore, peak levels of glutamate in the dialysate reached concentrations as high as 100 μmol/l reflecting millimolar ECF concentrations. In contrast, the increase in GABA

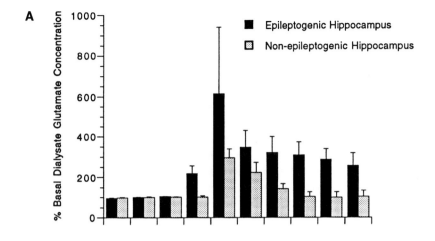

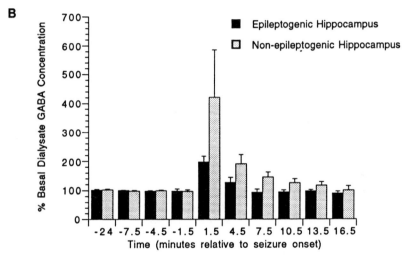

Fig. 6.1 Bilateral measurements of glutamate and γ-aminobutyric acid (GABA) during complex partial seizures iwth secondary generalization. Data represent the mean and s.e.m. of 6 seizures in 6 patients of glutamate (**A**), and GABA (**B**) as the percentage of basal concentrations in one sample collected over an interval ranging from 5 to 30 min (represented as – 24 min) and then at 3-min intervals from 9 min prior to seizure onset to 18 min following the onset. The times reflect the mid-point of the collection interval relative to the time of seizure onset, as determined by review of hard-copy EEG. The basal dialysate concentration (100%) was calculated as the mean of three consecutive samples collected from 30 to 3 min prior to seizure onset.

was much greater in the non-epileptogenic hippocampus with levels return-ing to baseline within several minutes following the seizure arrest (Fig. 6.1).

These studies suggest that the release of neurotransmitter amino acids is involved in seizure-related neurochemical changes in the human brain. Of major interest is the significant elevation in glutamate in the epileptogenic hippocampus prior to seizure onset. Since perfusion of glutamate into the hippocampus in vivo induces seizures, these data suggest that an increase in ECF glutamate may be a mechanism of spontaneous seizure generation. A hypothesis proposed by Chamberlin et al (1990) is that the neuronal synchronization characteristic of epileptiform activity requires an initial activation of a small, critical, number of neurons. This excitatory neuronal activity may be reflected in an increase in glutamate release prior to the seizure-like bursting and the extracellular glutamate may therefore act as a paracrine factor to produce synchronization.

The peak glutamate dialysate concentration, which reached 100 µmol/l during seizures in several patients, reflects a theoretical ECF glutamate concentration of approximately 0.5–1 mmol/l. Similar concentrations are toxic to neurons in vitro with very brief exposures (Frandsen & Schousboe 1987). Thus, the ictal concentrations of glutamate may indeed be sufficiently high to produce neurotoxicity. However, neurons in vivo are less vulnerable to glutamate than cells grown in vitro; presumably the efficiency of the high-affinity uptake of glutamate prevents accumulation of the excitatory amino acid within the synaptic cleft. Furthermore, although glutamate is the presumed mediator of excitotoxicity, other neurotransmitters may modulate its excitotoxic effects. In particular, GABA may act to counter the glutamate-induced excitation. Treatments that facilitate GABAergic neurotransmission have been shown to prevent excitotoxic neuronal injury in the hippocampus (Sternau et al 1989). Therefore, the balance between excitatory and inhibitory transmitters may be more relevant than the absolute level of ECF glutamate. During clinical seizures, the glutamate/GABA ratio is elevated in the epileptogenic hippocampus, particularly in the postseizure period when glutamate remains elevated as the GABA concentration returns to the preictal values. This mismatch in excitation may be causally related to the hippocampal damage characteristic of temporal lobe epilepsy, since a similar pattern is produced in normal animals by stimulation of excitatory input to the hippocampus (Sloviter 1987).

Basal GABA concentrations in the epileptogenic hippocampus are diminished relative to the non-epileptogenic side, suggesting that there may be altered release or reuptake of the transmitter despite the relative preservation of GABA neurons. Furthermore, the difference in GABA concentration between epileptogenic and control hippocampi is increased during seizures. In addition, glutamate-induced GABA release is diminished in the epileptogenic hippocampus and this release is not calcium-dependent (unpublished observations) and may be transporter-mediated (Pin & Bockaert 1989). The increase in ECF GABA during seizures may occur in part via a calcium-independent, transporter-mediated mechanism with a reduction in this specific release mechanism consistent with the seizure-release data.

The increase in extracellular glutamate in the epileptogenic hippocampus despite a significant loss of glutamatergic neurons may reflect decreased uptake. High-affinity uptake largely occurs via nerve terminals with glutamatergic deafferentation decreasing glutamate uptake in vivo (Storm-Mathisen 1977). Moreover, there is an increase in the release of glutamate (but not GABA) from glia cultured from epileptogenic tissue, suggesting that the increase in ECF glutamate may be partially of glial origin (Cornell-Bell et al 1992).

ADENOSINE

Although the evidence supporting glutamate and GABA as the mediators responsible for the generation and propagation of clinical seizures is increasing, the neurochemical mechanism by which seizures spontaneously terminate remains unknown. Adenosine has been postulated as an endogenous anticonvulsant (Lee et al 1984, Dragunow et al 1985, Stringer & Lothman 1990). This hypothesis proposes that, during a seizure, extracellular adenosine increases to concentrations which may suppress epileptic activity. An alternative hypothesis of the role of adenosine in modulating seizure activity is that tonically released adenosine maintains a high seizure threshold, and receptor antagonism or lowered extracellular concentrations of the nucleoside may lead to the generation of seizures (Phillis & Wu 1981, Chin 1989). Adenosine is released following neuronal depolarization (Bender et al 1981 Jonzon & Fredholm 1985), although the increase in extracellular concentrations of adenosine may in part originate from its extracellular generation by $5'$-nucleotidase from released adenosine triphosphate (ATP; Richardson et al 1987) or other nucleotides (Hoehn & White 1990).

Adenosine acts on at least two subtypes of purinergic receptors, A_1 and A_2, which are coupled negatively and positively to cyclic adenosine monophosphate (cAMP) generation, respectively (Daly 1982). Although both receptors mediate the central actions of adenosine, the depression of synaptic transmission in the hippocampus is mediated largely via A_1 receptors (Dunwiddie & Fredholm 1989). Autoradiography of A_1 receptors shows a wide distribution throughout the central nervous systems, with high concentrations in limbic regions, including the hippocampus (Lee et al 1986).

Studies of hippocampal slices have demonstrated potent anticonvulsant activity of adenosine and its analogs in these in vitro models of epilepsy (Dunwiddie 1980, Ault & Wang 1986). In vivo animal studies have shown that systemically administered adenosine protects against audiogenic seizures in sensitive mice (Maître et al 1974). In addition, inhibition of reuptake of adenosine with papaverine retards the development and reduces the severity and duration of seizures in the amygdala-kindled rat (Dragunow et al 1985). Moreover, adenosine antagonists, including the methylxanthines, caffeine and theophylline, lower the seizure threshold and may cause fatal convulsions at high doses (Chiu 1981, Perrson & Erjefalt 1982, Nakada et al 1983). Further evidence in support of adenosine's role in epilepsy includes studies showing rapid elevations in tissue levels of adenosine with bicuculline-induced seizures

(Sattin 1971, Schrader et al 1980, Winn et al 1980). Recently, During & Spencer (1992) performed microdialysis bilaterally during seizures in patients with clearly established unilateral hippocampal disease. Samples obtained during these seizures were quantified for adenosine concentration. The concentration of adenosine in the dialysates collected during these seizures is represented in Figure 6.2. Adenosine levels rose approximately 20-fold in the epileptogenic hippocampus and sevenfold in the contralateral hippocampus during the seizure. (The increase in adenosine ranged from 7.5-to 31-fold in the epileptogenic hippocampus, whereas the increase ranged from 5.8- to 8.4-fold in the contralateral hippocampus.) Dialysate adenosine remained elevated above the preictal concentrations throughout an 18 min postictal period. The increases in adenosine levels in the human hippocampus during seizures (by as much as 30-fold) are much greater than those generally reported for tissue levels in bicuclline-induced seizures in experimental animals (ranging from two- to sixfold increases; Sattin 1971, Schrader et al 1980). Furthermore, levels of extracellular adenosine remained elevated in the postictal period for at least 18 min.

The peak concentration of adenosine in hippocampal ECF during these seizures reaches approximately 65 µmol/l (During & Spencer 1992). As

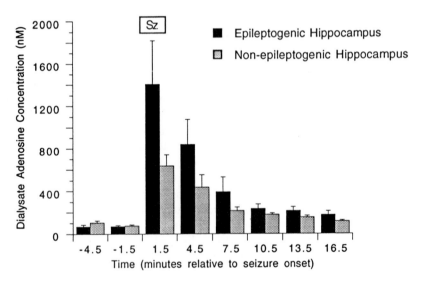

Fig. 6.2   Bilateral hippocampal extracellular fluid adenosine during complex partial seizures. Data represent the mean and s.e.m. of adenosine levels in hippocampal dialysates collected at 3-min intervals during four secondarily generalized seizures (in 4 patients). The box with Sz represents the seizures, with error bars representing the imprecision in determining time of onset and the range of seizure duration. Adenosine is increased above basal levels (– 4.5 and – 1.5 samples) during the 1.5-min interval and all subsequent samples. Adenosine levels are significantly higher in the epileptogenic hippocampus during the seizure collection (time 1.5) compared to the contralateral hippocampus ($P<0.05$; two-way analysis of variance with repeated measures and paired t-test).

concentrations of adenosine of 40–50 μmol/l consistently suppress neuronal activity in vitro (Kostopoulos et al 1989), the levels reached in the human hippocampus during a seizure are clearly in a range at which adenosine may exert inhibitory activity.

The ECF levels of adenosine are influenced by both efflux and uptake of the nucleoside as well as its extraneuronal metabolism. Changes in the adenosine concentration as determined by microdialysis may therefore reflect an alteration in uptake or extracellular generation from ATP (Richardson et al 1987) rather than release. In addition, during seizures there are major changes in ECF volume (Dietzel et al 1989) and probable changes in ECF diffusion kinetics. The increase in the concentration of adenosine may therefore reflect, in part, alterations in ECF volume and activity of cell-membrane transporters and not release per se.

Dragunow and colleagues (1985) originally hypothesized that adenosine is the brain's natural anticonvulsant, with seizures producing a rapid rise in extracellular levels of adenosine, with seizure arrest occurring when a critical concentration is reached. In support of this hypothesis is the report of a patient who developed status epilepticus following electroconvulsive therapy who had subconvulsant plasma levels of the adenosine antagonist, theophylline (Peters et al 1984). Furthermore, at higher concentrations theophylline produces potentially fatal status epilepticus in humans (Zwillich et al 1975). Both adenosine analogs and uptake inhibitors prolong the postictal refractory period (Burley & Ferrendelli 1984), and the human dialysis data of a sustained elevation in ECF adenosine are consistent with a role for adenosine in postictal refractoriness.

Further clinical support for a role of endogenous adenosine is the inhibitory activity of benzodiazepines and diphenylhydantoin on adenosine uptake (Phillis & Wu 1982, Phillis 1984), whereas carbamazepine binds to adenosine receptors (Skerrit et al 1982), although this does not appear to mediate its anticonvulsant effects (Marangos et al 1983).

LACTATE

An increase in cerebral activity is associated with an increase in local regional glucose utilization (Fox et al 1988). Glycolysis produces an increase in brain tissue concentrations of lactate (Ackerman & Lear 1989). Moreover, lactate is released from both neurons and glia in proportion to its intracellular generation via a lactate/proton cotransporter (Kuhr et al 1988, Walz & Mukerji). Perhaps the most dramatic increase in cerebral activity is that associated with seizures. During the synchronized neuronal activity charac-terizing a seizure there is a marked increase in cellular metabolism. In rats with bicuculline-induced seizures, the metabolic rate for oxygen increases by 200–300% (Meldrum & Nilsson 1976), whereas the increase in glycolysis may increase even more than the change in oxidative metabolism (King et al 1967, Duffy et al 1975, Chapman et al 1977). Similar increases in glucose utilization are observed with seizures induced by electroconvulsive shock, fluorothyl, pentylenetetrazol, bicuculline and kainic acid (Meldrum 1981, 1983). More recent studies of experimental animals using nuclear magnetic resonance (NMR) spectroscopy have shown that the rise in tissue lactate with seizures may persist for an hour or more (Petroff et al 1986; Pritchard et al 1987). However, the only published studies of brain lactate associated with seizures in humans is that of Woods & Chiu (1990) using ^{1}H spectroscopy following electroconvulsive therapy and Matthews et al (1990) also using proton spectroscopy. Woods & Chiu reported no significant change in tissue lactate, however, the spectroscopic lactate signal was obscured in part by an increased lipid signal. Their interpretation of the data was that there might be an increase in lactate metabolism or egress to account for the failure to demonstrate a significant increase in tissue lactate levels using NMR. Matthews et al did observe an increase in the lactate signal in the brain region involved in the seizure compared to the contralateral hemisphere, however, their study was confined to a single subject with partial status epilepticus.

An alternative method to NMR spectroscopy to quantitate lactate in brain regions is the method of lactography. This is a term coined by Kuhr & Korf and colleagues to describe the on-line measurement of extracellular lactate using microdialysis (Kuhr & Korf 1988a, 1988b, Kuhr et al 1988, Korf et al 1991). Furthermore, they have characterized this method as a valid indicator of regional glucose utilization and have shown coupling between neuronal activity and extracellular lactate generation including a rise in ECF lactate following a single electroconvulsive shock (Kuhr & Korf 1988a and 1988b). During et al (1994) used this method to perform hippocampal lactography in patients with complex partial seizures to determine dynamic changes in ECF lactate during spontaneous-onset clinical seizures.

Basal levels of lactate in the dialysate ranged from 50 to 300 µmol/l, reflecting an extracellular concentration of 0.1–0.75 mmol/l directly, correcting for in vitro recovery. However, as diffusion, extracellular metabolism and capillary exchange may affect in vivo recovery, this concentration range may significantly underestimate actual ECF levels (Morrison et al 1991).

In patients with secondarily generalized seizures, lactography was performed unilaterally over the peri-ictal period. Extracellular lactate levels increased significantly during all seizures and remained elevated, slowly returning to preictal levels over the 2-h monitoring period (Fig. 6.3).

During et al (1994) also studied patients with bilateral hippocampal lactography. In 1 patient, a spontaneous seizure commenced in the left hippocampus and did not propagate contralaterally. Lactate levels increased in the epileptogenic hippocampus (the site of seizure activity), but no change occurred in the contralateral hippocampus. In addition, several patients were studied during the interictal period with the concentration of extracellular lactate changing in parallel to the frequency of the interictal spikes. This report suggested that neuronal activity was tightly coupled with lactate generation with both seizure activity as well as the neuronal activity

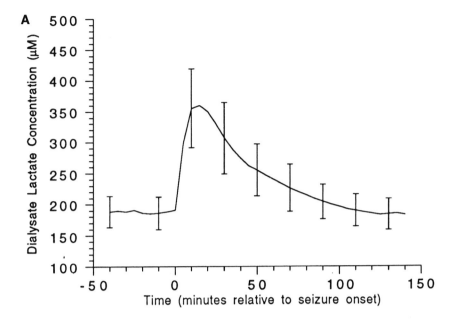

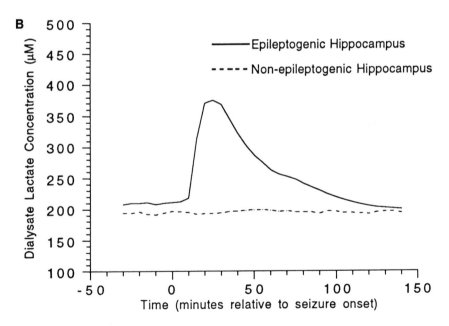

Fig. 6.3 Ictal lactography. **A** The data represent the mean and s.e.m. of hippocampal lactate concentrations of 4 patients obtained during four secondarily generalized seizures using unilateral lactography. **B** The data represent bilateral lactography in a patient in whom a hippocampal-onset seizure did not propagate to the contralateral hippocampus.

underlying interictal spikes directly correlating with extracellular lactate concentrations. Moreover, the increase in ECF lactate during seizures was limited to the site of seizure activity. In studies of experimental animals, tissue lactate increased by two- to fivefold within 10 s (Petroff et al 1986; Pritchard et al 1987). In contrast, in human hippocampal dialysates, lactate increased immediately but levels took 10–15 min to reach peak concentrations, similarly to the data obtained following a single electroconvulsive shock in rats (Kuhr & Korf 1988a, 1988b, 1988c). This delay in ECF lactate may reflect the carrier-mediated transport of lactate into ECF which is dependent on cellular energy (Kuhr et al 1988). The intracellular lactate concentration is primarily dependent on three variables — the cytoplasmic redox state, pH and the pyruvate concentration (Hohorst et al 1959). Seizures have been shown to produce a major change in the cytoplasmic redox state (Howse & Duffy 1975), thereby increasing lactate production. Kuhr & Korf (1988a) confirmed that ECF lactate is affected by these same factors, as disruption of the cytoplasmic redox state with 2,4–dinitrophenol increases lactate concentration both in tissue and in the ECF. Moreover, ECF lactate generation is directly coupled to glucose metabolism. Inhibition of glycolysis with 2-deoxyglucose reduces the amount of pyruvate available for metabolism and lowers tissue lactate (Miller et al 1986). Presumably, lactate levels drop as it is reconverted into pyruvate for subsequent use in aerobic metabolism. ECF lactate falls rapidly following local 2-deoxyglucose administration, suggesting that lactate measured using microdialysis reflects local tissue metabolism.

The rate of disappearance of ECF lactate following an electroconvulsive seizure in animals is equal to the fall in tissue lactate. In tissue culture, lactate is released from both neurons and glia in direct proportion to its intracellular generation (Walz & Mukerji 1988). Moreover, lactate is released via a lactate/proton cotransporter (Pauwels et al 1985). Although tissue lactate levels following clinical seizures have not been reliably measured, a similar relationship may exist in the human brain, with our data suggesting that tissue levels remain elevated for 60–90 min following a seizure. During anoxia and spreading depression, lactic acid release is the main cause of acidification of the ECF (Mutch & Hansen 1984). Moreover, it is well-established that brain ECF becomes acid during seizures (Dusser de Barenne et al 1938, Jasper & Erikson 1941, Tschirgi et al 1957, Caspers & Speckmann 1972), including during spontaneous clinical seizures (Meyer et al 1966). Our data would support the hypothesis that the drop in pH associated with seizures may be largely based on the increase in ECF lactate.

Engel & Ackerman (1980) demonstrated that, in amygdala-kindled rats, the frequency of interictal EEG spikes actually correlates with decreased seizure susceptibility. They proposed that interictal spikes reflect enhanced inhibitory mechanisms which may be necessary in chronic epilepsy to prevent a continuous convulsive state. We propose that lactate production which, in our study, was elevated for a prolonged period during the postictal phase and was also associated with interictal spike activity, may mediate the reduction in seizure susceptibility associated with frequent interictal spikes. The reduced excitability associated with extracellular lactate generation and acidification may be mediated in part by the diminished current associated with activation of N-methyl-D-aspartate (NMDA) receptors when extracellular pH falls (Tang et al 1990). Furthermore, seizure arrest may occur when ECF lactate increases to a critical concentration, with lactate acting as an indirect NMDA antagonist. This hypothesis however, assumes that the ionic mechanisms of interictal spikes and seizures are different, given the immunity of interictal spikes to the antiepileptic effect of elevated extracellular lactate. Although the precise mechanisms underlying both spontaneous seizures and interictal spikes remain unknown, several papers support our hypothesis that interictal spike generation is independent of seizure generation and that the mechanisms underlying these epileptic phenomena are clearly different. For example, there is no change in interictal spike frequency prior to seizures, whereas during the postictal refractory period (when lactate levels are still elevated; see Fig. 6.3) spike frequency is increased (Gotman & Marciani 1985, Katz et al 1991). These data suggest that, although both interical spikes and seizures originate from the same epileptogenic region, they are distinct phenomena with different ionic mechanisms (Gotman 1991). Indeed, Schweitzer et al (1992) have recently described interictal spike activity in rat hippocampal slices under low (0.5 mmol/l) calcium and moderately elevated potassium (5 mmol/l) concentrations, whereas when extracellular potassium was further increased to 9 mmol/l, interictal spikes completely disappeared, whereas spontaneous seizure-like events were observed.

ANTIEPILEPTIC DRUG MEASUREMENTS USING MICRODIALYSIS

In addition to measuring endogenous transmitters, modulators and metabolites, microdialysis has also been used to monitor antiepileptic drug (AED) levels in epilepsy. The general aim of the majority of these studies has been to determine the relationship between brain microdialysate levels of an AED and drug dose and specifically to determine whether plasma measurements are an accurate index of ECF concentrations. The first preliminary report suggested that carbamazepine could be measured in the dialysate following standard oral dosing and that the change in plasma levels over time was paralleled synchronously by a reciprocal change in brain as determined by hippocampal dialysis (During et al 1989). More definitive studies have subsequently determined both absolute drug levels in brain ECF (Scheyer et al 1994a), as well as pharmacokinetic data on the rate of entry into the brain and washout of AEDs, including phenytoin and carbamazepine (Scheyer et al 1993, 1994b). In addition, microdialysis has been used to characterize the mechanism of action of specific AEDs in the human brain. The novel AED, tiagabine, which in animal studies was shown to be an inhibitor of both the neuronal and glial GABA transporters, increased human hippocampal ECF GABA levels at clinically relevant doses (During et al 1992).

DISCUSSION

Despite the conflicting results in experimental animal studies regarding alterations in extracellular glutamate and aspartate with seizures, the human data reported to date are consistent in so far as electrographic seizures are associated with a local rise in ECF aspartate and glutamate. The most comprehensive study to date, that of During & Spencer (1993), also found a consistent pattern of a preictal rise in extracellular glutamate and a delayed and blunted ictal elevation in extracellular GABA in the epileptogenic hippocampi in their series of patients with temporal lobe epilepsy. Clinical microdialysis coupled to depth electrode EEG recordings might therefore be useful as a diagnostic aid and the biochemical data generated using this technique may help in defining the epileptogenic region for subsequent surgical resection.

Moreover, these studies provide direct evidence for a sustained increase in ECF glutamate to potentially neurotoxic concentrations during spontaneous seizures in the awake human brain. It is particularly interesting that glutamate concentrations rose before the seizure onset, suggesting that the increase in ECF glutamate may be a mechanism of seizure generation. Moreover, the diminished increase in GABA during seizures suggests that the decreased inhibition in the epileptogenic hippocampus may be secondary to a loss of a specific GABA release mechanism.

Several recent articles have addressed the potential neurochemical mediators of seizure arrest and postictal refractoriness. Specifically, During & Spencer (1992) provided direct evidence for seizure-induced increases in ECF concentrations of adenosine and its sustained elevation postictally in the human hippocampus. Moreover, the magnitude and duration of this seizure-induced release suggest that adenosine may play a pivotal role in both seizure arrest as well as postictal refractoriness, and that treatments which facilitate adenosine's action may be clinically useful.

During et al (1994) demonstrated a direct relationship of spike frequency to extracellular lactate, suggesting that neuronal activity stimulates lactate production in the setting of normal oxygenation during interictal periods. These results support animal data of physiological stimulation inducing non-oxidative glucose metabolism, despite abundant oxygen (Fellows et al 1993) as well as human positron emission tomography data of increased glucose consumption unaccompanied by oxidative metabolism during visual imagery tasks (Roland et al 1987). In addition, these authors reported an ictal rise in extracellular lactate limited to the site of seizure activity. Moreover, During et al (1994) raised the hypothesis that extracellular lactate generation during seizures may not merely be a metabolic bystander as a product of non-oxidative glycolysis but may have a direct relationship to neuronal excitability and, in so far as extracellular lactate generation reflects acidification of the ECF, the lactate rise during and following seizures may be an additional mechanism of seizure arrest and postictal refractoriness.

These initial in vivo neurochemical studies of human temporal lobe epilepsy have not only confirmed previous experimental animal studies but have also yielded significant novel insights into the neurochemical alterations associated with clinical seizures and suggested basic mechanisms of epileptogenesis. Ongoing microdialysis studies will continue to define the neurochemical substrates of seizure generation and arrest. Moreover, clinical microdialysis may also be useful as a diagnostic technique to help define the epileptogenic region and guide therapeutic strategies. Furthermore, the biochemical data generated by the coupling of microdialysis to depth electrodes is likely to aid significantly in the evaluation of epilepsy patients considered for surgical resection.

REFERENCES

Ackerman R F, Lear J L. 1989 Glycolysis-induced discordance between glucose metabolic rates measured with radio-labelled fluorodeoxyglucose and glucose. J Cereb Blood Flow Metab 9: 774–785

Adams R N, Marsden C A. 1982 Electrochemical detection methods for monoamine measurements in vitro and in vivo. In: Handbook of psychopharmacology, vol. 15 pp 1–74

Ault B, Wang C M. 1986 Adenosine inhibits epileptiform activity arising in hippocampal area CA3. Br J Pharmacol 87: 695–703

Bean A, During M J, Roth R H. 1990 Effects of dopamine autoreceptor stimulation on the release of colocalized transmitters: in vivo release of dopamine and neurotensin from rat prefrontal cortex. Neurosci Lett 108: 143–148

Bender A S, Wu P H, Phyllis J W. 1981 The rapid uptake and release of [^{3}H]adenosine by rat cerebral cortical synaptosomes. J Neurochem 36: 651–660

Benveniste H. 1989 Brain dialysis. J Neurochem 52: 1667–1679

Benveniste H, Diemer N H. 1987 Cellular reactions to implantation of a microdialysis tube in the rat hippocampus. Acta Neuropathol 74: 234–238

Biscoe T J, Straughan D W. 1966 Micro-electrophoretic studies of neurones in the cat hippocampus. J Physiol 183: 341–359

Bito L, Davson H, Levin E, Murray M, Snider N. 1966 The concentrations of free amino acids and other electrolytes in cerebrospinal fluid, in vivo dialysate of brain, and blood plasma of the dog. J Neurochem 13: 1057–1067

Burley E S, Ferrendelli J A. 1984 Regulatory effects of neurotransmitters on electroshock and pentylenetrazol seizures. Fed Proc 43: 2521–2524

Carlson H, Ronne-Engstrom E, Ungerstedt U, Hillerid L. 1992 Seizure related elevations of extracellular amino acids in human focal epilepsy. Neurosci Lett 140: 30–32

Caspers H, Speckmann E-J. 1972 Cerebral P_{O_2}, P_{CO_2} and pH: changes during convulsive activity and their significance for spontaneous arrest of seizures. Epilepsia 13: 699–725

Chamberlin N L, Traub R D, Dingledine R. 1990 Role of EPSPs in initiation of spontaneous synchronized burst firing in rat hippocampal neurons bathed in high potassium. J Neurophysiol 64: 1000–1006

Chapman A G, Meldrum B S, Siesjo B K. 1977 Cerebral metabolic changes during prolonged epileptic seizures in rats. J Neurochem 28: 1025–1035

Chastain J E, Samson F, Nelson S R, Pazdernik T L. 1989 Kainic acid-induced seizures: changes in brain extracellular ions as assessed by intracranial microdialysis. Life Sci 45: 811–817

Chin J H. 1989 Adenosine receptors in brain: neuromodulation and role in epilepsy. Ann Neurol 26: 695–698

Choi DW. 1988 Glutamate neurotoxicity and diseases of the nervous system. Neuron 1: 623–634

Chiu N. 1981 Caffeine- and aminophylline-induced seizures. Epilepsia 22: 85–94

Cornell-Bell A, Magge S, During MJ. 1992 Human astrocytes from hyperexcitable foci are themselves hyperexcitable. In: Simon RP, ed. Excitatory amino acids. New York: Thieme, pp 273–277

Croucher MJ, Collins JF, Meldrum BS. 1982 Anticonvulsant actions of excitatory amino acid antagonists. Science 216: 899–901

Daly JW. 1982 Adenosine receptors: targets for future drugs. J Med Chem 25: 197–207

Delgado JMR, DeFeudis FV, Roth RH, Ryugo DK, Mitruka BM. 1972 Dialytrode for long term intercerebral perfusion in awake monkeys. Arch Int Pharmacodyn 198: 9–21

Delgado-Escueta AV, Ward AA, Woodbury DM, Porter RJ. (eds) 1986 New wave of research in the epilepsies. Advances in neurology, vol. 44. New York: Raven Press, pp 3–55

Di Chiara G. 1990 In vivo brain dialysis of neurotransmitters. Trends Pharmacol Sci 11: 116–121

Dichter MA, Ayala GF. 1987 Cellular mechanisms of epilepsy: a status report. Science 237: 157–167

Dietzel I, Heinemann U, Lux HD. 1989 Relations between slow extracellular potential changes, glial potassium buffering, and electrolyte and cellular volume changes during neuronal hyperactivity in cat brain. Glia 2: 25–44

Do KQ, Klancnik JM, Gahwiler B, Perschak H, Weiser HG, Cuenod M. 1991 Release of excitatory amino acids: animal studies and epileptic foci studies in humans. In: Meldrum BS, Moroni F, Simon RP, Woods JH, eds. Excitatory amino acids. New York: Raven Press, pp 677–685

Dodd PR, Bradford HF. 1976 Release of amino acids from the maturing cobalt induced epileptic focus. Brain Res 111: 377–388

Dodd PR, Bradford HF, Abdul-Ghani AS, Cox DW, Continho-Netto J. 1980 Release of amino acids from chronic epileptic and sub-epileptic foci in vivo. Brain Res 193: 505–517

Dragunow M, Goddard GV, Laverty R. 1985 Is adenosine an endogenous anticonvulsant? Epilepsia 26: 480–487

Duffy TE, Howse DC, Plum F. 1975 Cerebral metabolism during experimental status epilepticus. J Neurochem 24: 925–934

Dunwiddie T V. 1980 Endogenously released adenosine regulates excitability in the vitro hippocampus. Epilepsia 21: 541–548

Dunwiddie TV, Fredholm BB. 1989 Adenosine A_1 receptors inhibit adenylate cyclase activity and neurotransmitter release and hyperpolarize neurons in rat hippocampus. J Pharmacol Exp Ther 249: 31–37

During MJ. 1991 In vivo neurochemistry of the conscious human brain: intrahippocampal microdialysis in epilepsy. In: Robinson TE, Justice JB Jr, eds. Microdialysis in the neurosciences. Amsterdam: Elsevier, pp 425–442

During MJ. 1992 Brain microdialysis in experimental and clinical neurology In Vecsei L, Freeze A, Swartz, KJ, Beal MF, eds Neurological disorders: novel experimental and therapeutic strategies. Chichester: Ellis Horwood, pp 249–273

During MJ, Spencer DD. 1990 Neurotransmitter release in the human hippocampus in vivo: physiological and pharmacological studies of complex partial epilepsy. Epilepsia 31: 623

During MJ, Spencer DD. 1992 Adenosine: a potential mediator of seizure arrest and postictal refractoriness. Ann Neurol 32: 618–624

During MJ, Spencer DD. 1993 Extracellular hippocampal glutamate and spontaneous seizure in the conscious human brain. Lancet 340: 1607–1610

During MJ, Anderson GM, Roth RH, Spencer DD. 1989 A human dialytrode: in vivo measurements of neuroactive substances in the human hippocampus with simultaneous depth EEG recordings. Soc Neurosci Abstr 15: 340.8

During MJ, Mattson RH Scheyer R, Spencer DD. The effect of tiagabine HCl on extracellular GABA levels in the human hippocampus. Epilepsia 33 (suppl 3): 83

During MJ, Fried I, Leone P, Katz A, Spencer DD. 1994 Direct measurement of extracellular lactate in the human hippocampus during spontaneous seizures. J Neurochem 62: 2356–2361

Dunwiddie TV. 1980 Endogenously released adenosine regulates excitability in the in vitro hippocampus. Epilepsia 21: 541–548

Dusser de Barenne JG, Marshall CS, McCulloch WS, Nims LF. 1938 Observations of the pH of arterial blood and the pH and electrical activity of the cerebral cortex. Am J Physiol

124: 631–636

Egawa M, Hoebel B G, Stone E A. 1988 Use of microdialysis to measure brain noradrenergic receptor function in vivo. Brain Res 458: 303–308

Engel J, Ackerman R F. 1980 Interictal EEG spikes correlate with decreased, rather than increased epileptogenicity in amygdaloid kindled rats. Brain Res 190: 543–548

Fellows L K, Boutelle M G, Fillenz M 1993 Physiological stimulation increases nonoxidative glucose metabolism in the brain of the freely moving rat. J Neurochem 60: 1258–1263

Fox P T, Raichle M E, Mintum D C, Derce C. 1988 Non-oxidative glucose consumption during focal physiological neural activity. Science 241: 462–464

Frandsen A, Schousboe A. 1987 Time and concentration dependency of the toxicity of excitatory amno acids on cerebral neurones in primary culture. Neurochem Int 10: 583–591

Fuxe K, Agnati L F. 1991 Volume transmission in the brain. New York: Raven Press

Gaddum J H. 1961 Push-pull cannulae. J Physiol 155: 1P–2P

Gotman J. 1991 Relationships between interictal spiking and seizures: human and experimental evidence. Can J Neurol Sci 18 (suppl 4): 573–576

Gotman J, Marciani M G. 1985 Electrographical spiking activity drug levels and seizure occurs in epileptic patients. Ann Neurol 17: 597–603

Hayashi T. 1952 A physiological study of epileptic seizures following cortical stimulation in animals and its application to human clinics. Jpn J Physiol 3: 46–64

Hoehn K, White T D. 1990 Glutamate-evoked release of endogenous adenosine from rat cortical synaptosomes is mediated by glutamate uptake and not by receptors. J Neurochem 54: 1716–1724

Hohorst H J, Kreutz F K, Bucher T. 1959 Uber metabolitge-halte metabolit-konzentrationen in der leber der ratte. Biochem Z 332: 18–46

Howse D C, Duffy T E. 1975 Control of the redox state of the pyridine nucleotides in the rat cerebral cortex. Effect of electroshock-induced seizures. J Neurochem 24: 935–940

Hsiao J K, Ball B A, Morrison P F, Mefford I N, Bungay P M. 1990 The effects of different semipermeable membranes on in vitro and in vivo performance of microdialysis probes. J Neurochem 54: 1449–1452

Jacobson I, Hamberger A. 1985 Kainic acid-induced changes of extracellular amino acid levels, evoked potentials and EEG activity in the rabbit olfactory bulb. Brain Res 348: 289–296

Jasper H, Erikson T C. 1941 Cerebral blood flow and pH in excessive cortical discharge induced by metrazol and electrical stimulation. J Neurophysiol 4: 333–347

Jobe P C 1984 Neurotransmitters and epilepsy: an overview. Fed Proc 43: 2503–2504

Jonzon B, Fredholm B B. 1985 Release of purines, noradrenaline, and GABA from rat hippocampal slices by field stimulation. J Neurochem 44: 217–224.

Katz A, Marks D A, McCarthy G, Spencer S S. 1991 Does interictal spiking change prior to seizures? EEG Clin Neurophysiol 79: 153–156

King L J. Lowry O H, Passoneau J V, Venson V. 1967 Effects of convulsants on energy reserves in the cerebral cortex. J Neurochem 14: 599–611

Korf J, DeBoer J, Postema F, Venema K, Flentge F. 1991 On-line real-time monitoring of extracellular lactate, ethanol, glucose and choline using microdialysis and enzyme reactors. In: Robinson T E, Justice J Jr, eds Techniques in the behavioral and neural sciences. Amsterdam: Elsevier (in press)

Kostopoulos G, Drapeau C, Avoli M, Olivier A, Villemeure J G. 1989 Endogenous adenosine can reduce epileptiform activity in the human epileptogenic cortex maintained in vitro. Neurosci Lett 106: 119–124

Kuhr W G, Korf J. 1988a Extracellular lactic acid as an indicator of brain metabolism: continuous on-line measurement in conscious, freely moving rats with intrastriatal dialysis. J Cerebral Blood Flow Metab 8: 130–137

Kuhr W G, Korf J. 1988b N-methyl-D-aspartate receptor involvement in lactate production following ischemia or convulsion in rats. Eur J Pharmacol 155: 145–149

Kuhr W G, Korf J. 1988c Direct coupling of intracerebral dialysis with flow injection analysis based on enzymatic/fluorescence detection of lactic acid. Anal Chim Acta 205: 53–59

Kuhr W G, van den Berg C J, Korf J. 1988 In vivo identification and quantitative evaluation of carrier-mediated transport of lactate at the cellular level in the striatum of conscious, freely-moving rats. J Cerebral Blood Flow Metab 8: 848–856

Lazarewicz, JW, Lehmann A, Hagberg H, Hamberger A. 1986a Effects of kainic acid on brain calcium fluxes studied in vivo and in vitro. J Neurochem 46: 494–498

Lazarewicz JW, Hagberg H, Hamberger A. 1986b Extracellular calcium in the hippocampus of unanesthetized rabbits monitored with dialysis-perfusion. J Neurosci Methods 15: 317–328

Lee KS, Schubert P, Heinemann U. 1984 The anticonvulsant action of adenosine: a postsynaptic, dendritic action by a possible endogenous anticonvulsant. Brain Res 321: 160–164

Lee KS, Schubert P, Reddington M, Kreutzberg GW. 1986 The distribution of adenosine A_1 receptors and 5'-nucleotidase in the hippocampal formation of several mammalian species. J Comp Neurol 246: 427–434

Lehmann A. 1987 Alterations in hippocampal extracellular amino acids and purine catabolites during limbic seizures induced by folate injection into the rabbit amgydala. Neuroscience 22: 573–578

Lehmann A, Hagberg H, Jacobson I, Hamberger A. 1985 Effects of status epilepticus on extracellular amino acids in the hippocampus. Brain Res 359: 147–151

MacIntosh FC, Oborin PE. 1953 Release of acetylcholine from intact cerebral cortex. In: Abstracts of the XIX international physiology congress, pp 580–581

Maître M, Ciesielski L, Lehmann A et al 1974 Protective effect of adenosine and nicotinamide against audiogenic seizures. Biochem Pharmacol 23: 2807–2816

Marangos PJ, Post RM, Patel J, Zander K, Parma A, Weiss S. 1983 Specific and potent interactions of carbamazepine with brain adenosine receptors. Eur J Pharmacol 93: 175–182

Matthews PM, Anderman F, Arnold DL. 1990 A proton magnetic resonance spectroscopy study of focal epilepsy in humans. Neurology 40: 985–989

Meldrum BS. 1981 Metabolic effects of prolonged epileptic seizures and the causation of epileptic brain damage. In Rose FC, ed. Metabolic disorders of the nervous system. London: Pitman Medical, pp 175–187

Meldrum BS. 1983 Metabolic factors during prolonged seizures and their relation to nerve cell death. Adv Neurol 34: 261–275

Meldrum BS, Corsellis JAN. 1984 Epilepsy. In: Adams JH, Corsellis JAN, Duchen LW, eds. Greenfield's neuropathology. New York: Wiley, pp 921–950.

Meldrum BS, Nilsson B. 1976 Cerebral blood flow and metabolic rate early and late in prolonged epileptic seizures induced in rats by bicuculline. Brain 99: 523–542

Meyer JS, Gotoh F, Tazaki Y. 1966 Cerebral metabolism during epileptic seizures in man. Electroencephalogr Clin Neurophysiol 21: 10–22

Millan MH, Obrenovitch TP, Sarna GS et al. 1991 Changes in rat brain extracellular glutamate concentration during seizures induced by systemic picrotoxin or focal bicuculline injection: an in vivo dialysis study with on-line enzymatic detection. Epilepsy Res 9: 86–91

Miller LP, Villeneuve JB, Braun LD, Oldendorf BA. 1986 Effect of pharmacological doses of 3-O-methyl-D-glucose and 2-deoxy-D-glucose on rat brain glucose and lactate. Stroke 17: 957–961

Morrison PF, Bungay PM, Hsiao JK, Ball BA, Mefford IN, Dedrick RL. 1991 Quantitative microdialysis: analysis of transients and application to pharmacokinetics. J Neurochem 57: 103–119

Mutch WAC, Hansen AJ. 1984 Extracellular pH changes during spreading depression and cerebral ischemia: mechanisms of brain pH regulation. J Cerebral Blood Flow Metab 4: 17–27

Nakada T, Kwee IL, Lerner AM, Remler MP. 1983 Theophylline-induced seizures: clinical and pathophysiological aspects. West J Med 138: 371–374

Pauwels, PJ, Opperdoes FR, Trouet A. 1985 Effects of antimycin, glucose deprivation, and serum on cultures of neurons, astrocytes, and neuroblastoma cells. J Neurochem 44: 143–148

Perrson CGA, Erjefalt I. 1982 Seizure activity in animals given enprofylline and theophylline, two xanthines with partly different mechanisms of action. Arch Int Pharmacodyn Ther 258: 267–282

Peters SG, Wochos DN, Peterson GC. 1984 Status epilepticus as a complication of concurrent electroconvulsive and theophylline therapy. Mayo Clin Proc 59: 568–570

Peterson DW, Collins JF, Bradford HF. 1983 The kindled amygdala model of epilepsy;

anticonvulsant action of amino acid antagonists. Brain Res 275: 169–172

Petroff OAC, Prichard JW, Ogino T, Avison M, Alger JR, Shulman RG. 1986 Combined ^{1}H and ^{31}P nuclear magnetic resonance spectroscopic studies of bicuculline-induced seizures in vivo. Ann Neurol 20: 185–193

Phillis JW. 1984 Interactions of the anticonvulsants diphenylhydantion and carbamazepine with adenosine on cerebral cortical neurons. Epilepsia 25: 765–772

Phillis JW, Wu PH. 1981 The role of adenosine and its nucleotides in central synaptic transmission. Prog Neurobiol 16: 187–239

Phillis JW, Wu PH. 1982 The effect of various centrally active drugs on adenosine uptake by the central nervous system. Comp Biochem Physiol 72C: 179–187

Pin JP, Bockaert J. 1989 Two distinct mechanisms, differentially affected by excitatory amino acids, trigger GABA release from fetal mouse striatal neurons in primary culture. J Neurosci 9: 648–655

Pritchard JW, Petroff OAC, Ogino T, Shulman RG. 1987 Cerebral lactate elevation by electroshock: a ^{1}H magnetic resonance study. Ann NY Acad Sci 508: 54–63

Richardson PJ, Brown SJ, Bailyes EM, Luzio JP. 1987 Ectoenzymes control adenosine modulation of immunoisolated cholinergic synapses. Nature 327: 232–234

Roland PE, Eriksson L, Stone-Elander S, Widen L. 1987 Does mental activity change the oxidative metabolism of the brain? J Neurosci 7: 2372–2389

Ronne-Engstrom E, Hillered L, Flink R, Spannare B, Ungerstedt U, Carlson H. 1992 Intracerebral microdialysis of extracellular amino acids in the human epileptic focus. J Cerebral Blood Flow Metab 12: 873–876

Sattin A. 1971 Increase in the content of adenosine 3′, 5′ monophosphate in mouse forebrain during seizures and prevention of the increase by methyl xanthine. J Neurochem 18: 1087–1096

Scheyer RD, During MJ, Hochholzer HM, Spencer DD, Mattson RH. 1993 Phenytoin concentrations in the human brain: a microdialysis study. Epilepsia 34 (suppl 6): 43

Scheyer RD, During MJ, Cramer, JA, Toftness BR, Hochholzer JM, Mattson RH. 1994a Simultaneous HPLC analysis of carbamazepine and carbamazepine epoxide in human brain microdialysate. J Liquid Chromatogr. 17: 1567–1576

Scheyer RD, During MJ, Spencer DD, Cramer JA, Mattson RH. 1994b Measurement of carbamazepine and carbamazepine epoxide in the human brain using in vivo microdialysis. Neurology 44: 1469–1472

Schrader J, Wahl M, Kuschinsky W, Kreutzberg GN. 1980 Increase of adenosine content in cerebral cortex of the rat during bicuculline-induced seizures. Pfluegers Arch 387: 245–251

Schweitzer JS, Patrylo PR, Dudek FE. 1992 Prolonged field bursts in the dentate gyrus: dependence on low calcium, high potassium, and nonsynaptic mechanisms. J Neurophysiol 68: 2016–2025

Skerrit J M, Daries L P, Johnston G A R. 1982 A purinergic component in the anticonvulsant action of carbamazepine? Eur J Pharmacol 82: 195–197

Sloviter RS. 1987 Decreased hippocampal inhibition and a selective loss of interneurons in experimental epilepsy. Science 235: 73–76

Snead OC. 1983 On the sacred disease: the neurochemistry of epilepsy. Int Rev Neurobiol 24: 93–180

Sternau LL, Lust WD, Ricci AJ, Ratcheson R. 1989 Role for GABA in selective vulnerability in gerbils. Stroke 20: 281–287

Storm-Mathisen J. 1977 Glutamic acid and excitatory nerve endings: reduction of glutamic acid uptake after axotomy. Brain Res 120: 379–386

Stringer JL, Lothman EW. 1990 A_1 adenosinergic modulation alters the duration of maximal dentate activation. Neurosci Lett 118: 231–234

Tang CM, Dichter M, Morad M. 1990 Modulation of the N-methyl-D-aspartate channel by extracellular H^+. Proc Natl Acad Sci USA 87: 6445–6459

Tschirgi RD, Inanga K, Taylor JL, Walker RM, Sonnenschein RR. 1957 Changes in cortical pH and blood flow accompanying spreading depression and convulsion. Am J Physiol 190: 557–562

Ungerstedt U. 1984 Measurement of neurotransmitter release by intracranial microdialysis. In: Marsden CA, ed. Measurement of neurotransmitter release in vivo. New York: Wiley, pp 81–106

Ungerstedt U, Pycock C. 1974 Functional correlates of dopamine neurotransmission. Bull Schweiz Akad Med Wiss 1278: 1–13

Ungerstedt U, Herrera-Marschitz M, Jungnelius U, Tossman U, Zetterstrom T. 1982

Dopamine synaptic mechanisms selected in studies combining behavioral recordings and brain dialysis. In: Kotisaka M, ed. Advances in dopamine research. New York: Pergamon Press, pp 219–231

Vezzani A, Ungerstedt U, French ED, Schwarcz R. 1985 In vivo brain dialysis of amino acids and simultaneous EEG measurement following intra-hippocampal quinolinic acid injection: evidence for a dissociation between neurochemical changes and seizures. J Neurochem 45: 335–344

Wade JV, Samson FE, Nelson SR, Pazdernik TL. 1987 Changes in extracellular amino acids during soman- and kainic acid-induced seizures. J Neurochem 49: 645–650

Walz W, Mukerji S. 1988 Lactate release from cultured astrocytes and neurons: a comparison. Glia 1: 366–370

Wasterlain CG, Morin AM, Dwyer BE. 1985 The epilepsies. In: Lajtha A ed. Handbook of Neurochemistry. New York: Plenum, pp 339–419

Westerink BHC, Damsa G, Rollema H, de Vries JB, Horn AS. 1987 Scope and limitations of in vivo microdialysis: a comparison of its application to various transmitter systems. Life Sci 41: 1763–1776

Westerink B H C, De Vries J M, Duran R. 1990 Use of microdialysis for monitoring tyrosine hydroxylase activity in the brain of conscious rats. J Neurochem 54: 381–387

Winn HR, Welsh JE, Rubio R, Berne RM. 1980 Changes in brain adenosine during bicuculline-induced seizures in rats. Effects of hypoxia and altered systemic blood pressure. Circ Res 47: 568–577

Woods BT, Chui T-M. 1990 In vivo ^{1}H spectroscopy of the human brain following electroconvulsive therapy. Ann Neurol 28: 745–749

Zwillich CW, Sutton FD, Neff TA et al. (1975) Theophylline-induced seizures in adults. Ann Intern Med 82: 784–787

7

New antiepileptic drugs

I. E. Leppik   A. Gil-Nagel

The increase in number of new antiepileptic drugs (AED) is the result of a number of factors. New drug development was spurred by the chance discovery of the effectiveness of valproate in animal models and its subsequent clinical use. Two approaches to the development of new drugs have evolved since. One has been the rational designing of compounds based on an increasingly sophisticated knowledge of basic mechanisms of action. The second is increased use of a variety of animal models of seizures or epilepsy syndromes to screen a large number of compounds. Both of these approaches have been significant departures from the previous method based on developing structural analogs of known effective drugs. Another factor has been the development of a rational approach to clinical testing based on sound principles of classification and statistical designs (Leppik et al 1993).

The ideal AED should have a number of properties.

1. It should be effective for a number of seizure types or epilepsy syndromes.
2. It should have a wide therapeutic range, i.e. a large difference between the least effective dose and the dose at which toxicity is experienced. Animal testing can often provide an estimation of the therapeutic range from the therapeutic index, which is derived by dividing the median toxic dose by the median effective dose.
3. It should not interact with other drugs, a characteristic of substances with low protein binding and lack of human metabolism.
4. There should not be any significant organ toxicity.
5. For compliance and ease of dosing the drug should have a 1 mg half-life, or in substances with a short elimination half-life, it should be available in a slow-absorption formulation, leading to a long period of activity.
6. Finally, it should be soluble, so parenteral formulations can be developed.

No standard AEDs or drugs in development have all the properties of the ideal drug. This review briefly examines the major features of the new drugs in early clinical use or still in development (Tables 7.1 and 7.2).

Table 7.1 New antiepileptic drugs and some of their pharmacokinetic properties

Drug	Sponsor	Elimination half-life (h)	Protein binding (%)	Water solubility	Adult dose (mg/day)
Felbamate	Wallace	11–18	35	Poor	2400–4800
Flunarizine	Janssen	500	99	Poor	10–15
Gabapentin	Parke-Davis	4–6	None	Very good	900–2400
Lamotrigine	Wellcome	15–60	55	Poor	100–600
Losigamone	Schwabe	4–5	60	Very poor	>1500
Oxcarbazepine	Ciba-Geigy	10–15 (metabolite)		Poor	300–1800
Ralitoline	Godecke	4–6	74	Poor	600–900
Remacemide	Fisons	4–6		Good	>600
Stiripentol	Biocodex	Variable	>90	Poor	2000–3000
Tiagabine	Abbott	5–14		Good	24–80
Topiramate	McNeil	19–23			600–1200
Vigabatrin	Marion Merrell Dow	Not relevant			2000–4000
Zonisamide	Dainippon	27–36		Poor	400–600

Table 7.2 Internations between new and standard antiepileptic drugs (AEDs)

New AED	Effect on standard AED		Effect by standard AED	
	Increases on	Decreases on	Increased by	Decreased by
Felbamate	PHT, VPA, PB, 10–11 epoxide	CBZ	VPA	PHT, CBZ
Flunarizine				PHT
Gabapentin				
Lamotrigine	VPA		VPA	PHT, CBZ
Oxcarbazepine				
Ralitoline				PHT, PB
Stiripentol	PHT, CBZ			
Topiramate				
Vigabatrin				
Zonisamide				

Abbreviations: AED, antiepileptic drug; CB2, carbamazepine; PB, phenobarbital; PHT, phenytoin; VPA, valproic acid.

FELBAMATE

Felbamate (FBM), chemical name 2-phenyl-1,3-propanediol dicarbamate, is a lipophilic water-insoluble dicarbamate. In animals, FBM is rapidly absorbed into tissues, including brain tissue (Adusumalli et al 1991). FBM effectively blocks seizures induced by maximal electroshock (MES), pentylenetetrazol (PTZ) and picrotoxin (chloride channel blocker), but confers no protection against bicuculline (γ-aminobutyric acid (GABA) receptor antagonist) and strychnine (glycine antagonist)-induced seizures (Swinyard et al 1986). FBM's mechanism of action may be due to an interaction with the strychnine-insensitive glycine site at the N-methyl-D-aspartate (NMDA) receptor

(McCabe et al 1993). In animal studies, FBM has a very favorable safety profile (Perhach et al 1986, Leppik & Graves 1989). Rats tolerated single doses of 3.0 g/kg without significant side-effects. These doses are significantly above the amount required for seizure protection in animal models. Because sufficiently large doses could not be physically administered to rodents, median lethal dose (LD_{50}) values could not be determined. No teratogenicity has been seen in animal models.

The first clinical study which supported the effectiveness of FBM in humans was a National Institutes of Health-sponsored, double-blind, placebo-controlled, add-on trial. FBM significantly reduced seizure frequency ($P = 0.007$; Leppik et al 1991). In this study, FBM was used as the third AED in patients receiving both phenytoin (PHT) and carbamazepine (CBZ). FBM has also been evaluated in patients with partial epilepsy undergoing presurgical evaluation (Bourgeois et al 1993). This study demonstrated that FBM could be titrated up to a daily dose of 3600 mg within 3 days with minimal adverse reactions in patients whose other AEDs had been discontinued or substantially reduced. FBM controlled seizures during the inpatient and follow-up outpatient periods.

A monotherapy trial of FBM in uncontrolled partial epilepsy demonstrated efficacy and a decreased rate of adverse effects compared to add-on studies (Sachdeo et al 1992). FBM also reduced the frequency of atonic seizures and improved the global assessment scores in children with Lennox–Gastaut syndrome (Felbamate Study Group 1993).

Orally administered FBM is well-absorbed in humans. In patients with epilepsy time to peak concentration was 1–4 h after the dose and the median elimination half-life was 14.6 h.

A major route of elimination (50–70%) is through the urine. FBM is also extensively metabolized by the liver via hydroxylation and conjugation. None of the metabolites appears to have anticonvulsant or neurotoxic properties (Swinyard et al 1986). However, hepatic elimination creates the potential for a number of drug–drug interactions. FBM has clinically significant interactions with PHT, CBZ, valproate (VPA), and phenobarbital (phenobarbitone; PB). When FBM is added, the levels of PHT, VPA and PB can increase by 20–40% or more. In contrast, CBZ concentrations decrease by about 20% when FBM is added but CBZ-epoxide levels increase approximately 50%. Although data are limited, FBM concentrations may be lowered by the concomitant use of other AEDs.

FBM is generally well-tolerated by patients with epilepsy. Of 977 adults treated with FBM in the clinical trials, 12% (120 patients) discontinued the drug because of side-effects. In studies with children FBM had to be discontinued in 6% (22 of 357) and the types of adverse effect were similar to those seen in adults (Physician Desk Reference (PDR) 1994). The most common side-effects of FBM have been insomnia, headache, weight loss, nausea, decreased appetite, dizziness, fatigue, ataxia and lethargy. Other reported side-effects include diarrhea, vomiting, fatigue and nervousness.

Side-effects are much more common in persons receiving polytherapy. With monotherapy, few adverse experiences have been reported and these have been mild and self-limited (Sachdeo et al 1992). Although there were no significant changes in laboratory tests in patients receiving FBM in clinical trials, aplastic anemia has recently been associated with FBM use. Ten cases (9 in the USA, 1 in Europe) were reported to the US Food and Drug Administration (FDA) in August 1994; 2 of these died. The FDA estimated the risk of aplastic anemia at 1 in 5000. As of December 1994 over 25 cases of aplastic anemia and 11 cases of hepatitis have been reported. Blood tests detect aplastic anemia or hepatitis only when they are established; they do not identify individuals at risk.

Felbamate is available in the USA as Felbatol in 400 and 600 mg tablets and suspension 600 mg/5 ml. In adult studies, doses have ranged from 1800 to 4800 mg/day. The usual maximal dosage in most studies has been 3600 mg/day. In general, higher doses are tolerated as monotherapy. In children, doses of 15–45 mg/kg have typically been used, although some pediatric epileptologists are using doses of 60 mg/kg per day, or higher, in intractable cases.

In one study, serum levels ranged between 20 and 45 µg/ml (Leppik et al 1991). However, in other studies patients tolerated concentrations as high as 100 µg/ml with monotherapy.

In December 1992, the US FDA advisory panel recommended that FBM be approved for use as monotherapy in adults with partial and generalized seizures and in children with the Lennox–Gastaut syndrome. Final approval for use in the USA was granted on 30 July 1993. Because of the cases of aplastic anemia, the FDA issued a warning to physicians on 1 August 1994 that FBM should not be used unless absolutely necessary.

GABAPENTIN

Gabapentin (GBP), chemical name 1-(aminomethyl) cyclohexaneacetic acid, is a GABA-related amino acid. It was designed to penetrate the blood–brain barrier readily. In animals, GBP effectively antagonizes seizures produced in the semicarbazide, isoniazid, bicuculline, picrotoxin, strychnine, NMDA, MES and maximal PTZ convulsant tests (Bartoszyk 1983, Bartoszyk et al 1986). This profile in animal models of epilepsy suggested that GBP had the potential to be a relatively broad-spectrum AED in humans. Its mechanism of action is unknown. In vitro studies with radiolabeled drug have revealed novel GBP binding sites in neocortex and hippocampus of rat brain (Hill et al 1993, Suman-Chauhan et al 1993, Taylor et al 1993). Extensive data from preclinical studies indicate that GBP has little toxicity. There were no deaths in acute toxicity studies at doses of up to 8000 mg/kg per day in rats and chronic studies showed tolerance with doses up to 500 mg/kg per day in monkeys (Foot & Wallace 1991). In male rats taking extremely high doses of GBP (14-fold larger than maximum human exposure), a weak carcinogenic response consisting of an increased frequency of pancreatic acinar carcinomas was noted following lifelong exposure. This effect was not seen in female rats of the same species or in any other animal tested, and the type of malignant cells noted was significantly different from human pancreatic tumors (Browne 1993). This is not considered to be a relevant risk for humans at therapeutic dosages. No teratogenicity has been reported in human in vitro cell cultures. It has been shown to be fetotoxic in rodents, causing delayed ossification, hydroureter and hydronephrosis (PDR 1994). Because animal studies are not always predictive of human response, GBP should not be used in pregnant women unless the benefit clearly justifies the potential risk.

The clinical efficacy of GBP has been established by a number of studies including three large masked, placebo-controlled studies and open-label studies (Browne 1993). In the first double-masked, parallel design study, 127 patients with refractory partial epilepsy (simple, complex or secondarily generalized) were randomized to placebo or GBP (1200 mg/day). Among treated patients, 26% had a greater than 50% reduction in seizure frequency versus 10% in the placebo group ($P = 0.042$; Andrews et al 1990). The second study involved 306 patients (Bruni et al 1991), and the third (US gabapentin study #5) enrolled 272 patients. Of the 705 participants in the three controlled studies, 53 received 600 mg/day of GBP, 111 received 900 mg/day, 214 received 1200 mg/day, 54 were treated with 1800 mg/day and the remainder received placebo. Outcome was measured by the response ratio (RR) which showed statistically significant superiority (improved seizure control) over placebo in all three studies using the intent-to-treat analysis (Browne 1993).

GBP is rapidly absorbed after oral administration, with peak serum levels reached in 2–4 h and elimination half-life of 5–7 h (Schmidt 1989). Its intestinal absorption follows a saturable transport mechanism, resulting in a lack of proportionality between increasing dose and drug levels in plasma (Stewart et al 1993). This quality may act as a protection in cases of overdoses; however, it can also be a limiting factor to achieve high plasma concentrations of the drug. GBP dose not bind to human serum albumin or other plasma proteins. The renal clearance of GBP equals the total clearance in normal volunteers — approximately 120–130 ml/min. In the elderly and patients with impaired renal function, GBP plasma clearance is reduced. The drug can be removed from plasma by hemodialysis. The dosage should be adjusted in patients with compromised renal function or undergoing hemodialysis. No metabolite has been detected in humans (Schmidt 1989). After single doses of 25–300 mg there is a linear correlation between dose and the 2-h concentration in patients on GBP monotherapy (Schmidt 1989). Following 1 week of 400 mg given three times daily to patients maintained on PHT, a maximum plasma concentration of 3.6–8.6 µg/ml and a concentration of 2–4.8 µg/ml were seen (Graves et al 1989).

In clinical use, adverse effects have been minor. Only 7% of the 2074 patients who received the drug in preclinical trials discontinued treatment because of adverse events (PDR 1994). The majority of side-effects involve the central nervous system and are reversed by decreasing or discontinuing the drug. They include somnolence (19.3%), dizziness (17.1%), ataxia (12.5%), fatigue (11.0%), nystagmus (8.3%), tremor (6.8%), diplopia (5.9%) and amblyopia (4.2%). Other relevant side-effects, which occurred in fewer than 3% of treated individuals are: depression, abnormal thinking, increased appetite resulting in weight gain, peripheral edema, vasodilatation, dyspepsia, constipation, dry mouth and throat, leukopenia, myalgia, pruritus and impotence (Andrews et al 1990, Crawford et al 1987; PDR 1994).

In follow-up studies of patients on GBP more than 1 year, there has been no evidence of chronic toxicity, including routine laboratory tests (Schmidt 1989). More recent studies have used doses of 2400 mg/day without problems, despite being added to existing AED therapy (Browne 1993).

Unlike other AEDs, GBP is not metabolized by the liver, does not induce hepatic enzymes, and is free of interactions with other drugs. It is almost completely eliminated by renal excretion of the parent compound. In human studies, GBP does not significantly affect antipyrine (Schmidt 1989) or PHT concentrations (Graves et al 1989). It may therefore be quite useful in patients who are on other medications as it can be added to existing AED regimens without modifying other drug doses. Concomitant administration of GBP with norethindrone acetate and ethinylestradiol did not affect the pharmacokinetics of any drug. Therefore increased failure of contraception in women receiving both GBP and oral contraceptives which contain norethindrone and ethinylestradiol is not expected. Cimetidine decreases clearance of GBP by 14%, but this is not expected to be of clinical significance. The antacid Maalox diminishes the bioavailability of GBP by about 20% therefore GBP should be taken at least 2 h after the administration of antacids.

At the present time, GBP has been mostly used as an add-on agent for patients with treatment-resistant partial and secondarily generalized tonic-clonic seizures, but studies of GBP as monotherapy are underway.

In most reported trials, GBP was initiated at doses of 300 mg/day and increased to 600–1800 mg/day. Recently, doses of 3600 mg/day have been used. Because it is well-tolerated, GBP can be titrated up to full therapeutic doses in 2–3 days (Foot & Wallace 1991). With its half-life of 5–7 h, t.i.d. administration is recommended. It can be given with or without food, although at higher doses, and especially when dose-related side-effects occur, taking GBP after meals may minimize adverse effects.

Gabapentin is marketed in Europe, and was approved by the FDA in December 1993, for use in adults with partial and secondarily generalized seizures. In the USA it is supplied as Neurontin, in 100, 300, and 400 mg capsules.

LAMOTRIGINE

Lamotrigine (LTG), chemical name 3,5-diamino-6-(2,3-dichlorophenyl)-1,2,4-triazine, is a phenyltriazine unrelated to currently available AEDs. It most likely exerts its anticonvulsant activity by inhibiting the release of excitatory amino acids, especially glutamate (Lamb et al 1985, Leach et al 1986). In the MES test, LTG has a potency that is similar to CBZ in rats and PHT in mice. In animal studies, LTG may act at voltage-sensitive sodium channels, stabilizing neuronal membranes and inhibiting neurotransmitter release, primarily glutamate. In animal studies, there is a wide gap between the effective and lethal doses in rodent species, indicating the potential for relatively low toxicity in humans. Chronic studies in rodents and primates at doses of up to 20–125 mg/kg per day have shown no toxic effects (Miller et al 1986). LTG has not exhibited teratogenicity in animal models.

Five double-blind, placebo-controlled, add-on trials have shown efficacy in partial and generalized tonic–clonic seizures (Sander et al 1990). Overall, results from these studies indicated that at least 22% of patients had a reduction of greater than 50% in their seizure frequency (Brodie 1992). LTG has also been evaluated in 11 patients with Lennox–Gastaut syndrome and appears to have some promise (Timmings & Richens 1992). It has also shown promising preliminary results in the treatment of primary generalized epilepsies (Timmings and Richens 1992).

LTG is rapidly and well-absorbed following oral administration; it is transported in the plasma 55% protein-bound. LTG is extensively metabolized and excreted predominantly as a glucuronide. In normal volunteers the mean terminal elimination half-life is 24 ± 5.7 h (range 21–50 h). In contrast, in patients who were on enzyme inducers such as PHT or CBZ, the mean half-life was 15 h (range 7.8–33 h). However, in patients on VPA, the $t_{1/2}$ increased to a mean of 59 h (range 30–89 h). Thus, the half-life of LTG is shortened by enzyme inducers such as PHT and CBZ, but markedly lengthened by VPA (Gram 1989). However, LTG does not appear to alter the pharmacokinetics of standard AEDs.

Serum concentrations ranging from 0.5 to 5 µg/ml have been reported after doses of 75–250 mg/day. In most published studies, LTG doses have been adjusted to maintain trough serum concentrations between 0.5 and 3 µg/ml. These concentrations have not produced toxicity. When VPA is added to LTG monotherapy, there may be a doubling or more of the LTG level because the elimination half-life of LTG is increased to approximately 60 h (Betts 1992).

Lamotrigine is well-tolerated (Binnie et al 1989, Jawad et al 1989, Loiseau et al 1990, Risner et al 1990, Sander et al 1990, Richens & Yuen 1991). The most common adverse effects are dose-related and include diplopia, drowsiness, dizziness, ataxia, headache, nausea and vomiting. Most adverse effects can be minimized by lowering LTG dosage. Approximately 3% of patients develop a rash, which usually begins shortly after drug initiation and resolves within days of drug discontinuation.

Lamotrigine does not seem to alter weight or laboratory measures such as complete blood count, biochemical profiles or folate levels (Betts 1992) and it only rarely alters the metabolism or serum levels of other AEDs (Wolf 1992). In combination with CBZ, LTG increased the CBZ-epoxide level approximately 10% in some studies, but this has not been a universal observation (Warner et al 1992).

LTG can usually be started at 50–100 mg/day and increased to 600 mg/day. Because VPA blocks the elimination of LTG, the initial dose of LTG and subsequent increments should be made more gradually in patients on VPA. Betts (1992) recommends starting LTG with 25 mg at bedtime and then increasing in 25 mg/day increments at 2-week intervals, monitoring closely for side-effects, which are common when the dose is higher than 100 mg/day. Seizure control is unlikely to improve with LTG doses of more than 200 mg/day in patients also taking VPA. If VPA is subsequently tapered or discontinued, the LTG dose may need to be increased and will likely be better tolerated.

Lamotrigine is marketed in the UK. In March 1993, the USA FDA advisory panel recommended approval of LTG as add-on therapy for treatment of partial seizures and secondarily generalized seizures in adults.

OXCARBAZEPINE

Oxcarbazepine (OXC; 10, 11-dihydro-10-oxo-carbamazepine) is a keto compound that is chemically related to CBZ (5-carbamyl^{5}H-dibenzazepine). Oxcarbazepine differs from CBZ in that it has a keto group in the 10,11 position. This keto group is responsible for its unusual metabolic fate. The compound was synthesized to produce a compound structurally related to CBZ; OXC has a similar therapeutic profile but improved tolerability compared with CBZ (Jensen & Dam 1990). In rodents, extremely high doses of OXC are tolerated in acute toxicity studies, with the oral LD_{50} estimated to be more than 5000 mg/kg. In a perinatal and postnatal study on OXC in female rats, doses of 25, 75 and 150 mg/kg were given orally from day 15 of pregnancy until weaning of the pups. OXC did not adversely affect growth or development of the progeny.

In a Scandinavian double-blind, multi-center study, 235 patients suffering from newly diagnosed epilepsy were randomly assigned to treatment with either OXC or CBZ (Dam et al 1989). Seizure frequency did not differ between the OXC and CBZ groups; efficacy was judged excellent or good in 96% of patients receiving OXC and 97% of those treated with CBZ.

OXC is as effective as CBZ for the treatment of partial and generalized tonic–clonic seizures in both monotherapy and polytherapy.

Following oral administration, nearly 100% of OXC is absorbed (Feldmann et al 1978). It is rapidly transformed into its active metabolite, 10,11-dihydro-10-hydroxy carbamazepine (MHD). Thus, plasma OXC levels are very low, while levels of MHD are higher and are associated with antiepileptic efficacy (Faigle & Menge 1990). MHD is therefore the true antiepileptic compound.

Among 791 patients in the Scandinavian study, 581 patients were exposed to either OXC or its primary metabolite MHD; 326 of the patients were treated in monotherapy. Treatment duration varied from 8 to 52 weeks; 143 patients were treated for more than 1 year. Because OXC is so extensively converted to MHD in humans, the pharmacokinetics are largely dependent on the plasma concentration of MHD (Feldmann et al 1978). The distribution volume of MHD is about 0.3–0.8 l/kg (Theisohn & Heinmann 1982).

Approximately 50% of MHD binds to plasma proteins (Kristensen et al 1983). Elimination is non-exponential, with a half-life of 8–12 h. In contrast to CBZ, there is no autoinduction of MHD (Jensen et al 1991).

In the Scandinavian multicenter trial of patients with newly diagnosed epilepsy (Dam et al 1989), the number of patients with side-effects (74 versus 68%) and the mean number of side-effects per patient (3.5 versus 2.8) tended to be lower during treatment with OXC as compared to carbamazepine. Although these differences were not statistically significant, there were significantly fewer adverse effects requiring drug discontinuation in the OXC group (Dam et al 1989). The most commonly reported side-effects of OXC were tiredness, headache, dizziness and ataxia. In 51 patients with a prior allergic skin rash on CBZ, only 27% developed a similar reaction with OXC (Jensen et al 1991). OXC, like its parent compound CBZ, can induce hyponatremia. This side-effect is of no clinical significance in the majority of patients, but on rare occasions it has been associated with a severe encephalopathy (Steinhoff et al 1992).

Since metabolism of OXC to MHD does not depend on the cytochrome P-450 system, one would not expect drug interactions to be a major problem with OXC. Drugs which are known to inhibit the metabolism of CBZ (leading to CBZ toxicity) such as propoxyphene, cimetidene and erythromycin, do not alter the pharmacokinetics of OXC or MHD (Jensen et al 1991).

In comparison to CBZ, the equivalent OXC dose is about 50% higher. The dose range in the large Scandinavian study was 300–1800 mg/day. In adults, OXC can be started at a dose of 100 mg t.i.d. and increased by 100–300 mg/day every 1–2 weeks, as tolerated. Although OXC was administered on a t.i.d. regimen, a simplification to a b.i.d. regimen may be possible in some patients. OXC is available in many European countries.

REMACEMIDE

Remacemide hydrochloride ((+/−) 2-amino-N-(1-methyl-1,2-diphenyl-lethyl)-acetamide monohydrochloride) is a diphenyl-ethyl-acetamide derivative. It is water-soluble. In animal models it is effective against MES seizures, and this activity persists for many hours. It is longer-acting in this model than PHT, CBZ and VPA. It is also effective against convulsions induced by N-methyl-D-aspartic acid; it does not have activity against convulsions elicited by picrotoxin, pentylenetetrazol, strychnine or bicuculline (Muir & Palmer 1991).

It is metabolized to a desglycinated derivative (FPL 12495AA) which is actually more potent against MES than the parent compound but also is associated with more cerebral toxicity. The LD_{50} in rats was 900 mg/kg. Doses of 80 mg/kg per day were well-tolerated in long-term toxicity studies. No teratogenicity was observed.

In volunteers, the drug was absorbed in 1–2 h after doses of up to 400 mg. Its elimination half-life was approximately 4 h. The apparent elimination half-life of the metabolite was 12–24 h. Preliminary evaluation of the pharmacokinetics of remacemide in persons with epilepsy indicates that concentrations of this drug are lower than those measured in normal volunteers, suggesting that there is induction of metabolism by concomitant antiepileptic medication. Clinical studies are underway.

TIAGABINE

Tiagabine, (R-)-N-(4,4-di-(3-methylthien-2-yl)but-3-enyl) nipecotic acid, is a potent inhibitor of GABA uptake into glial and neural elements. It is a potent anticonvulsant in several rodent models (Pierce et al 1991).

Tiagabine is rapidly absorbed, with the maximum concentration occurring 30–60 min after ingestion. The overall half-life in one study was 6.7 h, with a range of 4.5–13.4 h. Peak levels of 552 ng/ml have been measured after single doses of 24 mg.

One large study of 328 patients has shown a dose-level response in improved seizure control (Rowan et al 1993). Side-effects have been minor. Single doses of 2 and 8 mg have not produced any side-effects. At doses of 12 and 24 mg subjective symptoms of dizziness, lightheadedness and slow response were reported by a few subjects. Doses up to 80 mg/day have been used in a few patients who have tolerated it well. Multicenter studies are in progress.

TOPIRAMATE

Topiramate (2,3:4,5-bis-O-(1-methylethylidine)-beta-D-fructopyranose) is a sulfamate-substituted monosaccharide structurally different from other standard or experimental AEDs. It is active in the MES test but inactive in the PTZ test. Although its profile of action in animal models of epilepsy is similar to that of PHT, it is relatively less toxic with a protective index of approximately 12 (Rogawski & Porter 1990). It does not interact with PHT, VPA (Floren et al 1989) or CBZ (Wilensky et al 1989).

Topiramate, 800–1200 mg/day, is presently being tested in large multicenter trials. It appears to be effective in many patients although some neurotoxicity has been observed.

VIGABATRIN

Vigabatrin (γ-vinyl-GABA; GVG), chemical name dl-4-aminohex-5-enoic acid, a synthetic GABA derivative, is an enzyme-activated irreversible inhibitor of GABA transaminase (GABA-T). By blocking GABA breakdown, GVG increases the functional pool of GABA.

GVG is a racemic mixture; only the S(+)-enantiomer possesses pharmacologic activity. In rodents, GVG blocks MES- and strychnine-induced seizures. However, GVG is less potent in blocking seizures induced by bicuculline, picrotoxin and PTZ. The LD_{50} in rats is approximately 60 times higher than the maximum daily human dose (Richens 1989). In rodents, single high doses cause central nervous system depression and convulsions.

Repeated high doses of GVG cause alopecia, weight loss, anorexia and anemia in several animal species. GVG's slow progress in US clinical studies reflected concern over the development of central nervous system myelin vacuoles in some animal species. When administered chronically at doses of 50–100 mg/kg per day, intramyelinic edema develops in the cerebral white matter in mice, rats and dogs. These microvacuoles are most abundant in the cerebellum, but are also found in the reticular formation, optic tract, anterior commissure columns of the fornix, colliculi and hippocampus (Richens 1989). Magnetic resonance imaging brain scans and evoked potential studies in humans have not shown evidence of myelin abnormalities. Similarly, examination of either autopsy or surgically resected tissue from at least 37 GVG-treated patients revealed no evidence of myelin vacuolization (Butler 1989, Paljarvi et al 1990, Hammond et al 1992, Sivenius et al 1993).

GVG has mainly been used to treat refractory patients with partial epilepsy. In short-term double-blind studies, approximately 45% of patients have a good response (Mumford 1988). Sivenius and colleagues (1991) reported a 5-year follow-up of 75 patients with complex partial or secondarily generalized tonic–clonic seizures who started on VGB. At the end of the study, 19 (25%) had a greater than 50% seizure reduction at 5-year follow-up. The most common reason for withdrawal among those that initially benefited was loss of response. GVG has been widely studied in patients in Europe. The results in adults, as well as children, have been favorable (Ben-Menachem et al 1989, Appleton 1993). GVG is more effective in partial seizures than generalized-onset seizures (Livingston et al 1989). Tolerance does not seem to develop after long-term use (Browne et al 1989). GVG has also demonstrated efficacy in infantile spasms (Chiron et al 1991, Vles et al 1993).

After oral administration of GVG to normal volunteers, peak concentrations are attained within 2 h. The elimination half-life is between 5 and 7 h. Kinetics are linear between 1 and 3 g doses. Total clearance is approximately 1.7 ml/min per kg. Renal clearance comprises approximately 60–70% of total clearance (Schechter 1989). Absolute bioavailability is unknown; however, more than 80% of the dose is found in the urine (Richens 1989).

After 1.5 g p.o. of the racemic mixture, peak concentrations of the S(+)-enantiomer range from 50–100 mmol/l. Reduced renal clearance and an increased R/S ratio of GVG occur with compromised renal function (Richens 1989).

In 5 patients receiving other AEDs, the terminal elimination $t_{1/2}$ was 4.2–5.6 h (Browne et al 1989). Administration of food does not significantly alter the pharmacokinetic profile of GVG (Frisk-Holmberg et al 1989). PHT steady-state concentrations decrease with concomitant GVG administration (Richens 1989). When GVG 1.5 g b.i.d. was added to PHT monotherapy, PHT concentrations decreased from 59 ± 30 to 40 ± 13 mmol/l (Rimmer & Richens 1989). Phenytoin concentrations did not change until the patients had received 1.5 g GVG b.i.d. for 4 weeks.

GVG's short metabolic elimination half-life might lead to the expectation that multiple daily dosings are needed. However, the pharmacologic activity of GVG is determined by the resynthesis rate of GABA-T (Schechter 1989). Since inhibition of GABA-T precedes pharmacologic activity, there is a lag time before any anticonvulsant efficacy is observed. Conversely, after discontinuation of GVG, anticonvulsant activity may persist. In animals, it takes approximately 6 days to regain maximum enzyme activity when GVG is withdrawn (Gram 1988). Most clinical studies have used twice-daily dosing. One study (Ben-Menachem et al 1989) examined seizure frequency and cerebrospinal fluid concentrations of total GABA, free GABA, and homocarnosine following once-daily, every-other-day, and every-third-day dosing in 11 patients receiving other antiepileptic medications. As the interval is decreased, lumbar concentrations of the neurotransmitters increased.

In clinical trials, drowsiness, ataxia and headache are the most common side-effects (Browne et al 1987). Other side-effects include tremor, mood changes, abnormal behaviour, depression and psychosis (Sander et al 1991). In mentally retarded patients with epilepsy, the most commonly reported side-effects were tiredness, aggressiveness and ataxia (Matilainen et al 1988).

In one study of cognitive function and mood, 2 g/day of GVG — the lower end of the therapeutic dose range — was added to usual AEDs (McGuire et al 1992). In this setting, GVG was very well-tolerated and showed minimal side-effects. The only test which showed any significant change was a decreased response time on a test of central cognitive processing ability (arithmetic). In another study, GVG produced no impairment or some improvement in cognitive functions (Kalviainen et al 1990). Two studies found no mood changes after initiation of GVG therapy (Mumford et al 1990, McGuire et al 1992).

GVG is effective against partial seizures. Also, it may be effective in infantile Spasms (Vlies et al 1993). GVG is licenced in Europe. In the USA, clinical trials have been completed.

ZONISAMIDE

Zonisamide (ZNS) is a novel AED developed in Japan (Seino et al 1991). It suppresses MES but does not antagonize seizures induced by PTZ in mice.

ZNS blocks MES in rodents and dogs at minimal (~10 mg/ml) plasma concentrations. Its therapeutic range is much wider than that of PHT or CBZ, although its protective index is comparable to PHT and CBZ. In contrast to PHT and CBZ, ZNS's anti-MES effect is unchanged after repeated oral administration in rats. Neither metabolically nor pharmacodynamically mediated tolerance is observed to the anti-MES effect of ZNS (Taylor et al 1986).

A multicenter double-blind study compared ZNS and CBZ in patients who were uncontrolled with one to three AEDs or who were not previously treated (Seino et al 1991). Average monthly frequency of simple and complex partial seizures decreased from 14.9 to 3.4 in the ZNS group, and from 13.3 to 4.4 in the CBZ group. A similar reduction in mean monthly frequency (i.e. from 1.8 to 0.6 in the ZNS group) was also found for secondarily generalized tonic–clonic seizures. The percentage of patients showing a $\geq 50\%$ reduction in seizure frequency was 82% in the ZNS group and 71% in the CBZ group at week 16.

Seino and colleagues also compared the efficacy and safety of ZNS and VPA in 38 children with four or more convulsive or non-convulsive generalized seizures per month. The ZNS and VPA groups were treated for 8 weeks at mean daily doses of 7.3 and 27.6 mg/kg, respectively, at week 8. Both ZNS and VPA were effective in controlling generalized seizures, including tonic–clonic, tonic and atypical absence seizures. Loiseau et al (1987) performed a multicenter placebo-controlled double-blind study of ZNS in 139 patients with refractory partial and secondarily generalized seizures. Their overall evaluation after 12 weeks of treatment showed an improvement rate of 62% in the ZNS group and 19% in the placebo group ($P < 0.05$). In a multicenter open label trial performed in the USA, 167 adults with complex partial seizures had a median percentage reduction of 58% from baseline (Leppik et al 1993).

ZNS reduced the frequency of tonic–clonic and other seizure types in 2 patients with Unverricht–Lundborg (Baltic) syndrome of progressive myoclonic epilepsy (Henry et al 1988). Serum ZNS concentrations ranged from 27 to 43 µg/ml in patients whose seizure control and overall level of functioning improved (Henry et al 1988).

When ZNS was orally administered to healthy volunteers, the time to peak concentrations ranged between 2.4 and 6.0 h. Elimination half-lives were essentially independent of dose and ranged from 49.7 to 68.2 h (mean 60 h). In patients also treated with conventional AEDs, the half-life of ZNS after a single oral dose of 400 mg was 28.4 h (Sackellaves 1985). In humans, some ZNS is excreted in urine as unchanged drug and the rest is excreted as acetylated and glucuronide metabolites (Ito et al 1982). The usually effective serum range has been suggested to be about 20–40 µg/ml (Henry et al 1988).

Overall, ZNS appears to be well-tolerated. Among 1008 ZNS-treated patients (most receiving combination therapy) 517 (51%) reported side-effects and 185 (18%) discontinued therapy because of toxicity (Seino et al 1991).

Drowsiness was most commonly reported (24%), followed by ataxia (13%), anorexia (11%), gastrointestinal discomfort (7%), diminished spontaneity (6%) and mental slowing (5%). Among patients treated with ZNS only, side-effects were less frequent: drowsiness (9%), anorexia (7%), gastrointestinal discomfort (7%), decreased spontaneity (6%), headache (6%), and pruritus or rash (6%), (Seino et al 1991). Approximately 2% of the 1008 patients discontinued the drug because of abnormal liver function tests or leukopenia (Seino et al 1991).

In the USA and Europe, urinary calculi developed in some patients treated with ZNS, which caused further US clinical trials to be suspended. In Japan, however, only 2 out of 1008 patients had renal lithiasis.

In vitro studies show no protein-binding interactions between ZNS and PHT or PB (Ono et al 1988). The plasma half-life of ZNS is decreased when taken with CBZ or PHT (Sackellares et al 1985, Ojemann et al 1986), but steady-state ZNS plasma levels decrease only slightly when taken with CBZ or VPA (Seino et al 1991).

ZNS is available as a 100-mg tablet and as a powder. Doses in most studies have ranged from 6 to 11 mg/kg per day. In adults, ZNS is usually started at a dose of 100 mg h.s. or 100 mg b.i.d. Subsequent increases are approximately 100 mg/day every 1–2 weeks as tolerated. In some cases, t.i.d. dosing may help reduce adverse effects.

ZNS is available in Japan, and recently, clinical trials have resumed in the USA.

FLUNARIZINE

Flunarizine (FNZ), (E)-1-[bis(4-fluorophenyl)-methyl]-4-(3-phenyl-2-propenyl)-piperazine, is a difluorinated piperazine derivative (Overweg & Binnie 1990). This calcium-entry blocker was introduced clinically in several countries for its beneficial effects in peripheral and cerebral circulatory disorders, migraine prophylaxis and vertigo (Binnie 1989). FNZ antagonizes the tonic seizure component in the following seizure-induction tests: maximal PTZ, MES, allylglycine, bicuculline and audiogenic stimulation (Overweg & Binnie 1990). Eight double-blind, placebo-controlled, cross-over trials and seven open trials have evaluated 349 patients with favorable results (Overweg & Binnie 1990).

FNZ reaches peak levels within 2–4 h after oral administration in fasting normal subjects (Binnie 1989). Flunarizine has a long duration of action with a terminal half-life of 19 days (Heykants & Van Peer 1983). It is highly lipophilic, and more than 99% is protein-bound (Meuldermans et al 1978).

Mean steady-state concentrations after 3 months' treatment with 15 mg/day are 35.9 ng/ml. Therapy with 20 mg/day produces plasma levels between 17 and 135 ng/ml with a mean steady-state level of 59 ng/ml. Thus, there are marked individual differences in plasma FNZ levels (Heykants et al 1979).

Single high doses of FNZ are well-tolerated in adult rodents and dogs of both sexes. There is a wide safety margin (40–60-fold) between the effective (ED_{50}) and the lethal (LD_{50}) doses. FNZ has no primary embryotoxicity or teratogenicity in rats and rabbits.

The most frequently observed side-effect has been drowsiness, which occurred in 26% of patients in open trials but in only 8% in double-blind trials (Binnie et al 1985, Froscher et al 1988). Sedation appears to be dose-related, occurring most often with doses of 20 mg/day or higher and plasma levels of 50 μg/ml or higher (Binnie et al 1985). Other reported side-effects include headache, vertigo, and changes in appetite and weight, but there were no differences between placebo and treatment groups in some studies (Starreveld et al 1989). Parkinsonism, tardive dyskinesia, akathisia and depression may result from FNZ, or the related calcium-channel blocker, cinnarizine (Chouza et al 1986, Micheli et al 1987). These extrapyramidal reactions occurred in adults who were 45 years of age or older and were being treated for disorders other than epilepsy.

Clinical trials have not revealed significant enzyme induction or inhibition by FNZ (Binnie 1989). However, AED polytherapy may lower FNZ levels.

OTHER ANTIEPILEPTIC DRUGS IN TESTING

Losigamone, threo-5(2-chlorphenylhydroxymethyl)-4-methoxy-2(^{5}H)-fura-none, related to β-methoxybutenolides, is unusual in that it is related to naturally occurring compounds (Stein et al 1991). In animal models, it is effective against MES, metrazol, bicuculline, nicotine and picrotoxin seizures. Some evidence suggests that its activity may be mediated by GABA-gated chloride channels (Stein et al 1991). Little organ toxicity and no mutagenic activity were noted in animal studies. In one open-label, add-on study involving 15 patients treated for 24 weeks, 7 had a greater than 50% reduction in seizures. Side-effects included dizziness, headache and diplopia (Runge et al 1993). More clinical testing is needed to establish clinical efficacy.

Ralitoline, (Z)-N-(2-chloro-6-methyl-phenyl)-2-(3-methyl-4-oxo-2-thiazoli-dinone) acetamide, is a structurally novel compound derived from compounds known to modify ion transport mechanisms (Anhut et al 1991). It is three to six times more potent than PHT and CBZ in the MES model. It is also effective in chemically induced seizures. However, it is not active in PTZ seizures. Preliminary studies in patients are underway and appear promising.

Stiripentol, or 4,4-dimethyl-1-(3,4 methylene-dioxyphenyl)-1-penten-3-ol, is structurally unrelated to other AEDs. In animal models of seizures, it produces a dose-dependent inhibition of electrically and chemically induced convulsions in rats (Vincent 1991). It exhibits non-linear pharmacokinetics. Stiripentol has shown antiabsence activity in a strain of Wistar rats with a genetic petit mal epilepsy with spike-and-wave discharges. These were suppressed by intraperitoneal injections of stiripentol (Micheletti et al 1988). Stiripentol is extensively bound to plasma proteins with a free fraction of only

1%. Its pharmacokinetics have been extensively studied in patients with epilepsy (Levy et al 1984). It has significant interactions with other drugs, even in small doses (Levy et al 1988). In addition, use of stiripentol results in large increases in co-administered PHT and CBZ concentrations. In one study of 26 patients with intractable localization-related epilepsy, 3 became seizure-free and 7 had a greater than 50% reduction in seizures (Vincent 1991). In one study of children with atypical absence seizures, all 8 patients had a substantial decrease (49–95%) in numbers of absence seizures (Vincent 1991). Few side-effects have been reported, mainly gastric disturbances, insomnia, and weight loss. Therapeutic doses appear to be in the 2000–3000 mg/day range.

CONCLUSIONS

Several new compounds have been approved and others are undergoing extensive investigation in the USA, Europe and Japan. Many of them will be approved for clinical use during the next decade. Each has distinctive pharmacological properties.

New AEDs offer new opportunities for treating people with epilepsy. The three drugs recently approved in the USA — FBM, GBP and LTG — are effective against partial and secondarily generalized tonic–clonic seizures and are well-tolerated by the majority of patients. FBM is also effective in decreasing the frequency of atonic seizures in children with the Lennox–Gastaut syndrome. As with other AEDs, FBM, GBP and LTG are better tolerated when used as monotherapy. FBM has been approved for use as monotherapy but GBP and LTG are currently approved for add-on use only. Results of monotherapy efficacy trials will likely be available in the near future.

Although many of the new AEDs have been used for up to 5–10 years in a small number of people, the long-term safety of these drugs requires additional monitoring. Defining the actual frequency of rare but potentially serious adverse events will also require greater experience. As these drugs come into wider use, we should improve our ability to define patient groups that are most and least likely to benefit. Rational combinations of the new AEDs with older AEDs have begun to emerge based upon side-effects and tolerability. However, we need to establish the efficacy of these combinations as well as their safety.

Establishing the ultimate place of the new AEDs in our therapeutic armamentarium against epilepsy awaits carefully designed, controlled, double-blind studies comparing older and newer AEDs, as well as comparisons between new AEDs. Such studies should ideally incorporate not only traditional medical outcome measures such as seizure frequency and side-effects, but should also include quality-of-life measures (Devinsky 1993). More drugs are needed for the treatment of epilepsy syndromes in the pediatric age group.

KEY POINTS FOR CLINICAL PRACTICE

- The new AEDs have undergone more thorough preclinical and clinical testing than the standard drugs, but patient treatment years are less.
- FBM is effective for partial and secondarily generalized seizures and some types of seizures associated with the Lennox–Gastaut syndrome.
- FBM is best used as monotherapy; it inhibits PHT, VPA and CBZ 10,11-epoxide, but increases CBZ clearance.
- FBM has a higher incidence of aplastic anemia and hepatitis than other AEDs
- GBP has an active transport system for absorption and thus the fraction of the dose absorbed decreases at higher doses.
- GBP is renally excreted and has no drug–drug interactions.
- LTG has been used in the UK for many years and has the longest patient experience.
- LTG does not alter the kinetics of standard AEDs, but VPA and possibly FBM prolong its half-life.
- GVG has a novel mechanism of action and appears to be very potent against partial seizures. Its biological effectiveness is measured in days and greatly exceeds its plasma half-life.

ACKNOWLEDGEMENTS

The help of Liliane Dargis in preparing the manuscript is gratefully acknowledged. This research was supported in part by NIH NS16308.

REFERENCES

Adusumalli V E, Yang J T, Wong K K et al 1991 Felbamate pharmacokinetics in the rat, rabbit and dog. Drug Metab Dispos as 1: 1116–1125

Andrews J, Chadwick D, Bates D et al 1990 Gabapentin in partial epilepsy. Lancet i: 1114–1117

Anhut H, Satzinger G, von Hodenberg A. 1991 Ralitoline. In: Pisani F, Perucca E, Avanzini G, Richens A, eds. New antiepileptic drugs. Amsterdam: Elsevier Science, pp 141–145

Appleton R E. 1993 The role of vigabatrin in the management of infantile epileptic syndromes. Neurology 43 (suppl 5): S21–S23

Bartoszyk G D. 1983 Gabapentin and convulsions produced by excitatory amino acids. Naunyn-Schmiedebergs Arch Pharmacol 324: R24

Bartoszyk G D, Meyerson N, Reimann W et al. 1986 Gabapentin. In: Meldrum B S, Porter R J, eds. New anticonvulsant drugs. London: John Libbey, pp 147–163

Ben-Menachem E, Persson L I, Schechter P J et al. 1989 The effect of different vigabatrin treatment regimens on CSF biochemistry and seizure control in epileptic patients. Br J Clin Pharmacol 27: 79S–85S

Betts T. 1992 Clinical uses of lamotrigine. Seizure 1: 3–6

Binnie C D. 1989 Potential antiepileptic drugs: flunarizine and other calcium entry blockers. In: Levy R, Mattson R, Meldrum B, Penry J K, Dreifuss F E, eds. Antiepileptic drugs, 3rd edn. New York: Raven Press, pp 971–982

Binnie C D, de Beukelaar F, Meijer J W A et al. 1985 Open dose-ranging trial of flunarizine as add-on therapy in epilepsy. Epilepsia 26: 424–428

Binnie C, Debets R, Engelsman M et al. 1989 Double blind cross over trial of lamotrigine (Lamictal) as add-on therapy in intractable epilepsy. Epilepsy Res 4: 222–229

Bourgeois B, Leppik I E, Sackellares J C et al. 1993 Felbamate: a double-blind trial in patients undergoing presurgical evaluation of partial seizures. Neurology 43: 693–696

Brodie MJ. 1992 Lamotrigine. Lancet 339: 1397–1400

Browne, TR. 1993 Efficacy and safety of gabapentin. In: Chadwick D, ed. New trends in epilepsy management: the role of gabapentin. London: Royal Society of Medicine Services, pp 47–57

Browne TR, Mattson RH, Penry JK et al 1987 Vigabatrin for refractory complex partial seizures: multicentre single blind study with long term follow-up. Neurology 37: 184–189

Browne TR, Mattson RH, Penry JK et al 1989 A multicentre study of vigabatrin for drug-resistant epilepsy. Br J Clin Pharmacol 27: 95S–100S

Bruni J, Sanders M, Anhut H et al 1991 Efficacy and safety of gabapentin (neurontin): a multicenter, placebo-controlled, double-blind study. Neurology 41 (suppl 1): 330–331

Butler WH. 1989 The neuropathology of vigabatrin Epilepsia 30: S15–S17

Chiron D, Dulac O, Beaumont D et al. 1991 Therapeutic trial of vigabatrin in refractory infantile spasms. J Child Neurol 6: S52–S59

Chouza C, Caamano JL, Aljanati R et al. 1986 Parkinsonism, tardive dyskinesia, akathisia and depression induced by flunarizine. Lancet i: 1303–1304

Crawford P, Ghadiali E, Lane R et al. 1987 Gabapentin as an antiepileptic drug in man. J Neurol Neurosurg Psychiatry 50: 682–686

Dam M, Ekberg R, Loyning Y et al. (the Scandinavian oxcarbazepine study group). 1989 A double-blind study comparing oxcarbazepine and carbamazepine in patients with newly diagnosed, previously untreated epilepsy. Epilepsy Res 3: 70–76

Devinsky O. 1993 Clinical uses of the quality of life in epilepsy inventory (QOLIE). Epilepsia 34 (Suppl 4): S39–S44

Faigle JW, Menge GP. 1990 Pharmacokinetic and metabolic features of oxcarbazepine and their clinical significance: comparison with carbamazepine. Int Clin Psychopharmacol 5(suppl 1): 73–82

Felbamate study group in Lennox–Gastaut syndrome. 1993 Efficacy of felbamate in childhood epileptic encephalopathy (Lennox–Gastaut syndrome). N Engl J Med 328: 29–33

Feldmann KF, Brechbuhler S, Faigle JW, Imhof P. 1978 Pharmacokinetics and metabolism of GP 47 680, a compound related to carbamazepine, in animals and man. In: Meinardi H, Rowan AJ, eds. Advances in epileptology. Amsterdam: Swet & Zeitlinger, pp 290–294

Floren KL, Graves NM, Leppik IE et al. 1989 Pharmacokinetics of topiramate in patients with partial epilepsy receiving phenytoin or valproate. Epilepsia 30: 646

Foot M, Wallace J. 1991 Gabapentin. In: Pisani F, Perucca E, Avanzini G, Richens A, eds. New antiepileptic drugs. Holland: Elsevier Science, pp 109–114

Frisk-Holmberg M, Kerth P, Meyer PH. 1989 Effect of food on the absorption of vigabatrin. Br J Clin Pharmacol 27: 23S–25S

Froscher W, Bulau P, Burr W et al. 1988 Double-blind placebo controlled trial with flunarizine in therapy-resistant epileptic patients. Clin Neuropharmacol 11: 232–240

Gram L. 1988 Experimental studies and controlled clinical testing of valproate and vigabatrin. Acta Neurol Scan 78: 241–270

Gram L. 1989 Potential antiepileptic drugs: lamotrigine. In: Levy R, Mattson R, Meldrum B, Penry JK, Dreifuss FE, eds. Antiepileptic drugs, 3rd edn. New York: Raven Press, pp 947–953

Graves NM, Holmes GB, Leppik IE et al. 1989 Pharmacokinetics of gabapentin in patients treated with phenytoin. Pharmacotherapy 9: 196

Hammond EJ, Ballinger WE Jr, Lu L, Wilder BJ, Uthman BM, Reid SA. 1992 Absence of cortical white matter changes in three patients undergoing long-term vigabatrin therapy. Epilepsy Res 12: 261–265

Henry TR, Leppik IE, Gumnit RJ, Jacobs M. Progressive myoclonic epilepsy treated with zonisamide. Neurology 38: 928–931

Heykants J, Van Peer A. 1983 Steady-state pharmacokinetics of flunarizine in man are predictable from single-dose kinetics. Janssen Pharmaceutical, clinical research report R14950/58

Heykants J, De Cree J, Horig C. 1979 Steady-state plasma levels of flunarizine in chronically treated patients. Arzneimittel forsch/Drug Res 29: 1168–1171

Hill DR, Suman-Chauhan N, Woodruff GN. 1993 Localization of [^{3}H]gabapentin to a novel site in rat brain: autoradiographic studies. Eur J Pharmacol 244: 303–309

Ito T, Yamaguchi T, Miyazaki H et al 1982 Pharmacokinetic studies of AD-810, a new antiepileptic compound: phase I trials. Arzneimittel forsch 32: 1581–1586

Jawad S, Richens A, Goodwin G et al. 1989 Controlled trial of lamotrigine (Lamictal) for refractory partial seizures. Epilepsia 30: 356–363

Jensen P K, Dam M. 1990 Oxcarbazepine. In: Dam M, Gram L eds. Comprehensive epileptology. New York: Raven Press, pp 621–629

Jensen P K, Gram L, Schmutz M. 1991 Oxcarbazepine. In: Pisani F, Perucca E, Avanzini G, Richens A, eds. New antiepileptic drugs. Holland: Elsevier Science, pp 135–140

Kalviainen R, Aikia M, Saksa M et al. 1990 Cognitive effects of vigabatrin monotherapy. Acta Neurol Scand 82 (suppl 133): 13

Kristensen O, Klitgaard N A, Jönsson B, Sindrup S, 1983 PharmacoKinetics of 10-OH-carbazepine, the main metabolite of the antiepileptic oxcarbazepine, from serum and saliva concentrations. Acta Neurol Scand 68: 145–150

Lamb R J, Leach M J, Miller A A, Wheatley P L. 1985 Anticonvulsant profile in mice of lamotrigine, a novel anticonvulsant. Br J Pharmacol 85: 366P

Leach M, Harden C M, Miller A A. 1986 Pharmacological studies of lamotrigine, a novel potential antiepileptic drug: II. Neurochemical studies on the mechanism of action. Epilepsia 27: 490–497

Leppik I E, Graves N M. 1989 Potential antiepileptic drugs: felbamate. In: Levy R, Mattson R, Meldrum B, Penry J K, Dreifuss F E, eds. Antiepileptic drugs, 3rd edn. New York: Raven Press, pp 983–990

Leppik I E, Dreifuss F E, Pledger G W et al. 1991 Felbamate for partial seizures: results of a controlled clinical trial. Neurology 41: 1785–1789

Leppik I E, Willmore L G, Homan R W et al. 1993 Efficacy and safety of zonisamide: results of a multicenter study. Epilepsy Res 14: 165–173

Levy R H, Loiseau P, Guyot M et al. 1984 Michaelis–Menten kinetics of stiripentol in normal humans. Epilepsia 25: 486–491

Levy R H, Loiseau P, Guyot M et al. 1988 Effect of stiripentol dose on valproate metabolism. Epilepsia 29: 709

Livingston J H, Beaumont D, Arzimanoglou A et al. 1989 Vigabatrin in the treatment of epilepsy in children. Br J Clin Pharmacol 27: 109S–112S

Loiseau P, Schmidt P, Deisenhammer E et al. 1987 Zonisamide. 17th Epilepsy International Congress Abstracts 1987: 73.

Loiseau P, Yuen A W C, Duche B et al 1990 A randomized double blind placebo controlled cross over add-on trial of lamotrigine in patients with treatment-resistant partial seizures. Epilepsy Res 7: 136–145

McCabe R T, Wasterlain C G, Kucharaczyk N, Sofia R D, Vogel J R. 1993 Evidence for anticonvulsant and neuroprotectant action of felbamate mediated by strychnine-insensitive glycine receptors. J Pharmacol Exp Ther 264: 1248–1252

McGuire A M, Duncan J S, Trimble M R. 1992 Effects of vigabatrin on cognitive function and mood when used as add-on therapy in patients with intractable epilepsy. Epilepsy 33: 128–134

Matilainen R, Pitkanen A, Tuutiainen T et al. 1988 Effect of vigabatrin on epilepsy in mentally retarded patients: a 7-month follow-up study. Neurology 38: 743–747

Meuldermans W, Hendricks J, Hurkmans R et al 1978 A comparative study of the plasma protein binding and the distribution of flunarizine and cinnarizine in human blood. Clinical research report no. R14 950/30. Janssen Research Product Information Service

Micheletti G, Vergnes M, Lannes B et al. 1988 Effect of stiripentol on petit mal-like epilepsy in Wistar rat. Epilepsia 29: 709

Micheli F, Pardal M F, Gatto M et al. 1987 Flunarizine- and cinnarizine-induced extrapyramidal reaction. Neurology 37: 881–884

Miller A A, Sawyer D A, Roth B et al. 1986 In: Meldrum BS, Porter RJ, eds. New anticonvulsant drugs. London: John Libbey, pp 165–177

Muir K T, Palmer G C. Remacemide. In: Pisani F, Perucca E, Avanzini G, Richens A eds. New antiepileptic drugs. Amsterdam: Elsevier Science, pp 147–152

Mumford J P. 1988 A profile of vigabatrin. Br J Clin Pract 42 (suppl 61): 7–9

Mumford J P, Beaumont D, Gisselbrecht D. 1990 Cognitive function, mood and behaviour in vigabatrin treated patients. Acta Neurol Scand 82 (suppl 133): 15

Ojemann L M, Shastri R A, Wilensky A et al. 1986 Comparative pharmacokinetics of
zonisamide (CI-912) in epileptic patients on carbamazepine or phenytoin monotheraphy.
Drug Monit 293–296

Ono T, Yagi K, Seino M. 1988 Clin Psychiatry 30: 471–478 (In Japanese, quoted by Seino
M, Miyazaki H, Ito T. Zonisamide. In: Pisani F, Perucca E, Ayanzini G, Richens A, eds.
1991 New antiepileptic drugs. Elsevier Science, pp 169–174

Overweg J, Binnie C D. 1990 Flunarizine. In: Dam M, Gram L, eds. Comprehensive
epileptology. New York: Raven Press, pp 655–664

Paljarvi L, Vapalahti M, Sivenius J et al. 1990 Vigabatrin vacuoles in humans:
neuropathologic findings in 5 patients with vigabatrin treatment. Neurology 40: 157

Perhach J L, Weliky I, Newton J J et al. 1986 New anticonvulsant drugs. London: John
Libbey, pp 117–123

Physician Desk Reference. Felbatol (felbamate). 1994: 2473–2474

Pierce M W, Suzdak P D, Gustavson L E et al. 1991 Tiagabine. In: Pisani F, Perucca E,
Avanzini G, Richens A, eds. New antiepileptic drugs. Amsterdam: Elsevier Science,
pp 157–160

Richens A. 1989 Potential antiepileptic drugs. vigabatrin. In: Levy R, Mattson R, Meldrum
B, Penry J K, Dreifuss F E, eds. Antiepileptic drugs, 3rd edn. New York: Raven Press,
pp 937–946

Richens A, Yuen W. 1991 Overview of the clinical efficacy of lamotrigine. Epilepsia 31
(suppl 2): S13–S16

Rimmer E M, Richens A. 1989 Interaction between vigabatrin and phenytoin. Br J Clin
Pharmacol 27: 27S–33S

Risner M and the Lamictal study group. 1990 Multicentre double blind placebo controlled
add-on crossover study of lamotrigine (Lamactil) in epileptic outpatients with partial
seizures. Epilepsia 31: 619–620

Rogawski M A, Porter R J. 1990 Antiepileptic drugs: pharmacological mechanisms and
clinical efficacy with consideration of promising developmental stage compounds.
Pharmacol Rev 42: 223–285

Rowan J, Ahmann P, Wannamaker B et al. 1993 Safety and efficacy of three dose levels of
tiagabine HCl versus placebo as adjunctive treatment for complex partial seizures. Epilepsia
34 (suppl 2): 157

Runge U, Rabending G, Roder H et al. 1993 Losigamone: first results in patients with
drug-resistant focal epilepsy. Epilepsia 34 (suppl 2): 6

Sachdeo R, Kramer L D, Rosenberg A et al. 1992 Felbamate monotherapy: controlled trial
in patients with partial onset seizures. Ann Neurol 32: 386–392

Sackellares J C, Donofrio P D, Wagner J G et al. 1985 Pilot study of zonisamide (1, 2-
benzisoxazole-3-methanesulfonamide) in patients with refractory partial seizures. Epilepsia
26: 206–221

Sander J, Patsalos P, Oxley J et al. 1990 A randomized double blind placebo controlled
add-on trial of lamotrigine in patients with severe epilepsy. Epilepsy Res 6: 221–226

Sander J, Hart Y M, Trimble M R, Shorvon S D. 1991 Vigabatrin and psychosis. J Neurol
Neurosurg Psychiatry 54: 435–439

Schechter P J. 1989 Clinical pharmacology of vigabatrin. Br J Clin Pharmacol 27: 19S–22S

Schmidt D. 1989 Potential antiepileptic drugs: gabapentin. In: Levy R, Mattson R, Meldrum
B, Penry J K, Dreifuss F E, eds. Antiepileptic drugs, 3rd edn. New York: Raven Press,
pp 925–935

Seino M, Miyazaki H, Ito T. 1991 Zonisamide. In: Pisani F, Perucca E, Avanzini, G, Richens
A, eds. New antiepileptic drugs, Elsevier Science, pp 169–174

Sivenius J, Ylinen A, Murros K et al. 1991 Vigabatrin in drug-resistant epilepsy: a 5-year
follow-up study. Neurology 41: 562–565

Sivenius J, Paljarvi L, Vapalahti M, Nousiainen U, Riekkinen P J. 1993 Vigabatrin
(gamma-vinyl-GABA): neuropathologic evaluation in five patients. Epilepsia 34: 193–196

Starreveld E, de Beukelaar F, Wilson AF et al. 1989 Double-blind cross-over placebo
controlled study of flunarizine in patients with therapy resistant epilepsy. Can J Neurol Sci
16: 187–190

Stein U, Klessing K, Chatterjee S S. 1991 Losigamone. In: Pisani F, Perucca E, Avanzini G,
Richens A, eds. New antiepileptic drugs. Elsevier Science, pp 129–133

Steinhoff B J, Stoll K D, Stodieck S R, Paulus W. 1992 Hyponatremic coma under oxcarbazepine therapy. Epilepsy Res 11: 67–70

Stewart B H, Kugler A R, Thompson P R, Bockbrader H N. 1993 A saturable transport mechanism in the intestinal absorption of gabapentin is the underlying cause of the lack of proportionality between increasing dose and drug levels in plasma. Pharmacol Res 10: 276–281

Suman-Chauhan N, Webdale L, Hill D R, Woodruff G N. 1993 Characterisation of [^{3}H]gabapentin to a novel site in rat brain: homogenate binding studies. Eur J Pharmacol 244: 293–301

Swinyard E A, Sofia R D, Kupferberg H J. 1986 Comparative anticonvulsant activity and neurotoxicity of felbamate and four prototype antiepileptic drugs in mice and rats. Epilepsia 27: 27–34

Taylor C P, McLean J R, Bockbrader R A et al. 1986 In: Meldrum B S, Porter R J, eds. Zonisamide (AD-810, CI-912). New antiepileptic drugs. London: John Libbey, pp 277–294

Taylor C P, Vartanian M G, Yuen P W, Bigge C, Suman-Chauhan N, Hill DR. 1993 Potent and stereospecific anticonvulsant activity of 3-isobutyl GABA relates to in vitro binding at a novel site labeled by tritiated gabapentin. Epilepsy Res 14: 11–15

Theisohn M, Heinmann G. 1982 Disposition of the antiepileptic oxcarbazepine and its metabolites in healthy volunteers. Eur J Clin Pharmacol 22: 545–551

Timmings P L, Richens A. 1992 Lamotrigine as an add-on drug in the management of Lennox–Gastaut syndrome. Eur Neurol 32: 305–307

Timmings P L, Richens A. 1992 Lamotringe in primary generalised epilepsy. Lancet 339: 1300–1301

US Gabapentin Study Group No. 5. 1993 Gabapentin as add-on therapy in refractory partial epilepsy: a double-blind, placebo-controlled, parallel-group study. Neurology 43: 2292–2298

Vincent J C. 1991 Stiripentol. In: Pisani F, Perucca E, Avanzini G, Richens A, eds. New antiepileptic drugs. Holland: Elsevier Science, pp 153–156

Vles J S, van der Heyden A M, Ghijs A, Troost J. 1993 Vigabatrin in the treatment of infantile spasms. Neuropediatrics 24: 230–231

Theodore W H, Raubertas R F, Porter R J et al. 1991 Felbamate: a clinical trial for complex partial seizures. Epilepsia 32: 392–397

Warner T, Patsalos P N, Prevett M, Elyas A A, Duncan J S. 1992 Lamotrigine-induced carbamazepine toxicity: an interaction with carbamazepine 10,11-epoxide. Epilepsy Res 11: 147–150

Wilensky A J, Ojemann L M, Chmelir T et al 1989 Topiramate pharmacokinetics in epileptic patients receiving carbamazepine. Epilepsia 30: 645

Wolf P. 1992 Lamotrigine: preliminary clinical observations on pharmacokinetics and interactions with traditional antiepileptic drugs. J Epilepsy 5: 73–79.

8

Diagnosis, investigation and initiation of treatment in childhood epilepsies

F. Kirkham

Epilepsy is common in childhood, with a prevalence of approximately 5 per 1000 (Cowan et al 1989). The majority of patients respond to a single antiepileptic drug and have a good long-term outcome in terms of seizure control and intelligence, although school failure is a significant problem in many (Sturniolo & Galletti 1994). Seizures may remain intractable in up to 25% of paediatric patients and, with the advent of new drugs and the increased availability of surgical treatment, there has been considerable recent interest in the appropriate management of this population. In population-based studies, the number of seizures before treatment may be a predictor of long-term outcome (Camfield et al 1993), and there is therefore a good case for early diagnosis and treatment. On the other hand, it has been argued that, because epilepsy remits spontaneously in many patients, anticonvulsant treatment may be avoided altogether (Freeman et al 1987). Although idiopathic generalized and partial epilepsies form a substantial proportion of both of these groups, it has become increasingly clear that the international classification of epilepsies is inadequate to describe some of the individually rare but important epilepsy syndromes, particularly those lumped under symptomatic generalized. Their recognition, together with advances in neuroimaging and molecular genetics, has led to important advances in understanding pathophysiology and also to more rational investigation and treatment in some cases. One of the main difficulties is that the doctors to whom children and their parents present have usually seen very few, if any, seizures themselves and have little experience in electroencephalography. Medical education has almost certainly reduced the time between onset and treatment of infantile spasms, but other syndromes continue to cause considerable diagnostic uncertainty which may, in some cases, have adverse therapeutic consequences.

Although grossly oversimplified, this chapter describes a clinical approach to the diagnosis and initiation of treatment in some of the commoner epilepsies of childhood which present in outpatient clinics as well as in some of the rarer forms which are often misdiagnosed or mistreated. The emphasis is on the possibilities of, and difficulties with, early diagnosis in those epilepsies and syndromes in which appropriate treatment is effective and inappropriate treatment may be unnecessary or harmful. It should be emphasized that the syndrome approach used here has significant limitations and is under review by the International League against Epilepsy. It will probably be replaced or modified significantly in the foreseeable future.

CONVULSIONS (Table 8.1)

Febrile convulsions

Febrile convulsions are common in children between the ages of 1 and 5 years, occurring in 2–4% of that population. Risk factors include a family history in first- or second-degree relatives, neonatal problems, pre-existing developmental delay and day nursery care (Bethune et al 1993). The fever, usually above 38°C, is precipitated by viral infections in the majority. Meningitis must always be considered, although other clinical signs are usually present (Green et al 1993) and routine lumbar puncture is not necessary. A few febrile convulsions can occur in temporal association with immunization (Griffin et al 1991, Cherry et al 1993).

Recurrence occurs in up to one-third of children, most often between the ages of 12 and 24 months (Offringa et al 1994), particularly in those in whom the first convulsions were associated with rapidly increasing temperature, or occurred at a relatively lower temperature (Berg et al 1992). Age of onset at less than 18 months and family history in first-degree relatives are also risk factors. The majority of recurrent convulsions are generalized, and complex focal convulsions rarely follow simple attacks.

The risk for epilepsy in children who have had febrile convulsions is small — approximately 2–4%. The majority of those who have had short simple febrile convulsions who develop epilepsy have generalized tonic-clonic seizures alone, but febrile status epilepticus, particularly if focal, is associated with later development of hippocampal sclerosis and temporal lobe epilepsy (Kuks et al 1993). The question of whether the pathology predates or is causally associated, partly or wholly, with prolonged febrile convulsions remains controversial. If febrile convulsions do cause hippocampal sclerosis, this happens rarely (Camfield et al 1994). Occasionally children with febrile convulsions have a more complex epilepsy syndrome, e.g. severe myoclonic epilepsy of infancy, and this possibility should be considered in children presenting under the age of 1 year (Table 8.1). There is no evidence that febrile convulsions cause mental retardation or neurological sequelae, although subtle hemiparesis and facial palsy may occur after febrile status and may be useful localizing signs.

Parents and care givers should be educated about the management of fever. The great majority of febrile convulsions terminate spontaneously; diazepam administered rectally or intravenously is effective in the few remaining cases. Long-term prophylaxis for simple febrile convulsions is now not recommended because of limited efficacy, poor compliance and significant side-

Table 8.1 Convulsions

Presentation	Age	Clinical manifestations	Neurology/development	EEG	Imaging	Treatment	Long-term epilepsy	Most likely diagnosis	Comments
Convulsions with fever	1–5 years	Generalized tonic-clonic convulsions lasting a few minutes	Usually normal	Unnecessary (normal)	Unnecessary	None (possibly oral rectal diazepam during febrile illness)	2–4% mainly generalized. Partial epilepsy after prolonged convulsions	Simple febrile convulsion	Recurrence of febrile convulsions in one third
	1–5 years	Unilateral febrile convulsion	Postical Todd's paresis. Mild facial palsy later	May show focal abnormality	May show lesion	Oral/rectal diazepam for febrile illnesses	Partial epilepsy in some	Complex febrile convulsion	
	<1 year	Frequent febrile convulsions	Normal	Normal or generalized slowing	Normal	Sodium valproate	Common	Severe myoclonic epilepsy of infancy	
	1–2 years	Myoclonic and absence seizures	Ataxia and speech delay	Bursts of generalized spike-wave					
Convulsions without fever	Any	Generalized tonic-clonic seizures without fever	Normal	Normal background, generalized spikes, polyspikes, spike-waves, polyspike waves ≥3 Hz. ↑ by slow-wave sleep	Unnecessary (normal)	Sodium valproate after two convulsions	Occasional convulsions if untreated or after drug withdrawal	Primary generalized epilepsy	Check no partial or myoclonic seizures and that EEG is typical. Differential – secondary generalized especially frontal, benign rolandic, juvenile myoclonic
	1–12 years	Generalized tonic-clonic seizures without fever	Normal	Rolandic spikes	Usually normal, may show focal lesion	Carbamazepine	May remit but not necessarily	Benign rolandic or secondary generalized epilepsy	Less good prognosis than those presenting with typical rolandic seizures

effects, both cognitive and behavioural, particularly with phenobarbitone (Farwell et al 1990). There is no evidence that regular antipyretics reduce the risk of recurrence, but oral diazepam at a dose of 0.33 mg/kg 8-hourly during febrile episodes appears to do so (Rosman et al 1993). Many professionals believe that this is unnecessary in a condition with a benign prognosis, especially as significant side-effects were seen in about 40% of patients so treated. It may be more sensible to give rectal diazepam to be used to terminate a prolonged fit to the parents of children who have had complex initial febrile convulsions, particularly if they live a considerable distance from medical care; it is important that guidelines on dosage are discussed but, in fact, this practice appears to be safe and effective.

Unprovoked generalized convulsions

Only one-third of children presenting with their first unprovoked generalized convulsion will have another within the next 3 years (Shinnar et al 1990) and the risk of recurrence is even lower if there is no underlying aetiology and the electroencephalogram (EEG) is normal. Most physicians therefore withhold anticonvulsants after the first attack. Although the seizures are terrifying for parents, the risks of dying or sustaining brain damage during an attack are very low. There is no evidence that this type of attack has a detrimental effect on intelligence, and chronic anticonvulsant therapy may have comparatively more effect on school performance. It has therefore been argued that it may not be necessary to treat at all (Freeman et al 1987), although because there must be a small cumulative morbidity and mortality, the unpredictability of epilepsy is such a social handicap, and the main effect of anticonvulsants appears to be on motor and not on higher cognitive skills (Aldenkamp et al 1993), anticonvulsant prophylaxis is usually advocated in the medium term and can often be successfully withdrawn thereafter (Shinnar et al 1994), particularly in children whose first seizure occurs above the age of 3 years (Ehrhardt & Forsythe 1989). It may be possible to avoid drug therapy in those who are photosensitive provided that they can avoid seizure-inducing stimuli, e.g. computer games flickering on television screens at 50 Hz (Kasteleijn-Nolst Trénité 1994).

An EEG before anticonvulsant treatment may be very helpful in suggesting the correct syndromic diagnosis, which in turn may have implications for treatment and prognosis. For example, an EEG showing generalized spike-wave or polyspike wave either at rest or with photic stimulation or during hyperventilation would suggest a diagnosis of primary generalized epilepsy with a good prognosis. Focal slowing or rolandic spikes may sometimes be seen but do not necessarily imply that the seizures are secondary generalized; imaging should be considered if the seizures are frequent or intractable or if there are neurological signs, but epilepsy remits in the long term in most of these children. Frontal epilepsies may demonstrate rapid secondary generalization and it is worth inquiring about focal clonic jerking or complex gestural automatisms in patients who do not respond to anticonvulsant drugs; detailed video telemetry may be needed in doubtful cases without interictal EEG involvement. Juvenile myoclonic epilepsy (JME) of Janz is a common form (5–11% of all epilepsies) which is familial and shows linkage with human leukocyte antigen (HLA)-DRw13 on chromosome 6 (Obeid et al 1994), although the mode of inheritance remains controversial (Panayiotopoulos & Obeid 1989, Greenberg et al 1990). The EEG is characteristic in untreated patients with generalized interictal discharges, spike- or multispike-wave and fragmentation of the paroxysms; these features should suggest a diagnosis of JME if there is uncertainty about the clinical diagnosis, but in adolescents presenting with generalized tonic-clonic convulsions, it is also essential to ask carefully about myoclonus on awakening. The generalized tonic-clonic convulsions respond to sodium valproate in at least 80% of patients; clonazepam may be useful in controlling troublesome myoclonus. Carbamazepine, although without benefit as monotherapy, may occasionally be helpful in controlling generalized tonic-clonic convulsions in combination with sodium valproate (Knott & Panayiotopoulos 1994). As well as suggesting appropriate therapy, a correct diagnosis will avoid the mistake of withdrawing the patient's therapy, since the majority of patients relapse.

ABSENCE EPILEPSIES (Table 8.2)

At least four absence epilepsy syndromes are recognized (Porter 1993; Table 8.2). The diagnosis of childhood absence epilepsy is not difficult in an otherwise normal child presenting at the age of 6 with brief spells of staring, often associated with de novo or perseverative automatisms. Eye opening is characteristic and the diagnosis is usually confirmed by demonstrating 3/s spike-and-wave on EEG. Juvenile absence epilepsy is similar but presents around puberty. It is essential to ask eye witnesses about myoclonus of the arms during the absence, which would lead to a diagnosis of epilepsy with myoclonic absence, which is indistinguishable on EEG but has a poorer prognosis in terms of seizure control and intellect (Manonmani & Wallace 1994). Children with this epilepsy syndrome are commonly ataxic, particularly if seizure control is poor. Many have generalized tonic-clonic and atonic seizures in addition to frequent absences. In JME, absences may start in childhood (typically between 5 and 12 years) and may precede myoclonic and generalized tonic-clonic attacks by several years (Panayiotopoulos et al 1989). The diagnosis may be made in childhood as the seizures are typically shorter than those of childhood absence epilepsy and the EEG paroxysms consist of spike- and multispike-wave with fragmentation. Absence with eyelid myoclonia may represent a separate syndrome (Appleton et al 1993) as the EEG shows 3–5 Hz spike- and multispike-wave which disappears in darkness; sodium valproate appears to be the drug of choice.

Atypical absences are described in a number of other epileptic syndromes, including severe myoclonic epilepsy of infancy and Lennox–Gastaut syn-

Table 8.2 Absences

Presentation	Age	Clinical manifestations	Neurology/development	EEG	Imaging	Treatment	Long-term epilepsy	Most likely diagnosis	Comments
Absence	3–12 years	Blank stare with change of facial expression. Eye opening. De novo automatisms, e.g. rubbing face or hands. Perseverative automatisms, e.g. continuing to turn pages of book	Normal	Ictal 3/s spike-and-wave	Unnecessary (normal)	Ethosuximide, sodium valproate	Persistent absences 6% easily controlled. Generalized tonic-clinic seizures 40%	Childhood absence epilepsy	Reconsider electroclinical diagnosis if absences do not respond to ethosuximide or sodium valproate
	1–12 years	Absence with myoclonic movements of the shoulders, arms and legs during attack	Mental retardation common before onset of epilepsy	Ictal spike-and-wave 3/s. Interictal EEG normal	Normal usually	Sodium valproate, lamotrigine	Long-term epilepsy common, may evolve to Lennox–Gastaut	Epilepsy with myoclonic absences	Distinguish from typical absence by observing myoclonic jerks during attack
	2–5 years	Brief blank stare with some preservation of consciousness. Rapid eyelid myoclonia with retropulsive movements of eyeballs	Normal	High-amplitude spikes multi-spikes and slow waves 3–5 Hz on eye closure which disappear in darkness	Normal	Sodium valproate + either ethosuximide or benzodiazepine	Occasional tonic-clonic seizures	Eyelid myoclonia with absence	Photosensitive
	7–12 years	Blank stare with loss of facial expression. Automatisms	Normal	Spike-wave 3.5–4 Hz with frontal extension	Normal	Ethosuximide, sodium valproate	Generalized tonic-clonic attacks in most; respond to Rx	Juvenile absence epilepsy	Probably a continuum with childhood absence epilepsy
	3–18 years	Blank stare but often some preservation of consciousness. Automatisms	Normal	Multispike-wave with fragmentation	Normal	Sodium valproate, clonazepam	Relapses on withdrawal of sodium valproate	Juvenile myoclonic epilepsy	Absences precede myoclonic jerks in 10–25% of patients

drome. In addition, absences are commonly reported in children with learning difficulties, but it can be very difficult to distinguish epileptic absences from daydreaming. A sleep-deprived EEG may reveal spike-and-wave activity which would otherwise be missed (Borkowski et al 1992).

Treatment is not essential in childhood absence epilepsy as the long-term prognosis is good but if absences interfere with schoolwork, ethosuximide is almost always effective. The treatment of choice for the absences of JME is sodium valproate. Epilepsy with myoclonic absences is often resistant to anticonvulsant drugs and has been reported to evolve into the Lennox–Gastaut syndrome. It appears to respond to lamotrigine, usually used in combination with sodium valproate or a benzodiazepine (Manonmani & Wallace 1994).

PARTIAL EPILEPSIES (Table 8.3)

The clinical manifestations of partial epilepsies in childhood (Table 8.3) are often quite distinct from those seen in adults in a number of ways. First, there are a number of children who present with seizures which, to their parents, are extremely alarming, and which may be associated with very obvious EEG abnormalities, but which paradoxically have a benign prognosis in the long term (Loiseau et al 1988, Panayiotopoulos 1993; Holmes 1993). Secondly, it may be difficult to distinguish simple from complex partial seizures, particularly in infancy. Thirdly, unilateral clonic seizures are common in children both in the context of acute encephalopathies and as the presentation of partial epilepsy, with or without ipsilateral hemiparesis (Blume 1989). Fourthly, complex partial seizures do occur but may be rather different in infants and children. For example, in infancy the common manifestations are forced lateral deviation of the head and eyes and tonic stiffening of the arms in association with loss of consciousness (Duchowny 1987), whilst in young children temporal lobe attacks with typical motor arrest are accompanied by rather more simple automatisms, e.g. lip smacking and fiddling with the hands (Wyllie et al 1993), than those seen in adults, and it can be difficult to distinguish these clinically from absences, especially if the child cannot describe any aura.

An accurate seizure description is of the utmost importance in the management of childhood partial epilepsies, because the EEG, while usually helpful in confirming a clinical diagnosis or suggesting an alternative, it may in some circumstances be misleading. Children with rolandic seizures, with motor or sensory involvement of the oropharyngeal region, have an excellent long-term prognosis for seizure control (van der Meij et al 1992) even if there is concurrent organic brain disease. The same is not necessarily true for patients with focal motor or generalized seizures in association with centro-temporal or rolandic spikes. In up to half of children presenting with partial attacks arising from the temporal lobe, the EEG may be normal or show only non-epileptiform abnormalities such as focal slowing. Because, as has

Table 8.3 Partial seizures

Age	Clinical manifestations	Neurology/development	EEG	Imaging	Treatment	Long-term epilepsy	Most likely diagnosis	Comments
1–12 years	Focal seizure with motor and/or sensory manifestations in oropharyngeal region	Normal	Rolandic spikes	Unnecessary (normal)	None (carbamazepine)	2%	Benign rolandic epilepsy	Typical rolandic seizures
1–12 years	Unilateral jerking	Normal or abnormal	Rolandic spikes	Normal or occasionally focal lesion	Carbamazepine	Most remit in adolescence but epilepsy occurs	Benign rolandic or symptomatic partial epilepsy	Prognosis less good than for typical rolandic seizures
1–10 years	Nocturnal vomiting with eye deviation and loss of consciousness terminating with hemi- or generalized convulsions	Normal	Interictal occipital paroxysms with high-amplitude sharp and slow wave. Discharges may be elicited by visual fixation	Usually normal	None/carbamazepine	?	Benign childhood epilepsy with occipital paroxysms (early onset)	Recently delineated; natural history not yet determined
1–7 years	Daytime visual illusions and/or blindness followed by postical headache lasting seconds or minutes. Multicoloured circles and spots. Consciousness preserved	Usually normal. Perinatal problems or developmental delay suggest less good prognosis	Interictal occipital paroxysms of high-amplitude sharp and slow wave	Usually normal but sometimes lesion in otherwise typical electroclinical syndrome	Carbamazepine	5% if symptomatic partial epilepsy excluded	Benign childhood epilepsy with occipital paroxysms (late onset)	May be difficult to distinguish from symptomatic partial epilepsy arising from the occipital lobe

Table 8.3 Partial seizures (cont'd)

Age	Clinical manifestations	Neurology/development	EEG	Imaging	Treatment	Long-term epilepsy	Most likely diagnosis	Comments
2–9 years	Brief episodes of terror and screaming with pallor, sweating, abdominal pain, salivation, chewing, sometimes speech arrest, and loss of consciousness	Normal	High-amplitude sharp and slow-wave complexes located around the frontotemporal and parietotemporal electrodes	Normal	None/carbamazepine	?	Benign childhood epilepsy with affective symptoms	
2–9 years	Daytime versive seizures of the head and body, often without impairment of consciousness	Normal	Sharp and slow-wave complexes elicited by somatosensory stimulation giving single sharp and slow-wave complexes in the parietal paracentral electrodes	Normal	None/carbamazepine	?	Benign childhood epilepsy with somatosensory evoked spikes	
Any	Motor arrest followed by oroalimentary automatisms and postictal confusion with amnesia. Gradual recovery. Aura of autonomic or psychic symptoms, e.g. rising epigastric sensation	Normal or slight facial asymmetry	Temporal spikes, may be normal	Hippocampal sclerosis, tumour, focal cortical dysplasia of the temporal lobe	Carbamazepine, sodium valproate, vigabatrin, gabapentin, lamotrigine, phenytoin, temporal lobectomy	Spontaneous remission very rare. About 10% have a prolonged remission with anticonvulsants	Partial seizures arising from the temporal lobe	Surgery should be considered in childhood if intractable to all available anticonvulsants

Table 8.3 Partial seizures (*cont'd*)

Age	Clinical manifestations	Neurology/development	EEG	Imaging	Treatment	Long-term epilepsy	Most likely diagnosis	Comments
Any	Short seizures with prominent motor manifestation, e.g. tonic or postural and complex gestural automatisms. Nocturnal episodes of restlessness and confusion with repetitive abduction/adduction of the legs	Usually normal	Interictal often normal but may demonstrate frontal spikes or spike-wave. Ictal EEG shows frontal spike-wave but often obscured by movement artefact. Secondary bilateral synchrony with diffuse slow spike-wave may occur	May show tumour, abscess, injury or cortical dysplasia of frontal lobe. Commonly normal	Sodium valproate, carbamazepine, each as monotherapy. Vigabatrin, gabapentin, lamotrigine, phenytoin. Consider surgery for intractable cases	Remission may occur in familial syndrome. Overall remission unclear as previously under-diagnosed	Partial seizures arising from the frontal lobe	Rapid secondary generalization may occur. Otherwise may be very difficult to distinguish from psychogenic attacks. Poor outcome for surgery unless lesion removed
Any	Abnormal sensory symptomatology, often with loss of muscle tone	May be normal	May demonstrate parietal spikes	May demonstrate focal cortical dysplasia or other lesion	Sodium valproate. Carbamazepine, vigabatrin, gabapentin, lamotrigine. Consider surgery if intractable	Unknown	Partial seizures arising from the parietal lobe	Onset may be in childhood but poorly described
Any	Negative or positive visual manifestations with distortion and delusion	Often normal	May demonstrate occipital spikes	May demonstrate focal cortical dysplasia, calcification or other lesion	Sodium valproate, carbamazepine, vigabatrin, gabapentin, lamotrigine. Consider surgery if intractable	Unknown	Partial seizures arising from the occipital lobe	Onset may be in childhood. May be difficult to distinguish from benign occipital epilepsy electroclinically. Some have coeliac disease

Table 8.3 Partial seizures (*cont'd*)

Age	Clinical manifestations	Neurology/development	EEG	Imaging	Treatment	Long-term epilepsy	Most likely diagnosis	Comments
Any	Unilateral jerking with or without loss of consciousness at the beginning or after the jerking	Often abnormal	Focal spikes or slowing	Often abnormal, e.g. focal lesions, hemimegalencephaly	Sodium valproate, carbamazepine, vigabatrin, gabapentin, lamotrigine. Consider surgery to remove lesion	May remit with medical therapy. Outcome after surgery may be excellent if lesion removed	Unilateral clonic seizures	Common, particularly in infants
Any	Continuous jerking ± loss of consciousness continuing throughout sleep	Progressive hemiparesis	Abnormal background. Interictal and ictal discharges	(I) Lesion or (II) normal initially, then progressive atrophy of the hemisphere	Anticonvulsants (± high-dose steroids for II). Lesionectomy for I. Hemispherectomy usually required for II	Intractable epilepsy common in I and usual in II without surgery	Epilepsy partialis continua. If II, Consider Rasmussen's syndrome	Rasmussen's encephalitis is a pathological diagnosis but may be suggested by onset of severe intractable partial epilepsy in normal child
0–10 years	Laughing seizures. Multiple seizure types may develop later	May be normal or developmental delay. Precocious puberty	Interictal – generalized spike-slow wave. Ictal – generalized low-voltage rhythmic fast	Hypothalamic hamartoma	Drug therapy. Surgery difficult but may be curative	Usually intractable to medical therapy	Gelastic epilepsy	Differential diagnosis – temporal lobe epilepsy

been described above, clinical attacks may be atypical and inconspicuous, it is a common mistake to assume that the child does not therefore have epilepsy. In order to avoid late diagnosis which may be detrimental (Camfield et al 1993), it may be worth either admitting the child for observation or asking the parents to videotape characteristic attacks. In the extratemporal epilepsies, the diagnosis may be even more difficult because the interictal EEG may be completely normal. There has been an increasing recognition over the past few years that frontal lobe epilepsies may take very bizarre forms, and have, in the past, frequently been misdiagnosed as night terrors or behaviour disorders. Even with EEG telemetry, spikes and spike-wave paroxysms during ictal EEG of the brief, bizarre episodes of thrashing, pedalling, cycling and abduction/adduction may be obscured by, or confused with, muscle artefact (Stores et al 1991). A familial form with probable autosomal dominant inheritance has recently been described and has probably been underdiagnosed previously (Scheffer et al 1994). Patients with JME may have focal myoclonic attacks which may be misdiagnosed as simple partial seizures; some also have focal abnormalities on the EEG (Panayiotopoulos et al 1991). A careful history together with detailed review of the initial EEG with this diagnosis in mind may avoid inappropriate treatment with carbamazepine. Ictal laughter may suggest a hypothalamic hamartoma (Berkovic et al 1988).

In children presenting between the ages of 2 weeks and 15 months, benign partial syndromes are very rare if they are seen at all. Complex partial seizures may occur, although they can be very difficult to recognize. Secondary generalization is common and may lead to the recognition of a symptomatic partial epilepsy. Infants presenting with unilateral clonic seizures almost always have a lesion demonstrable on neuroimaging, e.g. porencephaly or hemimegalencephaly. Intractable epilepsy due to Sturge–Weber syndrome commonly presents with unilateral clonic seizures in the first year of life (Arzimanoglou & Aicardi 1992). Although these seizures may be scarcely noticeable initially, they are often associated with progressive hemiparesis and intellectual decline in the long term and should be managed aggressively, either medically or, frequently, surgically.

Older children presenting with partial epilepsies usually have relatively infrequent seizures even if they remain uncontrolled. Previously normal children presenting with very frequent partial seizures and associated cognitive decline may have Rasmussen's syndrome (see chapter 10). The classical presentation is with intractable unilateral clonic seizures, often so frequent as to constitute epilepsia partialis continua, in association with a progressive hemiparesis. Ipsilateral uveitis may give an early clue. An infectious aetiology is likely, perhaps a herpes virus such as cytomegalovirus, but this remains controversial. Treatment with anticonvulsants is very disappointing and, although antiviral agents or immunotherapy with high-dose intravenous and oral steroids and immunoglobulins (Hart et al 1994) may improve the situation, most patients eventually require hemispherectomy. Contralateral disease has been described, mainly in adults.

Recent improvements in imaging have revolutionized the diagnosis of the underlying pathology in the symptomatic partial epilepsies of children. Magnetic resonance imaging (MRI) is very sensitive to the pathologies found in intractable epilepsy in childhood (Kuzniecky et al 1993, Cross et al 1994) and is now the modality of choice if available; the diagnostic rate is very much higher than with computed tomographic (CT) scan (Minford & Forsythe 1992), which may miss tumours as well as more subtle lesions. CT scan may occasionally demonstrate lesions which are difficult to see on MRI, for example, occipital calcification associated with epilepsy and coeliac disease (Magaudda et al 1993). Because MRI is expensive and heavy sedation is required in order to demonstrate subtle lesions adequately in young children, it is important that the indications are carefully considered. In benign partial epilepsies CT and MRI scan are characteristically normal and may be avoided if the electroclinical syndrome is typical (e.g. benign rolandic epilepsy with centrotemporal spikes) (van der Meij et al 1992). If there is doubt, neuroimaging may be justified as a method of attempting syndrome diagnosis. For example, centrotemporal spikes may be associated with imaging abnormalities if the seizures are not typical — if they do not involve the oropharynx (van der Meij et al 1992) — and, although the seizures commonly remit, the prognosis is probably less favourable in this group. For children presenting with electroclinical evidence of occipital epilepsy, it may be very difficult to separate the idiopathic benign syndrome from symptomatic forms on electroclinical grounds at onset; CT and/or MRI scan may be helpful if seizures remain difficult to control (Cooper & Lee 1991). It is possible that the syndrome presenting in young children with nocturnal attacks is more obviously benign soon after presentation (Panayiotopoulos 1989), but because it is has almost certainly been underdiagnosed in the past, the natural history cannot yet be predicted with confidence.

Pathological examination of surgical specimens from patients with typical temporal lobe epilepsy reveals mesial temporal sclerosis, indolent glioma or neuronal migration defects of the lateral temporal cortex. Neocortical lesions are sometimes seen in association with mesial temporal sclerosis (dual pathology; Jay et al 1993). Mesial temporal sclerosis can be diagnosed on MRI oriented in the coronal plane at right angles to the body of the hippocampus, particularly if the lesions are unilateral and the asymmetry is obvious, in addition to the signal change within the body of the hippocampus (Jackson et al 1990; Fig. 8.1). T2 images are useful in confirming unilateral or in diagnosing bilateral hippocampal sclerosis (Jackson et al 1993). There are problems with analysing the volume of the hippocampus (Cook et al 1992) as there is a wide range of normal. Indolent gliomas may be seen on CT scan, although the images may be misinterpreted (Lee et al 1989); MRI is more sensitive and specific. Neuronal migration defects may be missed on MRI unless the technique is optimal and those who report the scans know where the likely lesion is. Some lesions demonstrable pathologically in epilepsy patients remain beyond the resolution of the present-day technology. Nevertheless,

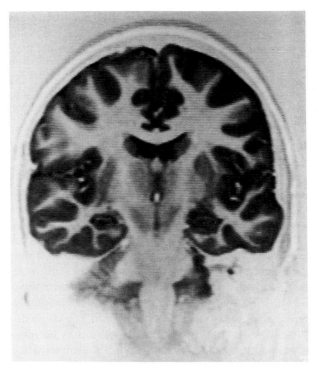

Fig 8.1 Magnetic resonance imaging (MRI) scan from a normally intelligent patient who presented at 9 months with a febrile convulsion of uncertain duration and had complex partial seizures from the age of 2¼ years. T1-weighted inversion recovery image in the coronal plane at right angles to the hippocampus shows that the right hippocampus is smaller and returns an abnormal signal, diagnostic of hippocampal sclerosis.

with high-resolution MRI scanning, it is possible to identify many focal lesions, including cortical dysplasia, polymicrogyria, schizencephaly and subcortical heterotopia. These lesions, which probably have a vascular basis, are commonly bilateral (Kuzniecky 1994). Localization of cortical defects may be suggested by the clinical presentation or on MRI by the demonstration of associated white matter abnormalities (Palmini et al 1994) or, if there is difficulty, by focal hypometabolism on positron emission tomography (PET) scanning (Lee et al 1994). In extratemporal epilepsy, PET is not abnormal if there is no lesion on MRI, except perhaps in very young children where the lack of myelin may mean that it is difficult to detect subtle cortical abnormalities. Interictal single-photon emission computed tomography (SPECT) is much less sensitive and specific than either PET or MRI when compared with electroencephalographic or pathological diagnosis of the focus, but ictal SPECT provides corroborative evidence of lateralization in the majority of children with temporal (Harvey et al 1993) and frontal (Harvey et al 1993) lobe epilepsy considered for surgery and may obviate the need for invasive EEG technique in some of these patients. Proton and phosphorous spectroscopy and functional imaging are magnetic resonance techniques with localizing potential in the future.

If a definite diagnosis of a benign syndrome is made at the time of presentation, treatment may be avoided unless seizures are embarrassing or otherwise troublesome. In practice, this may be difficult except in the case of classical rolandic seizures because the electroclinical picture in the other benign syndromes can show considerable overlap with symptomatic partial epilepsies (Table 8.3). Although a benign syndrome can be tentatively diagnosed if the EEG is classical and neuroimaging is normal, this can only be confirmed when the natural history has become clear, often many years later. For partial seizures requiring treatment, carbamazepine or sodium valproate monotherapy should be tried initially. As first-line treatment, sodium valproate may be preferred, because the available evidence from monotherapy trials in recently presenting and previously untreated patients suggests that it is of equal efficacy in controlling simple and complex partial and secondary generalized seizures and has fewer cognitive side-effects. In addition, because it has a wider spectrum of efficacy, epilepsy may be controlled even if an incorrect syndrome diagnosis has been made (Chadwick 1994). Carbamazepine is also a very useful drug and often reduces the frequency of symptomatic partial seizures. Severe hypersensitivity is well-recognized, and, although rare, it may be life-threatening and require treatment with steroids (Horneff et al 1992). Vigabatrin (Gram et al 1992) and gabapentin have shown efficacy in a number of patients when used as add-on therapy, and lamotrigine also has a role in intractable partial epilepsies in childhood, particularly if secondary generalization is a problem (Schlumberger et al 1994). Phenytoin and phenobarbitone may occasionally be useful in intractable cases, although the long-term side-effects preclude their widespread use nowadays.

If benign syndromes are excluded, partial epilepsies arising in childhood are symptomatic or cryptogenic, do not remit spontaneously and are commonly refractory to anticonvulsant medication (Harbord & Manson 1987; Kotagal et al 1987), particularly if associated with mental retardation (Huttenlocher & Hapke 1990). If seizures remain intractable despite adequate trials of all the available anticonvulsants either as monotherapy or with two drugs with adequate blood levels, surgery should be considered because, even if late remission is possible (Huttenlocher & Hapke 1990), psychosocial adjustment is often better if epilepsy does not continue into adolescence and adulthood. The demonstration of structural and functional abnormalities on imaging may obviate the need for invasive EEG monitoring in the majority of patients who are surgical candidates. In terms of seizure control, the results are very good for either classical or functional hemispherectomy in children with unilateral lesions and contralateral hemiplegia (Villemure & Rasmussen 1993; Davies et al 1993). There is some evidence for improved cognition

(Tinuper et al 1988), especially in terms of language and non-verbal communication (Caplan et al 1992). The operation should be considered early for intractable epilepsy associated with hemimegalencephaly and Sturge–Weber syndrome (Arzimanoglou & Aicardi 1992) and perhaps for Rasmussen's disease (Vining et al 1993). When carefully selected by neuroimaging and electrophysiological criteria, the majority of children undergoing temporal lobectomy become seizure-free or have only auras (Duchowny et al 1992; Fish et al 1993). The results are particularly good for those patients who originally presented with febrile convulsions (Abou-Khalil et al 1993). The prognosis for children with a resectable extratemporal lesion is reasonable (Morrell et al 1989, Adler et al 1991), but otherwise the results of surgery for frontal (Fish et al 1993), parietal and occipital lobe seizures are relatively disappointing. Nevertheless, resective surgery should be considered early even in young children if seizures are very frequent and there is evidence of intellectual arrest or deterioration (Duchowny et al 1990). If a lesion can be identified and removed, seizure control may be achieved even if the EEG abnormality is generalized (Chevrie et al 1988, Burnstine et al 1991). Multiple subpial transections may be considered for severe intractable partial epilepsies arising from eloquent areas (Morrell et al 1989).

EPILEPSIES ASSOCIATED WITH GENERALIZED EEG ABNORMALITIES AND COGNITIVE DISORDERS

Infantile spasms

Infantile spasms occur in 1 child in every 3000–4000 (Cowan & Hudson 1991), and are cryptogenic, i.e. with no obvious aetiology or previous risk factors and with normal prior development in between 20 and 50%; a substantial proportion of these cases may fulfil criteria for an idiopathic aetiology on a presumed genetic basis. CT scanning is abnormal in 60–70% of children with infantile spasms and is equally likely to be abnormal in clinically cryptogenic or symptomatic cases. Focal lesions, including cerebrovascular lesions and occasionally brain tumours, may be demonstrated as well as more diffuse congenital malformations. Diffuse atrophy is a common finding even before the initiation of adrenocorticotrophic hormone (ACTH) therapy (Howitz et al 1990). MRI may demonstrate focal or diffuse abnormalities, including neuronal migration defects, supratentorially or in the posterior fossa, although any advantage over CT scan in terms of sensitivity has not yet been formally assessed. Findings may be non-specific, e.g. periventricular hyperintensity or poor myelination. Perinatal lesions are not uncommon in infantile spasms and include porencephaly, periventricular leukomalacia and generalized atrophy. As well as destructive lesions, specimens from patients with infantile spasms may show cortical dysplasia. Gemistocytic ballooning, similar to that seen in tuberous sclerosis (Vintners et al 1994), is a common abnormality. These lesions may not be visible on

MRI, particularly in infancy when the lack of myelin means that there is less contrast between grey and white matter. It has been argued that focal hypometabolism on PET represents localized areas of cortical dysplasia (Chugani et al 1993), which may be a surgical target in intractable cases, but since PET may be transiently abnormal in the majority of patients with infantile spasms (Maeda et al 1994), great care must be taken over interpretation. As MRI resolution improves, more neuronal migration defects, focal and diffuse, may be diagnosed in vivo.

Clinically the spasms are usually symmetrical, even when there is a focal cortical lesion. Videotelemetry has revealed that some children have very subtle variants missed by the parents which usually either coexist with typical spasms or follow their apparent cessation with treatment (Donat & Wright 1991). Partial seizures occur before or simultaneously with the infantile spasms in 51% of symptomatic and 33% of cryptogenic cases. They are often associated with asymmetrical interictal EEG patterns. Focal slow activity in the EEG is commonly associated with a prenatal aetiology. The partial seizures may continue after the run of infantile spasms in some patients. In three-quarters of these patients focal cerebral lesions may be demonstrated.

ACTH has been the mainstay of treatment for infantile spasms for many years, although there has been controversy over the optimal dose and preparation. Natural ACTH is not available in many countries now and has been replaced by synthetic ACTH or tetracosactrin; 100 IU of ACTH is equivalent to 1 mg synthetic ACTH. There is some suggestion that neurological outcome may be better with an ACTH dose of at least 1.6 IU/kg per day. Very-high-dose ACTH may have an advantage in terms of seizure control, but a recent trial failed to show an advantage of 150 IU compared with 20–30 IU/m^2 per day (Hrachovy et al 1994). There is also an increased incidence of side-effects with higher doses of ACTH, including reversible hypertrophic obstructive cardiomyopathy and bacteraemia; the latter is often fatal. Non-depot ACTH appears to be as effective in terms of seizure control and less toxic (Kusse et al 1993). High-dose sodium valproate at a dose of 200 mg/kg per day with or without vitamin B$_6$ may be helpful in the management of intractable infantile spasms, although side-effects may be a serious problem. A combination of valproate in moderate dosage (40 mg/kg reached over a week) together with hydrocortisone (15 mg/kg per day) controlled spasms in 90% of cryptogenic and 65% of symptomatic cases; adding 0.1 mg/kg per day of ACTH in the resistant cases increased the response rate to 100% and 78% respectively (Dulac & Schlumberger 1994). Symptomatic patients with periventricular leukomalacia, porencephaly or a postnatal aetiology had a higher response rate than those with term asphyxia.

In tuberous sclerosis, vigabatrin is commonly preferred as the initial treatment since there is a very high response rate in this condition. It has been suggested that vigabatrin should be the drug of choice in other symptomatic infantile spasms and perhaps in cryptogenic cases as side-effects are less common than with ACTH (Vles et al 1993). This is controversial (Schmitt et al 1994), and because patients with cryptogenic spasms or those with lesions associated with prematurity may do well when treated with steroids, the regime of choice should probably include the safest available steroid preparation until controlled studies are available. Surgery is certainly indicated for brain tumours and may be curative in intractable infantile spasms due to porencephaly (Uthman et al 1991). More controversially, surgery has been offered recently for children with cryptogenic infantile spasms with subtle focal cortical dysplasias initially demonstrated using PET (see Chapter 9). Chugani et al (1993) emphasized that surgery should only be offered if there is corroborative EEG evidence and the spasms are medically intractable. Although seizure control may be obtained, there is as yet no evidence that cognitive outcome is improved, and these might be the cryptogenic cases who would otherwise be expected to do well (Hrachovy et al 1991).

The prognosis for symptomatic infantile spasms is poor. In a recent study the mean IQ for the symptomatic group was 48.4, whilst the mean IQ for children who had presented with cryptogenic infantile spasms was 71.2 (Koo et al 1993). Developmental outcome appears to be worse for patients presenting with infections, and for those with posterior fossa abnormalities, generalized atrophy or focal porencephaly involving the frontal regions. Partial seizures preceding the infantile spasms are also poor prognostically. A normal CT scan does not predict a good outcome, although an abnormal CT scan is associated with a poor one (Howitz et al 1990). The role of early treatment in stopping spasms and improving intellectual outcome is controversial but may be important (Koo et al 1993). There is, however, a 25% spontaneous remission by 12 months from onset, and 9% of untreated patients are normal at follow-up (Hrachovy et al 1991). Prognosis is best for children with cryptogenic infantile spasms who respond to ACTH (Koo et al 1993). There may be improved long-term outcome for patients with tuberous sclerosis and symptomatic infantile spasms with the rational use of anticonvulsants such as sodium valproate or vigabatrin, with or without steroids. Multicentre controlled trials are required to answer this question.

LENNOX–GASTAUT SYNDROME AND ITS DIFFERENTIAL DIAGNOSIS

This eponym is used to describe children with tonic seizures, atypical absences and generalized tonic-clonic seizures with an associated EEG abnormality of slow (1–2.5 Hz) spike-and-wave discharges. The classical syndrome, which some authors restrict to those with tonic seizures accompanied by runs of 10 Hz activity during sleep, is rare. Lennox–Gastaut syndrome may follow infantile spasms or may arise in toddlers or, occasionally, in older children. Cryptogenic and symptomatic (e.g. secondary to tuberous sclerosis) cases are recognized. The boundaries of the syndrome have historically been unclear (Donat 1992, Dulac & N'Guyen 1993), and patients have been included who would now be considered to fulfil the criteria for an alternative syndrome, e.g. those with slow spike-and-wave without multiple seizure types who may have Landau–Kleffner syndrome or continuous spike-wave in slow sleep, and those with multiple seizure types without slow spike-and-wave who have an alternative epilepsy syndrome, such as severe myoclonic epilepsy of infancy. Some children who have previously had infantile spasms, particularly those with tuberous sclerosis, develop intractable epilepsy associated with multiple spikes on EEG, rather than Lennox–Gastaut syndrome (Dulac & N'Guyen 1993). The distinction between Lennox–Gastaut syndrome, a symptomatic generalized epilepsy, and myoclonic-astatic epilepsy, remains controversial (Aicardi & Levy Gomes 1992). These epilepsies have been previously considered to be intractable, rendering the nosological debates of theoretical interest only, but this can no longer be justified now that the underlying pathology may be revealed in many cases and a correct electroclinical or perhaps underlying diagnosis may have important management implications.

Using PET, Chugani et al (1987) showed that patients with Lennox–Gastaut syndrome could be divided into those with normal scans, those with focal or unilateral abnormalities and those with diffuse abnormalities. The presumed basis of the focal abnormalities is cortical dysplasia, which may sometimes be explicitly recognized using MRI. A number of patients with classical Lennox–Gastaut syndrome have diffuse cortical dysplasias, although similar abnormalities may also be seen on MRI in patients with milder epilepsy and intelligence within the normal range (Palmini et al 1991; Fig. 8.2). Children with a pseudobulbar palsy, presenting with minor seizures in middle childhood evolving later to drop attacks may have bilateral central macrogyria on MRI. Hyperdense T2-weighted lesions of uncertain significance may be seen in the mesencephalon of patients with Lennox–Gastaut syndrome (Velasco et al 1993).

Anticonvulsant drugs rarely render patients with Lennox–Gastaut syndrome seizure-free, and in many cases they either have no effect or are positively harmful. Vitamin B_6 should be tried (Coker 1992). Sodium valproate is the most useful of the conventional drugs and should be tried as monotherapy (Hurst 1993); in view of the recognized risks of fatal liver damage probably associated with metabolic conditions (Dreifuss et al 1989, Chabrol et al 1994), it is wise to measure cerebrospinal fluid lactate and urinary amino and organic acids before commencing treatment. A trial of vigabatrin is warranted (Appleton 1993), particularly if the underlying diagnosis is tuberous sclerosis (Curatolo 1994). Care must be taken as this drug is less effective if there is secondary generalization and it may make myoclonic epilepsies worse (Lortie et al 1993). Carbamazepine has been associated with exacerbation of seizures in some cases (Snead & Hosey 1985, Horn et al 1986) but it may be worth trying provided that it is stopped if there is no benefit. A controlled trial of felbamate produced substantial benefit in a proportion of patients. Unfortunately, this drug has been recently withdrawn

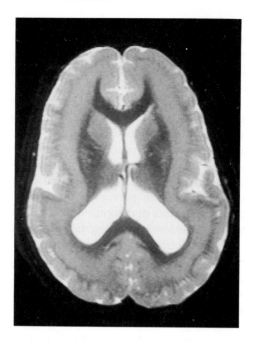

Fig. 8.2   Magnetic resonance imaging (MRI) scan from a patient who presented with infantile spasms at the age of 9 months, cured by adrenocorticotrophic hormone, and continued to have occasional complex partial seizures well-controlled by carbamazepine in association with moderate learning difficulties. T2-weighted image showing a diffuse neuronal migration disorder, often referred to as double cortex.

because of bone marrow aplasia and hepatotoxicity. Lamotrigine appears to be of benefit in Lennox–Gastaut syndrome (Schlumberger et al 1994) and the results of a controlled trial are awaited. Steroids may be useful during episodes of minor status and some patients respond to high-dose gammaglobulin (Gross-Tsur et al 1993). Corpus callosotomy may reduce the drop attacks (Reutens et al 1993) which are associated with considerable morbidity and mortality. If all available drugs have been tried and been proved ineffective this operation may be considered in childhood.

MYOCLONIC EPILEPSIES ASSOCIATED WITH COGNITIVE DECLINE

Severe myoclonic epilepsy of infancy affects between 1 in 20 000 and 1 in 40 000 children (Hurst 1990) and has almost certainly been underrecognized in the past. The onset is usually in the first year of life in a previously normal child and initially the seizures appear benign as they are commonly generalized or unilateral clonic in association with fever, although they may be very prolonged. The initial EEG is usually normal or shows only mild slowing of the background, and the developmental progression continues. However, although the child usually walks when expected, the gait is ataxic and speech delay becomes apparent during the second year. Myoclonic seizures and atypical absences then appear and eventually the EEG becomes abnormal. The clinical distinction from febrile convulsions and from progressive myoclonic and benign myoclonic epilepsies may be difficult initially, but the diagnosis may be made after two to three seizures (Yakoub et al 1992). The prognosis for severe myoclonic epilepsy of infancy is generally poor with a progressive decline in intellectual capacity and intractable seizures. Some patients may do rather better on sodium valproate with or without ethosuximide (Hurst 1987), and it is possible that apparent resistance to all anticonvulsants has been due to exacerbation by carbamazepine (Snead & Hosey 1985, Horn et al 1986).

Epilepsy with myoclonic absences often arises in a child previously recognized to be developmentally delayed; atonic attacks occur and may be troublesome (Manonmani & Wallace 1994). The nosological position of myoclonic-astatic epilepsy or Doose's syndrome remains controversial but, up to 50% of patients improve within a few years of onset while the remainder deteriorate intellectually and develop tonic seizures. A metabolic cause should be carefully excluded even if cognitive skills appear preserved. This is particularly important before initiating sodium valproate therapy, which is one of the more effective drugs in these relatively intractable syndromes (Chabrol et al 1994). Lamotrigine also appears to be useful (Manonmani & Wallace 1994), and a trial of vitamin B_6 is indicated (Coker 1992).

The main conditions causing progressive myoclonic epilepsies in young children are mitochondrial disorders and ceroid lipofuscinoses (Harbord et al 1991, Berkovic et al 1993). Baltic myoclonus and Lafora body disease tend to present in late childhood or adolescence.

LANDAU–KLEFFNER SYNDROME

The cardinal clinical feature of this syndrome is an acquired aphasia which is mainly a verbal auditory agnosia with severe receptive and variable expressive language problems. The typical history is of a child who has been previously completely normal developmentally and acquires an apparent deafness initially and then a few months later stops speaking. Seizures occur in the majority of cases but are usually nocturnal and easy to control with anticonvulsants. The diagnosis is confirmed by finding a severe EEG abnormality, particularly in sleep, but also in the waking state (Hirsch et al 1990). In patients with chronic Landau–Kleffner syndrome there is no evidence for a temporal association between the severity of the EEG abnormality, either awake or in sleep, and the severity of the aphasia.

Table 8.4 Epilepsies with multiple seizure types and/or cognitive decline

Age	Clinical manifestations	Neurology/ development	EEG	Imaging	Treatment	Long-term epilepsy	Most likely diagnosis	Comments
<1 year	Frequent febrile convulsions	None	Normal or generalized slowing	Normal	Sodium valproate	Common	Severe myoclonic epilepsy of infancy	
1–2 years	Myoclonic and absence seizures	Ataxia and speech delay	Bursts of generalized spike-wave					
2–5 years	Atypical absences, atonic seizures, tonic seizures, sometimes generalized tonic-clonic and partial seizures. May evolve from infantile spasms	Developmental delay at outset common but progressive deterioration may occur	During wakefulness, 1–2.5 Hz spike-and-wave. During sleep 10 Hz fast activity associated with tonic attacks	May show generalized or focal cortical dysplasia	Sodium valproate, benzodiazepines, lamotrigine. Vigabatrin if secondary to tuberous sclerosis. Avoid leaving on carbamazepine or vigabatrin for long periods of time without clear benefit. Try steroids and/or immunoglobulin. Corpus callosotomy indicated for severe drop attacks	Severe intractable epilepsy	Lennox–Gastaut syndrome	Differential: myoclonic epilepsies; epilepsy with multifocal spikes
1–2 years	Partial, tonic, atonic, tonic-clonic seizures. May follow infantile spasms, particularly in tuberous sclerosis	Usually abnormal	Multifocal spikes	Usually abnormal, e.g. tuberous sclerosis	Vigabatrin if tuberous sclerosis. Other anticonvulsants as monotherapy or in combination. Surgery may be possible if focal lesion	Usually intractable epilepsy	Severe multifocal epilepsy	Commoner than Lennox–Gastaut

Table 8.4 Epilepsies with multiple seizure types and/or cognitive decline (*cont'd*)

Age	Clinical manifestations	Neurology/ development	EEG	Imaging	Treatment	Long-term epilepsy	Most likely diagnosis	Comments
1–2 years	Myoclonic absences, atonic attacks, generalized tonic-clonic attacks	Ataxia and speech delay	3 Hz spike-and-wave during myoclonic absences	Normal	Sodium valproate, lamotrigine	Often intractable	Epilepsy with myoclonic absences	
2–4 years	Myoclonic-astatic seizures, generalized tonic-clonic seizures	Often normal before onset. Progressive deterioration in unfavourable cases	Generalized bursts of 2.5–3 Hz spike-and-wave	Normal	Sodium valproate, lamotrigine	50% improve within 2–3 years. Tonic seizures evolve in the rest	Myoclonic-astatic epilepsy of Doose	May be difficult to distinguish from Lennox–Gastaut syndrome. Exclude mitochondrial disorders
8–9 years	Absences, headnods, atonic drop attacks, generalized tonic-clonic, complex partial seizures	Pseudobulbar palsy. Developmental delay. Broad nose with notching	Interictal 8–10 Hz with theta either posteriorly or unilaterally. Spike or polyspike or sharp and slow wave	Bilateral central macrogyria	Anticonvulsants. Callosotomy	Intractable epilepsy	Bilateral central macrogyria with epilepsy, pseudobulbar palsy and mental retardation	

Table 8.4   Epilepsies with multiple seizure types and/or cognitive decline (cont'd)

Age	Clinical manifestations	Neurology/ development	EEG	Imaging	Treatment	Long-term epilepsy	Most likely diagnosis	Comments
0–10 years	Laughing seizures. Multiple seizure types may develop later	May be normal or developmental delay. Precocious puberty	Interictal – generalized spike-slow wave. Ictal – generalized low-voltage rhythmic fast	Hypothalamic hamartoma	Drug therapy. Surgery difficult but may be curative	Usually intractable to medical therapy	Gelastic epilepsy	Differential diagnosis – temporal lobe epilepsy
2–5 years	Loss of comprehension then later loss of expressive language. Occasional fits, often nocturnal	Normal before onset. Severe language problems	Generalized abnormality ↑ during sleep. Often 1.5–2.5 Hz slow spike-wave	Normal	Prednisolone, sodium valproate, ethosuximide	Epilepsy remits but severe language disorder in majority	Acquired epileptic aphasia (Landau–Kleffner)	Some overlap with continuous spike-wave in sleep
2–5 years	Behavioural and cognitive regression. Occasional fits often nocturnal	Normal before onset. Acquired frontal lobe disorder	Generalized 1.5–2.5 Hz spike-wave during slow sleep	Normal	Ethosuximide, prednisolone, sodium valproate	Epilepsy remits by teens but behavioural and cognitive problems in some	Continuous slow-wave in slow sleep	

Occasionally a structural lesion, such as a temporal lobe tumour or neurocystcercosis, may be found, but imaging in the majority of patients is either normal or reveals only minor changes of doubtful significance, asymmetry of ventricular size (e.g.). There was no evidence for a chronic encephalitis in 2 patients undergoing temporal lobectomy (Cole et al 1988). There appears to be a functional abnormality of the auditory cortex bilaterally, presumably related to the epileptiform discharges.

Anticonvulsant drugs have been tried in a number of patients with Landau–Kleffner syndrome, and seizures often respond well, although they also have a high spontaneous remission rate. Carbamazepine and phenytoin have both been reported to worsen the EEG and are not recommended. Sodium valproate, benzodiazepines and ethosuximide may have a transient beneficial effect on both the EEG abnormality and on the aphasia, but prolonged benefit is almost never seen (Marescaux et al 1990). A number of cases that respond to steroids have been reported; those who benefit most seem to be the patients who are diagnosed and treated early (Lerman et al 1991). Disappearance of the EEG abnormality is associated with recovery of the aphasia, but steroids may either need to be continued in the longer term or, if the patient is successfully weaned, may need to be given as subsequent courses if there is relapse. Surgery has been offered to some patients with chronic Landau–Kleffner syndrome and severe aphasia. The Morrell procedure of subpial transection may be beneficial in some but more data are needed before this procedure can be recommended. The prognosis for the epilepsy is almost always good with remission by the teens, although intractable complex partial seizures have been reported. The aphasia may recover completely, but in at least 40% of patients does not improve, even if the EEG abnormality eventually remits (Deonna et al 1989). The prognosis is worse in children who were a younger age at onset.

EPILEPSY WITH CONTINUOUS SPIKE-WAVE IN SLOW-WAVE SLEEP

Children with this condition usually present with cognitive and particularly behaviour problems. As well as autistic features, these children may have characteristics of a frontal lobe syndrome (Roulet Perez et al 1993). As in Landau–Kleffner syndrome, the epilepsy is usually mild and responds well to treatment, although consistent abolition of the EEG abnormality may be very difficult to achieve. Ethosuximide either as monotherapy or in combination with prednisolone may be effective (Roulet Perez et al 1993).

CONCLUSIONS

Short, simple febrile convulsions between the ages of 18 months and 5 years are almost always benign and do not warrant prophylactic treatment.

Unprovoked generalized convulsions recur in about two-thirds of children but further attacks are usually easily prevented with sodium valproate. An EEG before treatment may indicate whether or not the patient has primary generalized epilepsy. If the patient has been seizure-free for 2–3 years on anticonvulsants there is a good chance he or she will remain so off treatment. In adolescence, JME is an important differential diagnosis, made on clinical and electroencephalographic criteria, as treatment must be continued indefinitely.

There are at least four different absence epilepsy syndromes in childhood, which may be distinguished by careful observation of the length of the attack, the depth of loss of consciousness and accompanying phenomena such as eye opening and myoclonus. An EEG before treatment is very useful in distinguishing syndromes. Childhood and juvenile absence epilepsy responds well to ethosuximide but generalized tonic-clonic seizures occur and may require sodium valproate prophylaxis. JME should be treated with sodium valproate with or without clonazepam. Epilepsy with myoclonic absences may respond to sodium valproate but recent studies suggest that lamotrigine is also of benefit.

It is important to distinguish benign from symptomatic partial epilepsies using clinical and EEG criteria. A normal EEG does not exclude symptomatic partial epilepsy. Modern imaging techniques, particularly magnetic resonance, demonstrate a lesion in the majority of children with intractable partial seizures. Some of these lesions may be amenable to resective surgery leading to cure of the epilepsy.

Vigabatrin seems to be effective in infantile spasms secondary to tuberous sclerosis. In cryptogenic infantile spasms ACTH is still preferred until the results of controlled trials are available. In other symptomatic infantile spasms a regime of sodium valproate plus steroids is sometimes effective.

There is considerable overlap between some of the syndromes with multiple seizure types. It is possible to diagnose severe myoclonic epilepsy of infancy soon after onset in children presenting with frequent febrile convulsions under 1 year of age; MRI is usually normal. In some cases of Lennox–Gastaut syndrome MRI may show generalized or focal areas of cortical dysplasia. Metabolic conditions should be excluded as far as possible before commencing treatment with sodium valproate. Addition of benzodiazepines may be helpful. Lamotrigine may abolish seizures in some of the myoclonic epilepsies, e.g. epilepsy with myoclonic absences, and may reduce seizure frequency in some patients with Lennox–Gastaut syndrome. Vigabatrin should be tried in patients with tuberous sclerosis but may make myoclonic epilepsies worse, as may carbamazepine.

Epilepsy should be considered early in young children with language or behavioural regression. A sleep EEG may show diffuse slow spike-and-wave in Landau–Kleffner syndrome or in a related syndrome, continuous spike-wave in slow-wave sleep. Although the epilepsy in these syndromes usually remits, attempted treatment with sodium valproate, ethosuximide or steroids is warranted since behaviour and cognition may improve.

REFERENCES

Abou-Khali B, Andermann E, Andermann F, Olivier A, Quesney LP 1993 Temporal lobe epilepsy after prolonged febrile convulsions: excellent outcome after surgical treatment. Epilepsia 34: 878–883

Adler J, Erba G, Winston K R, Welch K, Lombroso C T 1991 Results of surgery for extratemporal partial epilepsy that began in childhood. Arch Neurol 48: 133–140

Aicardi J, Levy Gomes A 1992 Clinical and electroencephalographic symptomatology of the 'genuine' Lennox–Gastaut syndrome and its differentiation from other forms of epilepsy of early childhood. Epilepsy Res (suppl 6): 185–193

Aldenkamp A P, Alpherts W C, Blennow G et al 1993 Withdrawal of antiepileptic medication in children — effects on cognitive function: the Multicenter Holmfrid study. Neurology 43: 41–50

Appleton R E 1993 The role of vigabatrin in the management of infantile epileptic syndromes. Neurology 43 (suppl 5): S21–S23

Appleton R E, Panayiotopoulos C P, Acomb B A, Beirne M 1993 Eyelid myoclonia with typical absences: an epilepsy syndrome. J Neurol Neurosurg Psychiatry 56: 1312–1316

Arzimanoglou A, Aicardi J 1992 The epilepsy of Sturge–Weber syndrome: clinical features and treatment in 23 patients. Acta Neurol Scand (suppl 14): 18–22

Berg A T, Shinnar S, Hauser W A et al 1992 A prospective study of recurrent febrile seizures. N Engl J Med 327: 1122–1127

Berkovic S F, Andermann F, Melanson D et al 1988 Hypothalamic hamartomas and ictal laughter: evolution of a characteristic epileptic syndrome and diagnostic value of magnetic resonance imaging. Am Neurol 23: 429–439

Berkovic S F, Cochius J, Andermann E, Andermann F 1993 Progressive myoclonus epilepsies: clinical and genetic aspects. Epilepsia 34 (suppl 3): S19–S30

Bethune P, Gordon K, Dooley J, Camfield C, Camfield P 1993 Which child will have a febrile seizure? Am J Dis Child 147: 35–39

Blume W T 1989 Clinical profile of partial seizures beginning at less than four years of age. Epilepsia 30: 813–819

Borkowski W J Jr, Ellington R J, Sverdrup E K 1992 Effect of sleep deprivation on the EEG of learning-impaired children with absence seizures. Clin Electroencephalogr 23: 62–64

Burnstine T H, Vining E P, Uematsu S, Lesser R P 1991 Multifocal independent epileptiform discharges in children: ictal correlates and surgical therapy: Neurology 41: 1223–1228

Camfield C, Camfield P, Gordon K, Smith B, Dooley J 1993 Outcome of childhood epilepsy: a population-based study with a simple predictive scoring system for those treated with medication. J Pediatr 122: 861–868

Camfield P R, Camfield C S, Gordon K, Dooley J M 1994 What types of epilepsy are preceded by febrile seizures? A population based study of children. Dev Med Child Neurol 36: 887–892

Caplan R, Guthrie D, Shields W D et al 1992 Early onset intractable seizures: nonverbal communication after hemispherectomy. J Dev Behav Pediatr 13: 348–355

Chabrol B, Mancini J, Chretien D et al 1994 Valproate induced hepatic failure in a case of cytochrome c oxidase deficiency. Eur J Pediatr 153: 133–135

Chadwick D 1994 Valproate in the treatment of partial epilepsies. Epilepsia 35 (suppl 5): S96–S98

Cherry J D, Holtzman A E, Shields W D et al 1993 Pertussis immunization and characteristics related to first seizures in infants and children. J Pediatr 122: 900–903

Chevrie J J, Specola N, Aicardi J 1988 Secondary bilateral synchrony in unilateral pial angiomatosis: successful surgical treatment. J Neurol Neurosurg Psychiatry 51: 663–670

Chugani H T, Mazziotta J C, Engel J Jr, Phelps M E 1987 The Lennox–Gastaut syndrome: metabolic subtypes determined by 2-deoxy-2[^{18}F]fluoro-D-glucose positron emission tomography. Ann Neurol 21: 4–13

Chugani H T, Shewmon D A, Shields W D et al 1993 Surgery for intractable infantile spasms: neuroimaging perspectives. Epilepsia 34: 764–771

Coker S B 1992 Postneonatal vitamin B$_6$-dependent epilepsy. Paediatrics 90: 221–223

Cole A J, Andermann F, Taylor L et al 1988 The Landau–Kleffner syndrome of acquired epileptic aphasia: unusual clinical outcome, surgical experience, and absence of encephalitis. Neurology 38: 31–38

Cook M J, Fish D R, Shorvon S D, Straughan K, Stevens J M 1992 Hippocampal volumetric and morphometric studies in frontal and temporal lobe epilepsy. Brain 115: 1001–1015

Cowan L D, Hudson L S 1991 The epidemiology and natural history of infantile spasms. J Child Neurol 6: 355–364

Cowan L D, Bodensteiner J B, Leviton A, Doherty L 1989 Prevalence of the epilepsies in children and adolescents. Epilepsia 30: 94–106

Cross J H, Jackson G D, Neville B G et al 1994 Early detection of abnormalities in partial epilepsy using magnetic resonance. Arch Dis Child 69: 104–109

Curatolo P 1994 Vigabatrin for refractory partial seizures in children with tuberous sclerosis. Neuropaediatrics 25: 55

Davies K G, Maxwell R E, French L A 1993 Hemispherectomy for intractable seizures: long-term results in 17 patients followed for up to 38 years. J Neurosurg 78: 733–740

Deonna T, Peter C, Ziegler A L 1989 Adult follow-up of the acquired aphasia–epilepsy syndrome in childhood. Report of 7 cases. Neuropediatrics 20: 132–138

Donat J F 1992 The age-dependent epileptic encephalopathies. J Child Neurol 7: 7–21

Donat J F, Wright F S 1991 Unusual variants of infantile spasms. J Child Neurol 6: 313–318

Dreifuss F E, Langer D H, Moline K A, Maxwell J E 1989 Valproic acid hepatic fatalities. II. US experiences since 1984. Neurology 39: 201–207

Duchowny M S 1987 Complex partial seizures of infancy. Arch Neurol 44: 911–914

Duchowny M S, Resnick T J, Alvarez L A, Morrison G 1990 Focal resection for malignant partial seizures in infancy. Neurology 40: 980–984

Duchowny M, Levin B, Jayakar P et al 1992 Temporal lobectomy in early childhood. Epilepsia 33: 298–303

Dulac O, N'Guyen T 1993 The Lennox–Gastaut syndrome. Epilepsia 34 (suppl 7): S7–S17

Dulac O, Schlumberger E 1994 A simple, effective and well-tolerated treatment regime for West syndrome. Dev Med Child Neurol 36: 863–872

Ehrhardt P, Forsythe W I 1989 Prognosis after grand mal seizures: a study of 187 children with three-year remissions. Dev Med Child Neurol 31: 633–639

Farwell J R, Lee Y J, Hirtz D G, Sulzbacher S I, Ellenberg J H, Nelson K B 1990 Phenobarbital for febrile seizures — effects on intelligence and on seizure recurrence. N Engl J Med 322: 364–369

Fish D R, Smith S J, Quesney L F, Andermann F, Rasmussen T 1993 Surgical treatment of children with medically intractable or temporal lobe epilepsy: results and highlights of 40 years' experience. Epilepsia 34: 244–247

Freeman J M, Tibbles J, Camfield C, Camfield P 1987 Benign epilepsy of childhood: a speculation and its ramifications. Pediatrics 79: 864–868

Gilman J T, Duchowny M, Jayakar P, Resnick T J 1994 Medical intractability in children evaluated for epilepsy surgery. Neurology 44: 1341–1343

Gram L, Sabers A, Dulac O 1992 Treatment of pediatric epilepsies with gamma-vinyl GABA (vigabatrin). Epilepsia 33 (suppl 5): S26–S29

Green S M, Rothrock S G, Clem K J, Zurcher R F, Mellick L 1993 Can seizures be the sole manifestation of meningitis in febrile children? Pediatrics 92: 527–534

Greenberg D A, Durner M, Delgado-Escueta A V, Janz D 1990 Is juvenile myoclonic epilepsy an autosomal recessive disease? Ann Neurol 28: 110–111

Griffin M R, Ray W A, Mortimer E A, Fenichel G M, Schaffner W 1991 Risk of seizures after measles–mumps–rubella immunization. Pediatrics 88: 881–885

Gross-Tsur V, Shalev R S, Kazir E et al 1993 Intravenous high-dose gammaglobulins for intractable childhood epilepsy. Acta Neurol Scand 88: 204–209

Harbord M G, Manson J I 1987 Temporal lobe epilepsy in childhood: reappraisal of etiology and outcome. Pediatr Neurol 3: 263–268

Harbord M G, Hwang P A, Robinson B H et al 1991 Infant-onset progressive myoclonus epilepsy. J Child Neurol 6: 134–142

Hart Y M, Cortez M, Andermann F et al 1994 Medical treatment of Rasmussen's syndrome (chronic encephalitis and epilepsy): effect of high-dose steroids or immunogolobulins in 19 patients. Neurology 44: 1030–1036

Harvey A S, Bowe J M, Hopkins I J, Shield L K, Cook D J, Berkovic S F 1993a Ictal ^{99m}Tc-HMPAO single photon emission computed tomography in children with temporal lobe epilepsy. Epilepsia 34: 869–877

Harvey A S, Hopkins I J, Bowe J M, Cook D J, Shield L K, Berkovic S F 1993b Frontal lobe epilepsy: clinical seizure characteristics and localization with ictal ^{99m}Tc-HMPAO SPECT. Neurology 43: 1966–1980

Hirsch E, Marescaux C, Maquet P et al 1990 Landau–Kleffner syndrome: a clinical and EEG study of five cases. Epilepsia 31: 756–767

Holmes G L 1993 Benign focal epilepsies of childhood. Epilepsia 34 (suppl 3): S49–S61

Horn C S, Ater S B, Hurst D L 1986 Carbamazepine-exacerbated epilepsy in children and adolescents. Pediatr Neurol 2: 340–345

Horneff G, Lenard H G, Wahn V 1992 Severe adverse reaction to carbamazepine: significance of humoral and cellular reactions to the drug. Neuropediatrics 23: 272–275

Howitz P, Neergaard K, Pedersen H 1990 Cranial computed tomography in infantile spasms. Primary findings related to long-term mental prognosis. Acta Paediatr Scand 79: 1087–1091

Hrachovy R A, Glaze D G, Frost J D Jr 1991 A retrospective study of spontaneous remission and long-term outcome in patients with infantile spasms. Epilepsia 32: 212–214

Hrachovy R A, Frost J D Jr Glaze D G 1994 High-dose, long-duration versus low-dose, short-duration corticotropin therapy for infantile spasms. J Pediatr 124: 803–806

Hurst D L 1987 Severe myoclonic epilepsy of infancy. Pediatr Neurol 3: 269–272

Hurst D L 1990 Epidemiology of severe myoclonic epilepsy of infancy. Epilepsia 31: 397–400

Hurst D L 1993 The rapid change to monotherapy with valproic acid in children. J Child Neurol 8: 357–359

Huttenlocher P R, Hapke R J 1990 A follow-up study of intractable seizures in childhood. Ann Neurol 28: 699–705

Jackson G D, Berkovic S F, Tress B M, Kalnins R M, Fabinyi G C, Bladin P F 1990 Hippocampal sclerosis can be reliably detected by magnetic resonance imaging. Neurology 40: 1869–1875

Jackson G D, Connelly A, Duncan J S, Grunewald R A, Gadian D G 1993 Detection of hippocampal pathology in intractable partial epilepsy: increased sensitivity with quantitative magnetic resonance T2 relaxometry. Neurology 43: 1793–1799

Jay V, Becker L E, Otsubo H, Hwang P A, Hoffman H J, Harwood Nash D 1993 Pathology of temporal lobectomy for refractory seizures in children. Review of 20 cases including some unique malformative lesions. J Neurosurg 79: 53–61

Kasteleijn-Nolst Trénité D G A 1994 Video-game epilepsy. Lancet 344: 1102–1103

Knott C, Panayiotopoulos C P 1994 Carbamazepine in the treatment of generalised tonic clonic seizures in juvenile myoclonic epilepsy. J Neurol Neurosurg Psychiatry 57: 503

Koo B, Hwang P A, Logan W J 1993 Infantile spasms: outcome and prognostic factors of cryptogenic and symptomatic groups. Neurology 43: 2322–2327

Kotagal P, Rothner A D, Erenberg G, Cruse R P, Wyllie E 1987 Complex partial seizures of childhood onset. A five-year follow-up study. Arch Neurol 44: 1177–1180

Kuks J B, Cook M J, Fish D R, Stevens J M, Shorvon S D 1993 Hippocampal sclerosis in epilepsy and childhood febrile seizures. Lancet 342: 1391–1394

Kusse M C, Van Nieuwenhuizen O, van Huffelen A C, van der Mey W, Thijssen J H, van Ree J M 1993 The effect of non-depot ACTH(1–24) on infantile spasms. Dev Med Child Neurol 35: 1067–1073

Kuzniecky R I 1994 Magnetic resonance imaging in developmental disorders of the cerebral cortex. Epilepsia 35 (suppl 6): S44–S56

Kuzniecky R, Andermann F, Tampieri D et al 1989 Bilateral central macrogyria: epilepsy, pseudobulbar palsy, and mental retardation — a recognizable neuronal migration disorder. Ann Neurol 25: 547–554

Kuzniecky R, Murro A, King D et al 1993 Magnetic resonance imaging in childhood intractable partial epilepsies: pathologic correlations. Neurology 43: 681–687

Lee T K, Nakasu Y, Jeffree M A, Molyneux A J, Adams C B 1989 Indolent glioma: a cause of epilepsy. Arch Dis Child 64: 1666–1671

Lee N, Radtke R A, Gray L et al 1994 Neuronal migration disorders: positron emission tomography correlations. Ann Neurol 35: 290–297

Lerman P, Lerman-Sagie T, Kivity S 1991 Effect of early corticosteroid therapy for Landau–Kleffner syndrome. Dev Med Child Neurol 33: 257–260

Loiseau P, Duche B, Cordova S, Dartigues J F, Cohadon S 1988 Prognosis of benign childhood epilepsy with centrotemporal spikes: a follow-up study of 168 patients. Epilepsia 29: 229–235

Lortie A, Chiron C, Mimford J, Dulac O 1993 The potential for increasing seizure frequency, relapse, and appearance of new seizures types with vigabatrin. Neurology 43 (suppl 5); S24–S27

Maeda N, Watanabe K, Negoro T et al 1994 Evolutional changes of cortical hypometabolism in West's syndrome. Lancet 343: 1620–1623

Magaudda A, Dalla Bernardina B, De Marco P et al 1993 Bilateral occipital calcification, epilepsy and coeliac disease: clinical and neuroimaging features of a new syndrome. J Neurol Neurosurg Psychiatry 56: 885–889

Manonmani V, Wallace SJ 1994 Epilepsy with myoclonic absences. Arch Dis Child 70: 288–290

Marescaux C, Hirsch E, Finck S et al 1990 Landau–Kleffner syndrome: a pharmacologic study of five cases. Epilepsia 31: 768–777

Minford A M, Forsythe W I 1992 Computed tomography findings in partial seizures. Arch Dis Child 67: 693–696

Morrell F, Whisler W W, Bleck T P 1989 Multiple subpial transection: a new approach to the surgical treatment of focal epilepsy. J Neurosurg 70: 231–239

Obeid T, el Rab M O, Daif A K et al 1994 Is HLA-DRW13 (W6) associated with juvenile myoclonic epilepsy in Arab patients? Epilepsia 35: 319–321

Offringa M, Bossuyt P M, Lubsen J et al 1994 Risk factors for seizure recurrence in children with febrile seizures: a pooled analysis of individual patient data from five studies. J Pediatr 124: 574–584

Palmini A, Andermann F, Aicardi J et al 1991 Diffuse cortical dysplasia, or the 'double cortex' syndrome: the clinical and epileptic spectrum in 10 patients. Neurology 41: 1656–1662

Palmini A, Gambardella A, Andermann F et al 1994 Operative strategies for patients with cortical dysplastic lesions and intractable epilepsy. Epilepsia 35 Suppl 6: S57–S71

Panayiotopoulos C P 1989 Benign nocturnal childhood occipital epilepsy: a new syndrome with nocturnal seizures, tonic deviation of the eyes and vomiting. J Child Neurol 4: 43–49

Panayiotopoulos C P 1993 Benign childhood partial epilepsies: benign childhood seizure susceptibility syndromes. J Neurol Neurosurg Psychiatry 56: 2–5

Panayiotopoulos C P, Obeid T 1989 Juvenile myoclonic epilepsy: an autosomal recessive disease. Ann Neurol 25: 440–443

Panayiotopoulos C P, Obeid T, Waheed G 1989 Absences in juvenile myoclonic epilepsy: a clinical and video-electroencephalographic study. Ann Neurol 25: 391–397

Panayiotopoulos C P, Tahan R, Obeid T 1991 Juvenile myoclonic epilepsy: factors of error involved in the diagnosis and treatment. Epilepsia 32: 672–676

Porter R J 1993 The absence epilepsies. Epilepsia 34 (suppl 3): S42–S48

Reutens D C, Bye A M, Hopkins I J et al 1993 Corpus callosotomy for intractable epilepsy: seizure outcome and prognostic factors. Epilepsia 34: 904–909

Rosman N P, Colton T, Labazzo J et al 1993 A controlled trial of diazepam administered during febrile illnesses to prevent recurrence of febrile seizures. N Engl J Med 329: 79–84

Roulet Perez E, Davidoff V, Despland P A, Deonna T 1993 Mental and behavioural deterioration of children with epilepsy and CSWS: acquired epileptic frontal syndrome. Dev Med Child Neurol 35: 661–674

Scheffer I E, Bhatia K P, Lopes Cendes I et al 1994 Autosomal dominant frontal epilepsy misdiagnosed as sleep disorder. Lancet 343: 515–517

Schlumberger E, Chavez F, Palacios L, Rey E, Pajot N, Dulac O 1994 Lamotrigine in treatment of 120 children with epilepsy. Epilepsia 35: 359–367

Schmitt B, Wohlrab G, Boltshauser E 1994 Vigabatrin in newly diagnosed infantile spasms. Neuropediatrics 25: 54

Shinnar S, Berg A T, Moshe S L et al 1990 Risk of seizure recurrence following a first unprovoked seizure in childhood: a prospective study. Pediatrics 85: 1076–1085

Shinnar S, Berg A T, Moshe S L et al 1994 Discontinuing antiepileptic drugs in children with epilepsy: a prospective study. Ann Neurol 35: 534–545

Snead O C III, Hosey L C 1985 Exacerbation of seizures in children by carbamazepine. N Engl J Med 313: 916–921

Stores G, Zaiwalla Z, Bergel N 1991 Frontal lobe complex partial seizures in children: a form of epilepsy at particular risk of misdiagnosis. Dev Med Child Neurol 33: 998–1009

Sturniolo M G, Galletti F 1994 Idiopathic epilepsy and school achievement. Arch Dis Child 70: 424–428

Tinuper P, Andermann F, Villemure J G, Rasmussen T B, Quesney L F 1988 Functional hemispherectomy for treatment of epilepsy associated with hemiplegia: rationale, indications, results, and comparison with callosotomy. Ann Neurol 24: 27–34

Uthman B M, Reid S A, Wilder B J, Andriola M R, Beydoun A A 1991 Outcome for West syndrome following surgical treatment. Epilepsia 32: 668–671

van der Meij W, van Huffelen A C, Willemse, J, Schenk-Rootlieb A J, Meiners L C 1992 Rolandic spikes in the inter-ictal EEG of children: contribution to diagnosis, classification and prognosis of epilepsy. Dev Med Child Neurol 34: 893–903

Velasco A L, Boleaga B, Santos N, Velasco F, Velasco M 1993 Electroencephalographic and magnetic resonance correlations in children with intractable seizures of Lennox–Gastaut syndrome and epilepsia partialis continua. Epilepsia 34: 262–270

Villemure J G, Rasmussen T 1993 Functional hemispherectomy in children. Neuropediatrics 24: 53–55

Vining E P, Freeman J M, Brandt J, Carson B S, Uematsu S 1993 Progressive unilateral encephalopathy of childhood (Rasmussen's syndrome): a reappraisal. Epilepsia 34: 639–650

Vintners H V, De Rosa M J, Farrell M A 1994 Neuropathologic study of resected cerebral tissue from patients with infantile spasms. Epilepsia 34: 772–779

Vles JS, van der Heyden A M, Ghijs A, Troost J 1993 Vigabatrin in the treatment of infantile spasms. Neuropediatrics 24: 230–231

Wyllie E, Chee M, Granstrom M L et al 1993 Temporal lobe epilepsy in early childhood. Epilepsia 34: 859–868

Yakoub M, Dulac O, Jambaque I, Chiron C, Plouin P 1992 Early diagnosis of severe myoclonic epilepsy in infancy. Brain Dev 14: 299–303

9

Surgical treatment of infantile spasms

W. D. Shields

Infantile spasms is one of the 'catastrophic childhood' epilepsies. It is characterized by an early age of onset, resistance to standard antiepileptic drugs, and poor outcome with respect both to seizures and, perhaps more importantly, to development. Most children are left retarded, usually with an IQ less than 50 (Riikonen 1982). Infantile spasm is a relatively common disorder accounting for 3–15% of childhood-onset seizures (Hauser & Hesdorffer 1990). The peak age of onset of seizures is 5 months. Some patients begin having seizures within a few hours of birth; up to 15% begin after 1 year of age.

Infantile spasms are typically described as sustained, bilateral movements of the axial musculature and limbs with adduction of the arms. About 40% of the children have spasms with the trunk and legs both flexed, and about 20% of spasms are extensor. The remainder have a combination of the two types, usually with flexion of the head and extension of the legs. The spasms have been given a variety of names, including West syndrome, saalam spasms and jackknife seizures. The syndrome of infantile spasms was first described by West in a letter to the editor of the *Lancet* more than 150 years ago (West 1841). Dr West's description of the seizures was eloquent and as clear as any contemporary description:

To the Editor of the Lancet

Sir: I beg through your valuable and extensive circulating Journal, to call to the attention of the medical profession a very rare and singular species of convulsion peculiar to young children.

As the only case I have witnessed is in my own child, I shall be very grateful to any member of the profession who can give me any information on the subject, either privately or through your excellent Publication.

The child is now near a year old; was a remarkably fine, healthy child when born, and continued to thrive till he was four months old. It was at this time that I first observed slight bobbings of the head forward, which I then regarded as a trick, but were, in fact, the first indications of the disease; for these bobbings increased in frequency, and at length became so frequent and powerful, as to cause a complete heaving of the head forward towards his knees, and then immediately relaxing into the upright position, something similar to the attacks of emprosthotonus: these bowings and relaxings would be repeated alternately at intervals of a few seconds, and repeated from ten to twenty or more times at each attack, which attack would not continue for more than two or three minutes; he sometimes has two, three, or more attacks in the day; they come on whether sitting or lying; just before they come on he is all alive and in motion, making a strange noise, and then all of a sudden down goes his head and upwards his knees; he then appears frightened and screams out: at one time he lost flesh, looked pale and exhausted, but latterly he had regained his good looks, and independent of this affection, is a fine grown child ...

It was more than 100 years later that the advent of electroencephalogram (EEG) gave us the next important observation regarding infantile spasms the typical EEG disturbance called hypsarrhythmia. Gibbs & Gibbs (1952) characterized hypsarrhythmia as:

> random high voltage slow waves and spikes. These spikes vary from moment to moment, both in location and duration. At times they appear to be focal, and a few seconds later they seem to originate from multiple foci. Occasionally, the spike discharge becomes generalized, but it never appears as a rhythmically repetitive and highly organized pattern that could be confused with a discharge of the petit mal variant type. The abnormality is almost continuous.

Not every child with infantile spasms has hypsarrhythmia but, when it is present, it is virtually pathognomic of infantile spasms.

Because of the typically bilateral clinical appearance of the seizures and the diffuse EEG disturbances, infantile spasms have been classified in the generalized seizures category in the international classification system (Commission of Classification and Terminology of the International League Against Epilepsy 1989). By definition, this implies that the seizures are generalized from the onset and without focal origin. Because a key concept in current epilepsy surgery is to identify a single epileptic focus, the generalized nature of infantile spasms seems to preclude them from consideration for cortical resection. However, more recent evidence suggests that generalized infantile spasms may, on occasion, be the result of a localized cortical disturbance, and that resection of the abnormal cortex may be an effective treatment in such cases.

CAUSES

Patients with infantile spasms are customarily classified into one of three etiologic groups: symptomatic, cryptogenic and idiopathic. The *symptomatic* group includes patients in whom an underlying neurologic disorder has been identified, for example tuberous sclerosis or cortical dysplasia. Classification as *cryptogenic* indicates that no specific cause has been identified but the child was not developmentally normal prior to onset of seizures; thus, an underlying brain abnormality can be presumed. The final group, *idiopathic*, is reserved for infants who were neurologically normal prior to onset of infantile spasms and in whom no underlying cause can be identified. Because seizures begin exclusively during the early months of life and because there are many diverse causes, the syndrome of infantile spasms is thought to be an age-specific neurologic response at a time of critical brain development (Watanabe et al 1973, Riikonen 1983). There are numerous factors predisposing to infantile spasms such as birth trauma, hypoxic–ischemic encephalopathy, brain malformation, and genetic or metabolic diseases. The percentage of cases without an identifiable cause has been steadily decreasing over the years as technology has evolved. The ability to identify cortical abnormalities has been greatly enhanced by the development of neuroimaging devices, including magnetic resonance imaging (MRI) and positron emission tomography (PET). In the past, about one-half of the cases were reported as symptomatic. More recently, because of the improved technology, up to 80% are identified as symptomatic. Many of the underlying causes are clearly due to diffuse brain abnormalities but there are also reports of localized cortical disorders associated with infantile spasms (Table 9.1).

Table 9.1 Neurological disorders associated with infantile spasms

Diffuse or multifocal	Unifocal
Inborn errors of metabolism	Tumor
Hypoxic–ischemic encephalopathy	Stroke
Hypoglycemic brain damage	Developmental brain defects
Developmental brain defects	Tuberous sclerosis
Tuberous sclerosis	Neurofibromatosis
Neurofibromatosis	Aicardi syndrome
Aicardi syndrome	Focal cortical dysplasia
Miller–Dieker syndrome	Hemimegalencephaly
Acquired brain damage	Hamartoma
Trauma	Heterotopia
Infection	Acquired brain damage
	Trauma
	Infection

LOCALIZED CORTICAL ABNORMALITIES AND INFANTILE SPASMS

The University of California at Los Angeles (UCLA) pediatric epilepsy surgery program began in 1986 with the goals of improving the prospect for a more normal life for the unfortunate child afflicted with catastrophic childhood epilepsy and improving our understanding of pathophysiology of these seizure disorders. Three of our earliest surgical cases were young children with medically intractable partial seizures who had a past history of infantile spasms. A review of the literature revealed a few case reports of infantile spasm patients with focal brain abnormalities in whom a surgical procedure resulted in cessation of the infantile spasms. Infantile spasms ceased after surgical resection of a right temporal astrocytoma in 1 case

(Mimaki et al 1983), following resection of a choroid plexus papilloma in another (Branch & Dyken 1979), and by fenestration of porencephalic cysts in 4 cases (Palm et al 1988). Our own experience, plus the cases in the literature suggested that some children have infantile spasms due to a focal or regional cortical abnormality. Subsequent events in our program have confirmed this observation (Chugani et al 1990, 1993, Shields et al 1990, 1992, 1993), and other workers have now reported similar findings. Uthman et al (1991) reported that an 18-month-old child with infantile spasms was successfully treated by surgical resection of a porencephalic cyst. Similarly, Carrazana et al (1993) reported that 6 children with identified localized cortical disturbances associated with infantile spasms had good responses to surgery. Many of the localized disorders noted in a Table 9.1 are, in fact, amenable to surgical intervention.

Additional support for the view that generalized infantile spasms can be the consequence of focal brain disturbances comes from numerous papers describing early-onset partial seisures or focal cortical abnormalities in children with infantile spasms detected by EEG, computed tomography (CT), MRI and PET. It has long been recognized that other seizure types may be associated with infantile spasms, including partial seizures (Kellaway 1959, Jeavons & Bower 1964, Lombroso 1983, Yamamoto et al 1988). Carrazana et al (1993) recently reported 16 children in whom consistent partial seizures preceded the onset of the infantile spasms and Donat & Wright (1991) reported 11 patients with partial seizures that occurred simultaneously with infantile spasms. Indeed, even the characteristic hypsarrhythmia pattern may be asymmetric or unilateral (Hrachovy et al 1984). Careful observation may reveal focal disturbances more frequently than had been previously appreciated. Riikonen (1982), for example, found focal abnormalities in 110 of 149 cases. Focal abnormalities may be easier to detect in EEG's obtained early in the course of the illness. Once the hypsarrhythmic pattern is established it is easy to miss relatively subtle EEG abnormalities such as focal slowing or locally decreased activity. In addition, the relation between infantile spasms and partial seizure may become less apparent with time. Carrazana et al (1993) noted that the relation between partial seizures and infantile spasms was lost in 11 of 12 patients followed for more than 6 months. Thus, early identification of localized EEG abnormalities may be critical. Structural defects detected by CT or MRI are less common but may be more obvious than the EEG abnormalities (Singer et al 1982). Alvarez et al (1987) reported 3 children with porencephaly who developed infantile spasms and they proposed that the porencephaly was the cause of the spasms. Cusmai et al (1988) found CT evidence of focal abnormalities in 17 of 174 cases. They observed that the lesions associated with infantile spasms were mainly in the rolandic and the temporo-occipital areas, they postulated that this location favored the development of infantile spasms whereas lesions in the frontal areas favored onset of partial epilepsy at a later age. In a retrospective review of 37 infantile spasms patients, we observed definite localized abnormalities on CT or MRI in 17 cases (46%) and EEG evidence of focality in another 6 (16%). Only 38% of the cases had no localizing features (Shields et al 1990). The high percentage of focal features that we observed is probably an overestimation of the true incidence, because some patients were referred because they had a localizable lesion and were thus candidates for surgery. More recently, Sankar et al (1993) reported that MRI may be able to detect very subtle focal grey-matter disorders by developmental changes in the subjacent white matter. Perhaps the most sensitive neuroimaging tool for the detection of localized disturbances in these children is the PET scan. Chugani et al (1988, 1990) first reported that PET can detect cortical disturbances even when the MRI and CT are normal. Thus, many different modalities have been used to detect localized abnormalities. It often requires very careful evaluation of the available data but localized cortical abnormalities may be much more common in infantile spasms than previously appreciated.

MEDICAL INTRACTABILITY

As with other surgical approaches to epilepsy, children with infantile spasms must demonstrate medical intractability. In adults with complex partial epilepsy, it often takes 2 or more years to attempt all appropriate medical therapies. However, children with infantile spasms typically have many seizures each day so determining medical intractability takes only a few weeks or months (Shewmon et al 1990). Steroid therapy, most commonly adrenocorticotrophic hormone (ACTH), remains the treatment of choice. Most children with infantile spasms respond to ACTH with complete cessation of seizures and improvement in the EEG. The relapse rate, however, is significant. Overall, about 40% of patients either fail immediately or relapse at a later time. In such cases, other medical therapies should be attempted because some patients will respond. As a general rule, however, if the child fails ACTH therapy he/she is unlikely to respond to standard antiepileptic drugs. Patients are most likely to respond to benzodiazepines such as nitrazepam or clonazepam or to valproic acid. Vigabatrin, a new antiepileptic drug not yet available in the USA, shows great promise. In one series of 70 patients receiving vigabatrin as add-on therapy, 43% had complete suppression of spasms (Chiron et al 1990, 1991).

PROGNOSIS OF PATIENTS WITH INFANTILE SPASMS

In the 1841 letter to the editor regarding his son with infantile spasms, Dr West (1941) described the loss of developmental milestones which is now recognized as an integral characteristic.

> but he neither possesses the intellectual vivacity or the power of moving his limbs, of a child of his age; he never cries at the time of the attacks, or smiles or takes any notice, but looks placid and pitiful, yet his hearing and vision are good;

he has not power of holding himself upright or using his limbs, and his head falls without support.

Unfortunately, Dr West's description corresponds all too well to the typical child with infantile spasms. More than 90% of affected children will eventually prove to be mentally retarded, most with IQs less than 50 (Riikonen 1982). A child with infantile spasms is much more likely to develop normally if the seizures are idiopathic and if they respond readily to initial therapy with ACTH or other antiepileptic drugs. In such cases, approximately one-third will eventually prove to be mentally normal. In addition to a symptomatic cause and poor response to medical treatment, there are other factors that appear to predict a poor developmental outcome. Onset of seizures before age 4–6 months is one such predictor. In one study, 7 of 9 patients with onset at less than 6 months of age were severely handicapped on follow-up, whereas only 1 of 16 with onset after 6 months was severely affected. In that later-onset group, 9 of the 16 cases were in the normal or only mildly handicapped range. In another study, only 1 of 78 children with onset less than 4 months was normal, compared to 30 of 195 in the normal range if seizures began after 4 months of age. A second important factor is the presence of seizures other than infantile spasms. In three studies, 15% or fewer of the patients had a good developmental outcome if other types of seizures occurred prior to, or following, infantile spasms. If the infantile spasms occurred as the only seizure type, however, 31–85% of the patients had a good developmental outcome (Ohtahara et al, 1980, Matsumoto et al 1981, Riikonen 1982).

Thus, four factors predict a poor prognosis: first, symptomatic cause; secondly, continued seizures in spite of appropriate medical treatment; thirdly, onset of seizures before 4-6 months of age; and fourthly, other seizure types in addition to infantile spasms. For this subgroup of infantile spasm patients other therapies are clearly needed, and it is this population of infantile spasm patients who are most likely to be surgical candidates.

SURGICAL CONCEPTS

The notion that children with infantile spasms could be surgical candidates necessitates a reconsideration of the concepts that govern epilepsy surgery. The traditional approach to patients with medically intractable epilepsy has been to identify a single area of onset of the seizures and if it is surgically approachable, remove it. Surface EEG monitoring, MRI, PET and CT scans, depth electrodes and intracranial grid studies are all designed to identify a single restricted region of brain in which the epileptic seizures originate. This central principle of epilepsy surgery is not appropriate for children with infantile spasms because their seizures are generalized or multifocal in origin. To address this issue, the UCLA pediatric group has developed a different concept called the *zone of cortical abnormality* (ZCA) to distinguish it from the concept of the *epileptic focus*, used in traditional epilepsy surgery for partial seizures. In the ZCA concept, the purpose of the surgical evaluation is not to identify the site of origin of seizures, but rather to identify an area of the brain that is structurally or functionally abnormal. The EEG is still a very valuable aspect of the evaluation, but rather than concentrating on the ictal disturbances, the interictal abnormalities may be more revealing. There may be areas of diminished beta activity or increased delta activity typically associated with structural pathology. The MRI scan may show gross or perhaps very subtle cortical disturbances, and the PET scan typically shows cortical hypometabolism in an area of localized abnormality. Similarly, the CT scan may be abnormal in the same area. If multiple lines of evidence suggest that one area of the brain is structurally abnormal, the patient can then be considered for surgery. In essence, the goal of the evaluation is to identify a localized cortical abnormality and resect it. Using these concepts, we have operated on more than 20 children with infantile spasms and cortical resection has become an accepted method of therapy for a selected subset of these patients at UCLA.

SURGICAL CANDIDATES

Children may be considered for surgery when the infantile spasms are refractory to ACTH and prednisone plus trials of conventional antiepileptic drugs. If there is clear evidence of a generalized brain disorder, especially diffuse brain injury from hypoxic–ischemic encephalopathy or a progressive degenerative, metabolic or storage disease, the patient is not considered further. In fact, as will be reviewed later, the majority of refractory infantile spasms patients have clear evidence of localized brain abormality before the formal surgical evaluation. Most of our patients had either partial seizures that antedated the onset of infantile spasms or had focal abnormalities on EEGs that were performed before hypsarrhythmia developed. We have evaluated several patients who did not have pre-existing evidence of localized brain defect and have not been able to identify a ZCA in the vast majority of such patients.

SURGICAL EVALUATION

Evidence for ZCA is sought by first reviewing the seizure history to determine whether partial seizures preceded or followed the infantile spasms, and by examining present and past EEGs to identify focal abnormalities. A careful neurologic examination may reveal evidence of localized abnormality. These may be as obvious as a hemiparesis or as subtle as a mild visual field defect. CT and MRI scans are also reviewed for evidence of a focal lesion. If the MRI scans are of inadequate quality, they are repeated. Children whose history or neuroimaging studies indicate diffuse damage affecting both cerebral hemispheres are not further considered for surgery. The surgical evaluation begins with in-hospital, 24-h-a-day closed-circuit television/electroencephalography

(CCTV/EEG) to characterize and quantify seizures. Because the children have very frequent seizures, the duration of CCTV/EEG is usually much shorter than the typical epilepsy surgery evaluation. During the hospitalization, a PET scan is performed to gauge the metabolic activity of the brain, with special attention to the identification of focal hypometabolism.

SURGICAL CRITERIA

Children are recommended for surgery if there is a confluence of historical, EEG, CCTV/EEG, CT, MRI and PET data indicating the presence of a ZCA (a single lobe, contiguous multilobes or one hemisphere). No single abnormal test is sufficient to recommend surgery. A surgical decision is made using the following criteria: (Shields et al 1992).

EEGs and preoperative CCTV/EEG

1. If the child had partial seizures prior to infantile spasms, the area of onset is identified by reviewing past EEGs.

2. If the child has partial seizures associated with infantile spasms at the time of surgical evaluation, the CCTV/EEG is reviewed to identify the area of onset of partial seizures.

3. If the child has generalized or multifocal-onset seizures at the time of surgical evaluation, the CCTV/EEG is analyzed for the presence of interictal abnormalities suggestive of a localized abnormality (focal slowing, a predominant focus of interictal epileptiform discharges, locally decreased β activity, or unilateral subclinical electrodecremental events).

Imaging studies

1. The CT or MRI scans are examined for evidence of a ZCA. The abnormalities may be quite subtle (e.g. thickened cortex, sulci oriented in a wrong direction). If a ZCA is observed, it must correlate with the EEG focus. However, a completely normal CT or MRI scan is not a contraindication to surgery.

2. The PET study should demonstrate a focal or hemispheric hypometabolic area (or hypermetabolic if it is an ictal study rather than interictal) which correlates with other evidence of a ZCA.

3. The brain outside the area of possible resection should appear to be relatively normal on CT, MRI and PET (excluding generalized atrophy due to ACTH therapy).

Neurologic examination

If a focal neurologic deficit is detected on examination, it must correlate with the ZCA being considered for resection.

Assessment of anticipated neurologic deficit

The cortical resection should not create an unacceptable new neurologic deficit. There is, however, no absolute definition of unacceptable. A judgmental decision is made in consultation with the parents, based upon severity of the seizures, the extent of developmental failure, and the prognosis if the seizures remain uncontrolled, compared with the effects of the anticipated deficit. For example, children considered for hemispherectomy are required to manifest some evidence of hemiparesis prior to surgery (the minimum is poor motor control of the affected hand).

RESULTS OF SURGERY

Between 1986 and 1990 the UCLA group operated on 20 children with infantile spasms; they have now been followed for at least 3 years. By definition, all 20 patients had failed ACTH or prednisone plus numerous antiepileptic drugs. All patients were evaluated at UCLA and approved for surgery at the epilepsy surgery group conference using the previously discussed criteria. Nineteen of the patients were operated on at UCLA and 1 patient was operated on elsewhere. We will first review the characteristics of the surgical patients and then discuss the outcome with respect to seizure control and finally review the neuropathology of the resected tissue.

Characteristics of the surgical patients

Of the 20 patients, 13 were girls and 7 were boys. Five had a recognized underlying disorder that predisposed to infantile spasms. Two had tuberous sclerosis, and 1 each had neurofibromatosis, perinatal middle cerebral artery infarction and perinatal herpes simplex encephalitis. As will be noted in the neuroimaging section, several others had recognizable cortical abnormalities on neuroimaging but did not have a specific underlying disease.

Medical history

The average age of onset of infantile spasms is 5 months. In the 20 children undergoing surgery, the average age at onset was 2.5 ± 2.2 months with a range from birth to 8 months of age. Only 3 patients had onset of seizures later than 6 months of age. The average age at the time of surgery was 19 ± 15 months with a median age of 15 months and a range from 4.25 to 60 months of age. Thus, most patients had been having seizures for more than 1 year at the time surgery was performed. The shortest interval was 4.25 months. Fourteen children had had other seizures before the onset of infantile spasms. Twelve of the 14 had previous partial seizures and 1 each had tonic and autonomic seizures. Only 6 patients had infantile spasms as the initial seizure disorder. The EEG at the time of diagnosis of infantile spasms revealed hypsarrhythmia in 18 multifocal independent spike/wave discharges in one, and unknown in 1 (we have not yet been able to review the early EEGs in that patient).

CCTV/EEG at time of evaluation for surgery

The CCTV/EEG assessment has been an essential component of the surgical evaluation and was helpful in identifying the ZCA in all our operated patients. Fifteen patients were having clinical infantile spasms at the time of surgical evaluation but 5 had evolved to intractable partial seizures only. None of the patients had hypsarrhythmia at the time of surgery, but 3 had modified hypsarrhythmia. The ictal EEG was localizing in 9 patients, either because of a localized onset to the seizures or lateralized electrodecrements during spasms. Interictal EEG recording were more helpful than ictal ones: 16 of the patients had focal or lateralized slow activity, 5 had asymmetric β activity, and 2 had decreased sleep spindles over the area of the ZCA. Twelve of the patients had strongly localized interictal epileptiform discharges.

Neuroimaging

MRI/CT

Of our 20 patients, MRI scans were normal in 7. The remaining 13 had a variety of abnormalities, including 10 with developmental defects. Many of them were quite obvious: 1 had hemimegalencephaly while another had a very thickened cortical mantle with a narrow white-matter band beneath. Others had more subtle abnormalities such as loss of definition of the normal gray–white junction. Two patients had a history of brain injuries. One child had a perinatal middle cerebral artery infarction and the other developed herpes simplex II infection at 3 weeks of age. One child had a parietal lobe tumor associated with tuberous sclerosis. Two children had abnormalities that appeared not to be related to a ZCA: 1 had a cerebellar arachnoid cyst and the other had bilateral choroid plexus cysts. Thus, in 11 of the 20 patients, the ZCA was apparent on the MRI scan.

PET

PET was performed in 19 of the 20 cases, and was abnormal in all. The interictal PET usually demonstrated hypometabolism in the ZCA. In addition to utilizing interictal hypometabolism to indicate the ZCA, we use PET to provide information about the integrity of the normal areas of the brain. A few patients have appeared to have modest hypometabolism in other areas of the brain. This raised the possibility that the identified ZCA was merely the most abnormal part of an otherwise diffusely abnormal brain. For example, the child with a history of herpex simplex encephalitis had marked hypometabolism in the right hemisphere. This correlated with an MRI scan which indicated that the infection had largely destroyed the right hemisphere. However, a CT scan showed slight calcification in the basal ganglia on the left, and the PET scan demonstrated a mild decrease in metabolism in the left frontal area. The child underwent a right hemispherectomy and the seizures were completely controlled; her development, however, has remained markedly delayed. This case is in striking contrast to another patient who had apparently normal metabolic activity in the 'good' hemisphere and has not only been seizure-free but has made excellent developmental gains in the 1½ years since hemispherectomy. Thus, PET is not only invaluable in identifying the ZCA but seems to be helpful in identifying those patients whose potential for good development is optimal. This information is useful in presurgical counseling of the patient's parents.

Surgical procedures

At the conclusion of the evaluation, the patients were all presented at our epilepsy surgery conference and approved for surgery by the combined adult and pediatric epilepsy surgery teams. Seven of the 20 patients had hemispherectomies (5 right, 2 left). Ten patients had parietal–occipital–temporal resections (7 right, 3 left). Of the 3 remaining patients 1 had a parietal lobe tumor, 1 had a large central resection, and the other patient had a frontal–temporal resection.

Seizure frequency pre- and postoperatively

At the time of surgery, 19 of the 20 patients were having at least 10 seizures per day. One child had between 1 and 10 seizures per day. Preoperative seizure frequency was determined by CCTV/EEG monitoring. To address the special circumstances associated with infantile spasms, we have devised a seizure frequency classification system. The traditional method of determining the effect of surgery — percentage reduction in seizure frequency — has little meaning in many of these children. For example, if a child has 100 infantile spasms per day and surgery reduces the frequency by 90% to 10 infantile spasms per day, there is statistical but not meaningful clinical benefit. On the other hand, if the patient had 10 infantile spasms per day and surgery reduced the frequency and changed the character of the seizures such that the child was having 1 complex partial seizure per day, the child would likely have benefited significantly from the surgery, even though the percentage reduction was similar to the previous example. The frequency classification system addresses this problem by grouping seizure frequency into six classes ranging from class 1 (more than 10 seizures per day) to class 6 (seizure-free). Details of the classification system are presented in Figure 9.1 along with the preoperative and postoperative seizure frequencies in our 20 patients. All but 1 patient had at least 10 seizures per day (class 1) preoperatively; 1 patient was

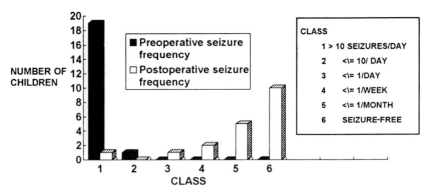

Fig 9.1   Frequency of seizures pre- and postsurgery in 20 children with infantile spasms.

class 2 with between 1 and 10 seizures per day. As can be seen in Figure 9.1, 10 of the patients are completely seizure-free (class 6) postoperatively. Two patients failed to benefit at all from surgery and remain in class 1. One of these continues to have 10 or more seizures per day. The other child continued to have very frequent seizures postoperatively and subsequently died without explanation. The death was not related to the surgery. One additional patient is having between 1 seizure per day and 1 seizure per week. Thus, of the 20 patients, 15 can be considered to have benefited greatly from the surgery, becoming either seizure-free or markedly improved, with less than 1 seizure per month. Two additional patients may have benefited modestly from surgery, with postoperative seizure frequency between 1 seizure per week and 1 seizure per month. Thus, cortical resection is an effective treatment for most children who have an identifiable zone of cortical abnormality associated with infantile spasms.

Neuropathology

The neuropathologic examination of resected tissue from these patients was helpful in improving our understanding of the cortical abnormalities associated with infantile spasms. In a report from our group, Vinters et al (1992) reported on the first 13 of the infantile spasm patients. They observed that neuropathological abnormalities could be divided into two groups: malformative lesions and destructive lesions. Ten of the 13 patients had dysplastic or hamartomatous lesions, 4 had cystic–gliotic encephalopathy (2 had both), and 1 patient had normal-appearing cerebral cortex and subcortical white matter. The additional 7 cases discussed in this chapter had similar abnormalities, including 1 child with tuberous sclerosis who had a parietal lobe glioma. Cytoarchitectural abnormalities were found even in patients with normal CT and MRI scans. However, all of these children had abnormal PET scans with localized areas of hypometabolism. Therefore, 19 of these patients represent the symptomatic category of infantile spasms, even though some would have been classified as cryptogenic without neuropathological data.

EARLY EVIDENCE OF A ZCA

Nineteen of the 20 patients had evidence of a ZCA before they came to UCLA for surgical evaluation. Twelve had partial seizures, 13 had localized interictal or ictal EEG abnormalities, 11 had abnormal neuroimaging studies, and 9 had abnormalities on neurologic examination. Only 1 child had no preliminary evidence for a ZCA. That child was found to have a localized hypometabolic abnormality in the left frontal area on PET scan. Subsequent CCTV/EEG studies corroborated the presence of a ZCA, and this child had a surgical resection. However, she did not respond to surgery and continued to have seizures unabated, eventually dying unexpectedly. Thus, the vast majority of refractory infantile spasm patients who are surgical candidates have early evidence of localized cortical disturbance. Children with clear evidence of generalized disease should not be considered for surgical evaluation.

CONCLUSIONS

Infantile spasm is a difficult and frustrating disorder to treat. Some children who fail traditional medical therapies are candidates for surgical intervention. The number of children with medically refractory infantile spasms who have a ZCA has not been established. Based on our experience, we believe the number to be about 20% of those who fail medical therapy.

As previously noted, the factors that predict a poor outcome to medical treatment appear to define the population who are surgical candidates. The four factors are:

1. Symptomatic cause. Neuropathologic observations on resected tissue indicate that operated children have a high likelihood of having underlying cerebral abnormalities and should all be considered to be symptomatic cases.

2. Persistent seizures in spite of appropriate medical therapies. By definition, all of our cases had medically resistant seizure disorders or they would not have been considered for surgery.

3. Early onset of seizures. The mean age of onset of seizures in our group was 2½ months of age. Onset at less than 4–6 months of age is considered a risk factor for poor outcome.

4. Seizure types other than infantile spasms. Most of these patients had other seizure types in addition to the infantile spasms. Fourteen had other seizure types prior to the onset of infantile spasms; 5 had evolved to partial seizures at the time of surgery.

KEY POINTS FOR CLINICAL PRACTICE

- Some children with medically refractory infantile spasms have a localizable brain defect called the ZCA. Evidence of a ZCA is generally apparent early in the course of the infantile spasms.
- Children with ZCA may have generalized seizures, although many have partial seizures which either precede or are concurrent with the infantile spasms.
- Children with a ZCA may have normal CT and MRI scans. However, developmental changes are important, and repeated MRI scans may reveal localized abnormalities that reflect cerebral pathology.
- The ZCA is often best identified using interictal EEG and PET data.
- Removal of the ZCA may result in control of medically refractory seizures, including generalized infantile spasms.

REFERENCES

Alvarez L A, Shinnar S, Moshe S L. 1987 Infantile spasms due to unilateral cerebral infarcts. Pediatrics 6: 1024–1026

Branch C E, Dyken P R. 1979 Choroid plexus papilloma and infantile spasms. Ann Neurol 5: 302–304

Carrazana E J, Lombroso C T, Mikati M et al. 1993 Facilitation of infantile spasms by partial seizures. Epilepsia 34: 97–109

Chiron C, Dulac O, Luna D et al. 1990 Vigabatrin in infantile spasms. Lancet 1: 363–364

Chiron C, Dulac O, Beaumont D et al. 1991 Therapeutic trial of vigabatrin in refractory infantile spasms. J Child Neurol 6 (suppl 2): 2S52–2S59

Chugani H T, Shewmon D A, Peacock W J et al. 1988 Surgical treatment of intractable neonatal seizures: The role of positron emission tomography. Neurology 38: 1178–1188

Chugani H T, Shewmon D A, Shields W D et al. 1990 Infantile spasms. I. PET identifies focal cortical dysgenesis in cryptogenic causes for surgical teatment. Ann Neurol 27: 406–413

Chugani H T, Shewmon D A, Shields W D et al. 1993 Surgery for intractable infantile spasms: Neuroimaging perspectives. Epilepsia 34: 764–771

Commission of Classification and Terminology of the International League Against Epilepsy. 1989. Proposal for revised classification of epilepsies and epileptic syndromes. Epilepsia 30: 389–399

Cusmai R, Dulac O, Diebler C. 1988 Lesions focales dans les spasmes infantales. Neurophysiol Clin 18: 235–241

Donat J F, Wright F S. 1991 Simultaneous infantile spasms and partial seizures. J Child Neurol 6: 246–250

Gibbs F A, Gibbs E L. 1952 Atlas of electroencephalography: epilepsy. Cambridge, MA: Addison-Wesley, p 2

Hauser W A, Hesdorffer D C. 1990 Epilepsy frequency, causes and consequences. New York: Demos Publications p 334

Hrachovy R A, Frost J D, Kellaway P. 1984 Hypoarrhythmia: variations on the theme. Epilepsia 25: 317–325

Jeavons P M, Bower B D. 1964 Infantile spasms: a review of the literature and a study of 112 cases. Clin Dev Med 15: 8–25

Kellaway P. 1959 Neurologic status of patients with hypsarrhythmia. In: Gibbs RA, ed. Molecules and mental health. New York: Lippincott, pp 134–149

Lombroso C T. 1983 A prospective study of infantile spasms: clinical and therapeutic considerations. Epilepsia 24: 135–158

Matsumoto A, Watanabe K, Negoro T et al. 1981 Long-term prognosis after infantile spasms: A statistical study of prognostic factors in 200 cases. Dev Med Child Neurol 23: 51–65

Mimaki T, Ono J, Yabuuchi H. 1983 Temporal lobe astrocytoma with infantile spasms. Ann Neurol 14: 695–696

Palm D G, Brandt M, Korinthenberg R. 1988 West syndrome and Lennox–Gastaut syndrome in children with porencephalic cysts: Long term follow-up after neurosurgical treatment. In: Niedermayer E, Degen Eds. The Lennox–Gastaut Syndrome. New York: Alan R. Liss, pp 419–426

Ohtahara S, Yamatogi Y, Ohtsuka Y, et al 1980 Prognosis of West syndrome with special reference to Lennox syndrome: a developmental study. In: Advances in epileptology. Eds Wada J, Penry J K .New York: Raven Press pp 149–154

Riikonen R. 1982 A long-term follow-up study of 214 children with the syndrome of infantile spasms. Neuropediatrics 13: 14–23

Riikonen R. 1983 Infantile spasms: some new theoretical aspects. Epilepsia 24: 159–168

Sankar R, Curran J, Kevill J, Vinters H V. 1993 Inference of microscopic cortical dysplasia in children with infantile spasms by time dependent white matter changes on MRI. Am Soc Neuroradiol 31: 259

Shewmon D A, Shields W D, Chugani H T, Peacock W J. 1990 Contrasts between pediatric and adult epilepsy surgery: rationale and strategy for focal resection. J. Epilepsy, 3 (suppl): 141–155

Shields W D, Shewmon D A, Chugani H T, Peacock W J. 1990 The role of surgery in the treatment of infantile spasms. J Epilepsy 3 (suppl); 321–324

Shields W D, Shewmon D A, Chugani H T, Peacock W J. 1992 Treatment of infantile spasms: medical of surgical? Epilepsia 33 (suppl 4): 25–30

Shields W D, Duchowny M S, Holmes G L. 1993 Operable syndromes of infancy and early childhood. In: Surgical treatment of the epilepsies. Engle J Jr, Ed. New York: Raven Press, pp 35–48

Singer W D, Haller J S, Sullivan L R et al. 1982 The value of neuroradiology in infantile spasms. Pediatrics 100: 47–50

Uthman B M, Reid S A, Wilder B J, et al 1991 Outcome for West syndrome following surgical treatment. Epilepsia 32: 668–671

Vinters H V, Fisher R S, Cornford M et al 1992 Neuropathologic substrates of infantile spasms: studies based on surgically resected cerebral cortical tissue. Child Nerv System 8: 8–17

Watanabe K, Iwawse K, Hara K. 1973 The evolution of EEG features in infantile spasms; a prospective study. Dev Med Child Neurol 15: 584–596

West W J. 1841 On a peculiar form of infantile convulsions. Lancet 1: 724–725

Yamamoto N, Watanabe K, Negoro I et al. 1988 Partial seizures evolving to infantile spasms. Epilepsia 29: 34–40

10

Chronic encephalitis and epilepsy (Rasmussen's syndrome): recent developments

Y. Hart   F. Andermann   T. B. Rasmussen

The original description of chronic encephalitis and epilepsy was made by Rasmussen et al in 1958, when they reported 3 young children with focal seizures due to chronic localized encephalitis. The children were aged between 18 months and 8 years at the onset of their illness and presented with severe focal motor seizures, sometimes with secondary generalization, followed by the development of progressive hemiparesis. Intellectual impairment was also noted. Following failure of medical treatment, surgery was carried out in an attempt to control the seizures. Two of the children, in whom serial pneumoencephalograms showed progressive unilateral hemispheric atrophy, underwent hemispherectomy and became seizure-free thereafter, while the third, who had a frontal lobectomy, continued to have very frequent seizures and died 9 months after the onset of his illness. Pathological examination in all 3 showed changes of chronic encephalitis, with perivascular cuffing, microglial nodules, spongy degeneration, and a pronounced astrocytic reaction. These changes were limited to one cerebral hemisphere in the child undergoing autopsy. It is of note that 2 of the children had suffered a minor infective episode shortly before the development of their neurological illness.

Since that time chronic encephalitis and epilepsy (Rasmussen's encephalitis) has been recognized as a distinct syndrome and described in more than 100 patients (Gupta et al 1974, Piatt et al, 1988, Rasmussen & Andermann 1991, Honovar et al 1992). Its salient features include the development of intractable partial seizures, usually in childhood; progressive neurological deterioration with hemiparesis, dysphasia if the dominant hemisphere is involved, and intellectual deterioration; progressive cerebral atrophy, mainly unilateral; and the characteristic pathologic picture of chronic encephalitis. It therefore does not encompass patients undergoing temporal lobe surgery for epilepsy who, as occasionally occurs, are found on pathologic examination to have mild encephalitic changes but who do not show progressive neurological deterioration (Aguilar & Rasmussen 1960, Jensen & Klinken 1976, Laxer 1991). Despite extensive study, the cause of Rasmussen's encephalitis is still unknown, as is the reason for its typically unilateral nature, and treatment remains unsatisfactory. In this chapter we review the progress made in our understanding of this unusual syndrome.

THE CLINICAL SPECTRUM

Although rare, chronic encephalitis and epilepsy have been described by authors from many different countries (Gupta et al 1974, Bancaud et al 1982, Piatt et al 1988, Harvey et al, 1992 Honovar et al 1992, Fukuda et al 1992). In the majority of cases, the onset is in childhood, most commonly between the ages of 1 and 10 years, and the incidence appears to be similar in males and females.

Most children have a normal birth and development prior to the onset of the condition. In up to 50% of the patients there is a history of an infectious episode in the 6 months before presentation, usually of a minor nature such as influenza or an upper respiratory or gastrointestinal infection, but occasionally more severe. The first sign of the chronic encephalitis itself is most commonly the development of partial seizures, with or without secondary generalization. The seizure bringing the child to medical attention is often a generalized tonic–clonic seizure, but subsequently simple partial motor seizures are the seizure type most frequently seen. These often involve jerking of the arm, and sometimes the leg, face or entire hemibody. Complex partial seizures, usually involving staring or the development of a trance-like state, and secondarily generalized tonic–clonic seizures, are also common, and many children have a mixture of seizure types. The seizures are typically very frequent (often occurring several times per day) and refractory to medical treatment. In about half the patients epilepsia partialis continua supervenes within a few years of the onset. Generalized convulsive status epilepticus occurs in about 20% of patients (Oguni et al 1992).

In the early stages of the disease, the diagnosis of chronic encephalitis may not be apparent, and suspicion of the diagnosis is raised with the development of progressive neurologic deterioration, beginning in the first year in 40% of patients, in the second or third year in 40%, and 4–15 years after the onset in 20% (Rasmussen & Andermann 1991). The earliest sign of this is commonly the development of a slowly progressive hemiparesis, the weakness often first being noted after a cluster of seizures or in the context of epilepsia partialis continua. Visual field defects may also occur. In association with these physical signs, the child typically develops evidence of intellectual deterioration which is often associated with behavioral disturbance. The duration of the neurologic deterioration is usually limited to a period varying from a few months to about 10 years, following which stabilization of the neurologic status occurs. By this time the patient usually has a significant hemiparesis and moderate mental impairment, but the seizures are often less severe and less frequent than in the early stages. Despite the severity of the condition, death due to the disease process itself is uncommon (Rasmussen & Andermann 1991).

There have been several reports of patients who, though presenting with symptoms and signs suggestive of Rasmussen's encephalitis, have had atypical features. These include patients developing the disease in adulthood or adolescence, and patients with a typical clinical course but unusual pathology.

Thirteen patients developing the condition in adult life or adolescence have been described (Gray et al 1987, Hart et al 1993a, McLachlan et al 1993). Gray et al (1987) reported a 29-year-old man who presented with myoclonus of the left side of the face rapidly progressing to involve the left arm. The seizures were initially responsive to carbamazepine. Four months later the patient developed choroiditis of the right eye which resolved with steroid treatment. He subsequently developed epilepsia partialis continua of the left arm and leg, and also complex partial and secondarily generalized seizures, accompanied by increasing left hemiparesis and mental slowing. Serial electroencephalograms (EEGs) showed gradual spread of epileptiform activity, and computed tomography (CT) scans showed progressive right hemispheric atrophy. Cerebrospinal fluid analysis showed mildly raised protein and white-cell count. The patient's condition steadily deteriorated, he became bed-ridden and died 2 years after presentation. Pathologic changes were limited to the right hemisphere. Microscopic examination showed thickened leptomeninges containing inflammatory mononuclear cells, while the cortex, particularly in the region of the precentral gyrus, showed neuronal loss, vacuolization, capillary proliferation and gliosis. Microglial nodules and perivascular cuffing were also noted throughout the cortex.

McLachlan et al (1993) described 3 patients with symptoms beginning at the ages of 36, 24 and 16 years. In the first patient, the onset of the illness was marked by the development of mild but progressive right hemiparesis: her first seizure occurred 10 months after the onset and was followed by a transient left hemiparesis. She then developed recurrent focal motor seizures of the left face and hand, with progressive left hemiparesis, dysarthria, dysphagia, pseudobulbar affect, gait ataxia and mild cognitive decline. Her seizure frequency improved following two surgical procedures but her neurologic deficit continued to progress for 3 months afterwards and she required long-term nursing home care. The second patient, a 24-year-old woman, presented with seizures consisting of flashing lights in the right upper visual field or twitching of the right side of the face. Later she developed secondarily generalized seizures, right hemiparesis and dysphasia. After two attempts at resective surgery her seizures improved and her neurologic condition stabilized, but she was ataxic to the extent that she could not walk without assistance. The final patient described by McLachlan et al, a 16-year-old student, also had seizures with visual symptomatology and secondary generalization. Four years after the onset she developed epilepsia partialis continua and weakness of the left leg. There was some improvement in her seizure frequency following a small focal resection but they gradually increased and she had progressive neurologic deterioration: as with the other 2 patients, cognitive impairment was also present. Cerebrospinal fluid analysis was normal in all 3 of these patients. Magnetic resonance imaging (MRI) scan was performed in 2: in the first patient, it showed increased signal in the right mesial temporal, insula and orbitofrontal regions, while in the second patient it remained normal 5 years after the onset. However, 1 year later there was increased T2 signal in the left parietal, temporal and occipital areas. The diagnosis of chronic encephalitis was confirmed on pathologic examination in all 3, and cytomegalovirus genome was isolated in each case by in situ hybridization.

Hart et al (1993a) reported 9 patients with the onset of seizures in adulthood or adolescence. Their patients fell into three groups. Four adults, aged 21–40 years at onset, had a syndrome similar to that occurring in children but with less progression of the neurologic deficit. In 1 of these patients, the disease process later became bilateral. The second group included 3 patients with onset of disease in adolescence and with a course rather similar to that in children. The third group included 2 adults presenting acutely with seizures, in whom pneumoencephalogram suggested the presence of tumour. The diagnosis of chronic encephalitis was made at biopsy, and mild neurologic deterioration subsequently occurred. However, the seizures followed a rather benign course in these 2 patients. Three of the patients described by Hart et al (1993a) had occipital involvement, and 2 had bilateral involvement. One of the latter patients had an altogether unusual course, with progressive dementia in the absence of hemiparesis. The diagnosis was not suspected prior to her death, although the pathologic findings were typical. The other had a typical course initially with apparently unilateral involvement, but subsequently went on to develop a progressive contralateral hemiparesis.

These patients resembled those presenting in childhood in that they had partial seizures and progressive neurologic impairment, which took the form of progressive hemiparesis and intellectual deterioration. However, within this small group of older patients, occipital involvement occurred more commonly than would be expected, being seen in 5 of 13 patients, compared with only 3 out of 42 in the Montreal series developing epilepsy under 12 years of age. The incidence of bilateral pathology was also higher than expected among the adult patients described: 2 of the patients described by Hart et al (1993a), and 2 of those reported by McLachlan et al (1993), had features indicating bilateral involvement, which is unusual in the childhood form of the disease. In some of the patients the course was more benign than that commonly seen in children. It is unclear at this stage whether these older patients have the same condition that occurs in childhood, perhaps less malignant from the onset, or whether they represent a heterogeneous group with similar clinical and pathologic features.

A few patients have been reported who presented with symptoms and signs typical of Rasmussen's encephalitis, but in whom pathologic examination showed the presence of a second abnormality in addition to changes of chronic encephalitis (Robitaille 1991, Hart et al 1993b). One such patient had the forme fruste of tuberous sclerosis, another had tuberous sclerosis with mild but typical cutaneous features, and 2 had multiple cavernous haemangiomas. Such patients constituted almost 10% of the Montreal series, and are an additional reason why medical treatment may not be effective. The association of the second pathology with chronic encephalitis raises important issues with regard to the etiology of chronic encephalitis and epilepsy, and the study of such patients may help clarify this.

RESULTS OF INVESTIGATIONS

The results of investigations in chronic encephalitis often show non-specific abnormalities and offer little help with diagnosis in the early stages, before the characteristic clinical course becomes apparent. At a later stage, the most striking and characteristic abnormalities are usually those seen on neuroimaging. When chronic encephalitis was first described, pneumo-encephalography was the most sophisticated means of neuroimaging available. Seventeen of the 23 patients undergoing this procedure in the Montreal series showed atrophy of one cerebral hemisphere, while diffuse atrophy was found in 5 patients and 1 had a normal pneumoencephalogram (Tampieri et al 1991). When repeated examinations were carried out, the characteristic radiologic feature of Rasmussen's encephalitis, namely progressive enlargement of the remainder of the ventricular system and of the subarachnoid space on that side, became apparent.

Since the advent of CT scanning and MRI, more detailed evaluation of the changes taking place has been possible, but the characteristic feature remains that of progressive unilateral cerebral atrophy (Fig. 10.1). In the Montreal series, 11 of 15 patients examined by CT scanning had evidence of hemiatrophy, while 2 had diffuse cerebral atrophy, and 2 seen at an early stage of the disease had normal scans (Tampieri et al 1991). Progression of the hemiatrophy, which usually started in the temporoinsular region, occurred

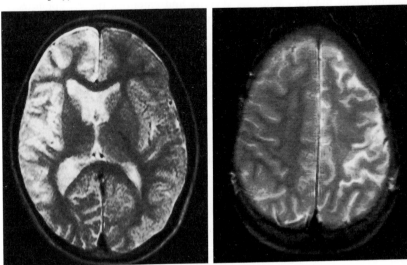

Fig. 10.1   A MRI Scan of a child with Rasmussen's encephalitis showing hemispheral atrophy and abnormal signal in the right hemisphere. **B** Left hemispheral atrophy.

rapidly and often became severe within 2 years. Little has been written about MRI in chronic encephalitis. Tampieri et al (1991) reported 2 patients: hemiatrophy was shown in both, and an abnormal, high-intensity signal in keeping with gliosis in 1 child, best visualized using the proton-density sequence. McLachlan et al (1993) performed MRI scans in 2 patients who developed Rasmussen's encephalitis in adult life, and found multifocal areas of increased T_2 signal in the affected hemisphere. Tien et al (1992) examined 4 patients with Rasmussen's encephalitis using CT scans, xenon CT scans, magnetic resonance scans and positron emission tomography (PET), although not all of the patients had each investigation. The 2 patients undergoing xenon CT cerebral blood flow (CBF) studies showed selectively decreased CBF to the affected hemisphere even when CT studies were relatively normal: another patient undergoing PET showed decreased ^{18}F-fluorodeoxyglucose (FDG) tracer uptake in the affected hemisphere. In contrast, Hajek et al (1991) reported an increase in FDG uptake in a child with chronic encephalitis and epilepsia partialis continua. Proton magnetic resonance spectroscopy has also been carried out in a few patients with chronic encephalitis. Matthews et al (1990) demonstrated decreased levels of N-acetylaspartate (NAA) in the diseased region of the brain. They also showed a high local lactate concentration around the motor strip in a 10-year-old girl with epilepsia partialis continua involving the right arm. Peeling & Sutherland (1993), who performed ^{1}H magnetic resonance spectroscopy in extracts of human epileptic neocortex from patients with chronic encephalitis and temporal lobe epilepsy, were not able to demonstrate differences in metabolite levels in tissue from actively spiking or non-spiking neocortical sites in temporal lobe epilepsy patients, but found that the metabolite concentrations did vary with the severity and extent of the encephalitis. In tissue showing mild encephalitis with mild histologic abnormalities, the metabolite levels differed little from those found for non-encephalitic neocortical tissue, while tissue showing marked abnormalities and extensive encephalitis had decreased NAA, glutamate, cholines and inositol. This raises the possibility that in vivo ^{1}H magnetic resonance spectroscopy may be of use in diagnosing the extent of chronic localized encephalitis.

English et al (1989) investigated 5 patients with Rasmussen's syndrome with single photon emission computed tomography (SPECT) using ^{99m}Tc-hexamethylpropylenamine oxime (HMPAO), which reflects cerebral perfusion. In all patients SPECT imaging demonstrated an area of hypoperfusion/hypometabolism which corresponded to the anatomical localization of the epileptogenic foci found by clinical assessment, EEG and CT. The area of abnormality was more extensive than that seen on CT, and in 2 patients who had sequential studies, it correlated with the patient's changing clinical condition. Burke et al (1992) described a patient with Rasmussen's syndrome with normal MRI and cerebrospinal fluid (CSF), in whom grossly abnormal results of ^{99m}Tc HMPAO SPECT brain imaging were found, and speculated that SPECT may be helpful in making the diagnosis in the early stages. It could also serve as a guide to accurate brain biopsy.

With regard to the results of CSF analysis, about half of the CSF examinations carried out in the Montreal series were normal (Rasmussen & Andermann 1991). Any abnormalities which did occur were usually mild: the white blood cell count ranged from 16 to 70 lymphocytes per cubic milliliter, the protein ranged from 50 to 98 mg%, and the colloidal gold curve showed either a first-zone or mid-zone elevation. In only 15% of the abnormal CSF specimens, however, were all three of these elements abnormal. In some patients in the Montreal series in whom several samples of CSF were examined over a period of weeks to years, the fluid could be abnormal on one occasion and normal on another (Rasmussen & Andermann 1991). The finding of oligoclonal bands in the CSF has varied between studies. Grenier et al (1991) performed CSF electrophoresis in 6 patients and did not find any oligoclonal bands, although a monoclonal band was detected in 1. However, Dulac et al (1991) report oligoclonal bands in 3 of 5 patients, and a pleocytosis in 1. Honovar et al (1992) examined CSF from 8 patients prior to surgery: it was normal in 7, but in 1 there was a slight increase in CSF protein, though not in cells. No comment was made about the presence or absence of oligoclonal bands.

Early in the course of Rasmussen's encephalitis the EEG often shows markedly disturbed background activity over both hemispheres, even though some or most of the clinical seizures are well-lateralized (Rasmussen & Andermann 1991). Subsequently the EEG abnormalities tend to become better lateralized to the involved hemisphere. The most prominent abnormalities, however, are generalized slow-wave abnormalities, with focal spiking less prominent, even in the presence of frequent, well-localized or lateralized seizures (So & Gloor 1991). Other investigators have reported slow-wave abnormalities mainly on the affected side (Piatt et al 1988), although they found that independent epileptic discharges were also not infrequently recorded from the other side.

PATHOLOGY

The pathologic changes seen in Rasmussen's encephalitis are not specific, and the features vary, probably according to the duration and activity of the disease. In the early stages, the chronic encephalitis is characterized by microglial nodules, often found near perivascular cuffs of small lymphocytes and monocytes, and frequently displaying neuronophagia and perivascular chronic inflammation (Robitaille 1991; Fig. 10.2). In the most active cases, the round cells fill the Virchow–Robin spaces and extend beyond the pia into the neuropil. Spongiosis may be observed in association with inflammatory changes, but does not have the widespread neuropil distribution seen in true spongiform encephalopathies. Multifocal neuronal loss occurs within inflamed cortex, predominating in superficial and intermediate cortex, and foci of neuronal loss tend to coalesce into wider and larger areas of complete structural collapse, surrounded by active inflammatory changes within

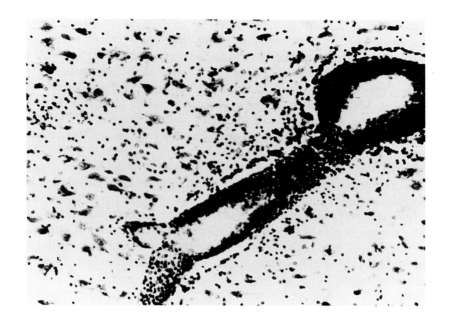

Fig. 10.2   Perivascular infiltrate and microglical nodules in the brain of a child with Rasmussen's encephalitis.

preserved cortex. Abundant astrocytosis occurs, involving entire cortical segments and gyri. Deep white matter is very seldom inflamed.

A classification of the pathology according to disease activity has been devised by Robitaille (1991). Specimens showing active disease (group 1) are characterized by an ongoing inflammatory process in which microglial nodules, with or without neuronophagia, are numerous and accompanied by perivascular round cells and glial scarring. Group 2, active and remote disease, includes brain tissue showing several microglial nodules, with perivascular round-cell cuffs and at least one gyral segment of complete necrosis and cavitation involving full-thickness cortex. Cases displaying neuronal loss and gliosis with moderately abundant perivascular round cells and few microglial nodules are included in group 3, remote disease, while group 4, comprising cases showing non-specific changes, includes tissues free of or with very few microglial nodules and mild perivascular inflammation, combined with various degrees of neuronal loss and scarring.

Farrell et al (1992) described similar pathologic changes in 3 patients with chronic encephalitis undergoing surgery for intractable epilepsy. Macroscopic examination of the resected tissue was normal, but microscopic examination showed extensive cortical and subcortical predominantly lymphocytic infiltration centered on blood vessels, and neuronophagia. Microglial nodules were conspicuous. There was severe neuronal loss with astrocytic gliosis. The inflammatory process extended into white matter in 2 patients and in 1 was associated with extensive myelin loss, astrocytic gliosis and axonal depletion located in a periventricular distribution. In one case, ill-defined basophilic clumps were present in the cytoplasm, and rare measles-like neuronal intranuclear inclusions were seen on electron microscopy.

THE ETIOLOGY OF CHRONIC ENCEPHALITIS AND EPILEPSY

There has been much interest in Rasmussen's encephalitis and its possible causes, partly stimulated by its unusual presentation and unilateral involvement, but despite extensive study, the etiology remains unknown. Possible mechanisms for the condition include a chronic viral infection, an acute viral infection leading to a local immune response, and an independent autoimmune process, unrelated to any known infection (Asher & Gajdusek 1991, Grenier et al 1991).

There are several factors suggesting a viral etiology for Rasmussen's syndrome. Up to half the patients developing this condition experience a minor infective episode in the 6 months before its onset. With the frequent occurrence of epilepsia partialis continua, the condition bears a considerable resemblance to Kozhevnikov's epilepsy in Russian spring–summer encephalitis (Omorokov 1991). A recent report has noted the association of ipsilateral uveitis with Rasmussen's syndrome in 3 patients (Harvey et al 1992) and choroiditis was reported in the patient of Gray et al (1987). The abnormalities sometimes seen in the CSF and the pathologic features are also suggestive of a viral infection. The presence of virus crystals resembling those of enteroviruses was described on electron microscopy in the brain cells of a child with chronic encephalitis and epilepsy by Friedman et al (1977). There has been much recent interest in the use of immunohistochemical and molecular biological techniques to identify viral antigens and nucleic acid sequences, but the results have been contradictory. Power et al (1990) detected cytomegalovirus (CMV) in 7 out of 10 samples using in situ hybridization, and Walter & Renella (1989) detected Epstein–Barr virus (EBV) genome in 2. Vinters et al (1993) found low levels of CMV and EBV genes by polymerase chain reaction (PCR) in most brain specimens from encephalitis patients, although they felt that the levels were too low to suggest a causal association. CMV genome was also demonstrated by in situ hybridization in resected tissue from all 3 adult patients with Rasmussen's encephalitis described by McLachlan et al (1993). In contrast, Mizuno et al (1985) were unable to detect viral antigens in either of their 2 patients, and Farrell et al (1992) obtained negative results with immunostaining using anti-CMV antibodies in their 3 patients with Rasmussen's encephalitis. In situ hybridization studies using a biotinylated probe to CMV were also negative in this group. Honovar et al (1992) were likewise unable to detect EBV virus or CMV genomic material using in situ hybridization.

Immunopathogenetic mechanisms have been suggested by Andrews et al (1990), who performed extensive testing in a child with Rasmussen's encephalitis. They found elevated serum antinuclear antibody titers, CSF oligoclonal bands, and elevated immunoglobulin G (IgG): albumin ratio, IgG index, and IgG synthesis rate. Pathologic study of a subtotal hemispherectomy specimen revealed widespread cerebral vasculitis with immunofluorescence staining for IgG, IgM, IgA, C3 and C1q, and ultra-structural evidence of vascular injury in addition to severe cortical atrophy with marked neuronal loss.

Interest has recently developed in the possible role of the glutamate receptor GluR3 in Rasmussen's encephalitis, following the description by Rogers et al (1994) of the development of features suggestive of Rasmussen's encephalitis in rabbits immunized with GluR3 protein. They also showed serum antibodies to GluR3 by protein immunoblot analysis and by immunoreactivity to transfected cells expressing GluR3 in children with the disease, and subsequently treated one of the affected children by repeated plasma exchanges, noting a transient reduction in the serum titres of GluR3 antibodies in association with decreased seizure frequency and improved neurologic function.

TREATMENT

The diagnosis of chronic encephalitis and epilepsy implies the prospect of a steady neurological deterioration, with increasing hemiparesis and cognitive impairment, for which treatment remains unsatisfactory. The seizures are almost invariably refractory to treatment with the antiepileptic drugs currently available. Dubeau & Sherwin (1991), reviewing the medical treatment of 25 patients with chronic encephalitis and epilepsy, found that 72% had at some time developed symptoms or signs related to drug toxicity during the vain attempt to achieve seizure control. The majority of patients were on polytherapy and high doses of drugs. No particular drug was found to be more efficacious than the others in controlling partial motor seizures, particularly epilepsia partialis continua. At the present time no medical treatment has been proven to be helpful in modifying the course of the disease, although the search is continuing. With regard to surgical treatment, focal resection is rarely of benefit (Rasmussen & McCann 1968, Dalos et al 1986, Honovar et al 1992). Although hemispherectomy is often effective in controlling the seizures, the morbidity associated with it is usually considered unacceptable unless a moderate hemiparesis is already present.

The knowledge that a diagnosis of Rasmussen's encephalitis implies a relentless neurological deterioration that does not respond to antiepileptic drugs has prompted trials of treatment with various agents. These have included steroids, intravenous gammaglobulin, and antiviral therapy, the choice reflecting the presumed causative mechanism. Unfortunately, it is difficult to gauge the effectiveness of such therapies. The incidence of Rasmussen's encephalitis is very low, and most centers thus gain little experience in its treatment even over a long period of time. Ideally, assessment should be by means of a double-blind placebo-controlled trial, but the organization of such a study creates both practical and ethical problems in a condition which is so rare, usually occurs in young children, and has a grave prognosis. The search for an agent effective in the treatment of Rasmussen's encephalitis is also hampered by a lack of useful measures to assess the activity of the condition. Seizure frequency has been used in some studies, and may reflect the severity of the disease, but also shows spontaneous variations. Radiologically, increasing ventricular size and hemispheric atrophy are seen with progression of the disease, but measurement is not usually undertaken and the relationship of these features to disease activity has not been formally assessed. The same reservations apply to the signal changes seen on MRI. The use of magnetic resonance spectroscopy is still being assessed. Electrographic changes are non-specific and are not generally helpful in evaluating severity. Some patients have oligoclonal bands in the CSF, and a few have an increase in the cell count, but in others no abnormality is seen. The situation is further complicated by the fact that some patients appear to show a relapsing and remitting course (Dulac et al 1992).

Antiviral drugs have been used in a few patients. One of the 3 adult patients described by McLachlan et al (1993) was treated with acyclovir, with no benefit, while another received a course of gancyclovir (an agent active against CMV) after surgery and improved, though the extent to which this was due to the surgery was not clear. CMV was detected in brain tissue resected from both of these patients.

Dulac et al (1992) reported treatment with high-dose steroids in 7 patients, all with epilepsia partialis continua and motor deficit prior to the onset of therapy. They were followed for a mean of 43 months. All showed a good response initially after 1–18 months of treatment. Thereafter, 5 of the patients had transient exacerbations of the disease, the intensity decreasing during follow-up, so that a relapsing and remitting course was seen. A sixth patient remained stable after the initial improvement, while the seventh had continuing epilepsia partialis continua with increasing neurological deficit.

Hart et al (1994) treated 19 patients with chronic encephalitis and epilepsy with high-dose steroids, immunoglobulins, or both. Ten of 17 patients receiving high-dose steroids, and 8 of 9 patients receiving intravenous immunoglobulins, had some reduction of seizure frequency in the short term. However, improvement of the hemiparesis was slight and usually related to seizure control. The effect of these drugs in ameliorating the end-point of the disease in the long term remains unclear. Walsh (1991) reported 2 patients with Rasmussen's encephalitis treated with intravenous immunoglobulins: both showed improvement in their seizure control.

A high proportion of patients with chronic encephalitis and epilepsy are eventually treated surgically as a result of failure of medical treatment. Initially complete hemispherectomy was used with good effect. However, it became apparent that one-quarter to one-third of patients subsequently developed the complication of superficial cerebral hemosiderosis, with its symptoms of hydrocephalus and gradual neurologic deterioration (Oppen-heimer & Griffith 1966). The techniques of modified hemispherectomy (Adams 1983), in which, following a standard anatomic hemispherectomy, the dura is stripped from the skull and sutured to the falx and tentorium, creating a large extradural space and a small hemispherectomy cavity, and functional hemispherectomy (Tinuper et al 1988), in which the central region, including the parasagittal tissue and cingular gyrus, is resected while the remainder of the frontal lobe and the parieto-occipital regions are left in place but disconnected from the rest of the brain, were therefore developed in an attempt to eliminate this complication.

The optimum time at which to carry out hemispherectomy is a matter for debate. Many believe that such a procedure, with its inevitable hemiparesis, is unacceptable in the early stages of the condition before a fixed neurologic deficit has already occurred. Others argue that a permanent hemiparesis is a small price to pay for stopping the seizures, eliminating the need for medication and allowing progressive intellectual improvement unhampered by the intractable seizures and their therapy, and feel that surgery should be performed early (Freeman & Vining 1991). It is clear that neither approach offers an ideal solution, and that there remains an urgent need for increased understanding of the etiology of the condition, and for medical treatment to prevent its progression.

Other procedures have also been used in this condition, but with limited success. Honovar et al (1992) described 19 patients with Rasmussen's syndrome treated surgically. Seven underwent small local resection, with no amelioration of their symptoms; 2 underwent diagnostic biopsy and multiple subpial transection (Morrell et al 1989) with greater benefit, while the remaining 10 patients underwent partial or complete hemispherectomies (Adams 1983). Corpus callosotomy has also been reported in 2 patients with chronic encephalitis (Spencer & Spencer 1991). One had frequent secondarily generalized seizures resulting in falls, which were stopped by the surgery. The other, a girl with complex partial seizures with secondary generalization, had improvement in her seizure frequency following callosotomy, but deteriora-tion in her cognitive abilities, possibly as a result of the fact that surgery was delayed until she was in her late teens.

THE FUTURE

It is clear from the foregoing that, more than 30 years after its first description, much remains to be learned about the etiology of Rasmussen's encephalitis, and further immunological and viral studies are urgently required. Until progress is made on this front, the development of effective medical treatment early in the disease both to control the seizures and prevent the relentless neurological deterioration will remain difficult. It is likely that studies of empirical treatment already under way will continue, and because of the rarity of the condition and its variable course, it is important that multicenter studies of treatment be undertaken. Until such time as effective medical treatment is discovered, functional hemispherectomy will remain an important procedure in halting the progression of the illness.

KEY POINTS FOR CLINICAL PRACTICE

- The diagnosis should be considered in children who develop epilepsia partialis continua, and who also have or subsequently develop progressive neurological deficit, progressive hemispheric atrophy on neuroimaging, the presence of oligoclonal or monoclonal bands in the CSF, or biopsy evidence of chronic encephalitis. Other causes of epilepsia partialis continua should be excluded. The diagnosis should also be considered in children with focal seizures and biopsy evidence of chronic encephalitis, particularly if other features are present.

- Biopsy is not crucial in children prior to immunosuppressive treatment with steroids or immunoglobulins if they have the typical features of the disease, but should be obtained in adults.

- Antiepileptic therapy is usually not very effective in controlling the seizures: the aim should be to keep seizures to the minimum to prevent such complications as status epilepticus, while avoiding toxicity.

- There is a need for controlled trials of medical treatment, and consideration should be given to using a standardized protocol in children in whom the use of immunoglobulins or high-dose steroids is contemplated.

- Functional hemispherectomy is effective in controlling seizures but causes morbidity. The optimum time to perform such surgery is not clear, but its potential benefits and risks should be kept under continuous consideration from the time of onset of hemiparesis.

REFERENCES

Adams C B T. 1983 Hemispherectomy — a modification. J Neurol Neurosurg Psychiatry 46: 617–619

Aguilar M J, Rasmussen T. 1960 Role of encephalitis in pathogenesis of epilepsy. Arch Neurol 2: 633–676

Andrews J M, Thompson J A, Pysher T J, Walker M L, Hammond M E. 1990 Chronic encephalitis, epilepsy, and cerebrovascular immune complex deposits. Ann Neurol 28: 88–90

Asher D M, Gajdusek D C. 1991 Virologic studies in chronic encephalitis. In: Andermann F, ed. Chronic encephalitis and epilepsy — Rasmussen's syndrome. Boston: Butterworth-Heinemann, pp 147–158

Bancaud J, Bonis A, Trottier S et al 1982 L'épilepsie partielle continue: syndrome et maladie. Rev Neurol 138: 803–814

Burke G J, Fifer S A, Yoder J. 1992 Early detection of Rasmussen's syndrome by brain SPECT imaging. Clin Nucl Med 17: 730–731

Dalos N, Vining E P G, Carson B, Freeman J M. 1986 Rasmussen's encephalitis: clinical recognition and surgical management. Epilepsia 27: 594

Dubeau F, Sherwin A L. 1991 Pharmacologic principles in the management of chronic encephalitis. In: Andermann F, ed. Chronic encephalitis and epilepsy — Rasmussen's syndrome. Boston: Butterworth-Heinemann, pp 179–192

Dulac O, Robain O, Chiron C et al. 1991 High-dose steroid treatment of epilepsia partialis continua due to chronic focal encephalitis. In: Andermann F, ed. Chronic encephalitis and epilepsy — Rasmussen's syndrome. Boston: Butterworth-Heinemann, pp 193–199

Dulac O, Chinchilla D, Plouin P et al. 1992 Follow-up of Rasmussen's syndrome treated by high-dose steroids. Epilepsia 33: 128

English R, Soper N, Shepstone B J, Hockaday J M, Stores G 1989. Five patients with Rasmussen's syndrome investigated by single-photon-emission computed tomography. Nucl Med Commun 10: 5–14

Farrell M A, DeRosa M J, Curran J G et al. 1992 Neuropathologic findings in cortical resections (including hemispherectomies) performed for the treatment of intractable childhood epilepsy. Acta Neuropathol 83: 246–259

Freeman J M, Vining E P G 1991. Hemispherectomy — the ultimate focal resection. In: Lüders HO, ed. Epilepsy surgery. New York: Raven Press, pp 111–118

Friedman H, Ch'ien L, Parham D. 1977 Virus in brain of child with hemiplegia, hemiconvulsions and epilepsy. Lancet ii: 666

Fukuda T, Oguni H, Yanagaki S et al. 1992 Chronic localized encephalitis (Rasmussen's syndrome) preceded by ipsilateral uveitis — a case report. Epilepsia (in press)

Gray F, Serdaru M, Baron H et al. 1987 Chronic localised encephalitis (Rasmussen's) in an adult with epilepsia paritalis continua. J Neurol Neurosurg Psychiatry 50: 747–751

Grenier Y, Antel J P, Osterland C K. 1991 Immunologic studies in chronic encephalitis of Rasmussen. In: Andermann F, ed. Chronic encephalitis and epilepsy — Rasmussen's syndrome. Boston: Butterworth-Heinemann, pp 125–134

Gupta P C, Roy S, Tandon P N. 1974 Progressive epilepsy due to chronic persistent encephalitis. Report of four cases. J Neurol Sci 22: 105–120

Hajek M, Antonini A, Leenders K L, Wieser H-G. 1991 Epilepsia partialis continua studied by PET. Epilepsy Res 9: 44–48

Hart Y M, Andermann F, Rasmussen T B et al. 1993a Adolescent or adult variant of Rasmussen's syndrome. Epilepsia 34: 37

Hart Y M, Andermann F, Rasmussen T et al. 1993b Double pathology in Rasmussen's syndrome of chronic encephalitis and epilepsy. Epilepsia 34: 14

Hart Y M, Cortez M, Andermann F et al. 1994 The medical treatment of Rasmussen's syndrome (chronic encephalitis and epilepsy): Éffect of high dose steroids or immunoglobulins in 19 patients. Neurology 44: 1030–1036

Harvey A S, Andermann F, Hopkins I J et al. 1992 Chronic encephalitis (Rasmussen's syndrome) and ipsilateral uveitis. Ann Neurol 32: 826–829

Honovar M, Janota I, Polkey C E. 1992 Rasmussen's encephalitis in surgery for epilepsy. Dev Med Child Neurol 34: 3–14

Jensen I, Klinken L. 1976 Temporal lobe epilepsy and neuropathology. Acta Neurol Scand 54: 391–414

Laxer K. 1991 Temporal lobe epilepsy with inflammatory pathologic changes. In: Andermann F, ed. Chronic encephalitis and epilepsy; Rasmussen's syndrome. Boston: Butterworth--Heinemann, pp 135–140

McLachlan R S, Girvin J P, Blume W T, Reichman H. 1993 Rasmussen's chronic encephalitis in adults. Arch Neurol 50: 269–274

Matthews P M, Andermann F, Arnold D L. 1990 A proton magnetic resonance spectroscopy study of focal epilepsy in humans. Neurology 40: 985–989.

Mizuno Y, Chou S M, Estes M L et al. 1985 Chronic localized encephalitis (Rasmussen's) with focal cerebral seizures revisited. J Neuropathol Exp Neurol 44: 351

Morrell F, Whisler W W, Bleck T P. 1989 Multiple subpial transection: a new approach to the surgical treatment of focal epilepsy. J Neurosurg 70: 231–239

Oguni H, Andermann F, Rasmussen T B. 1992 The syndrome of chronic encephalitis and epilepsy: a study based on the MNI series of 48 cases. Adv Neurol 57: 419–433

Omorokov L I, translated by Asher D. 1991 Kozhevnikov's epilepsy in Siberia. Reprinted in: Andermann F, ed. Chronic encephalitis and epilepsy — Rasmussen's syndrome. Boston: Butterworth-Heinemann, pp 263–269

Oppenheimer D R, Griffith H B. 1966 Persistent intracranial bleeding as a complication of hemispherectomy. J Neurol Neurosurg Psychiatry 9: 229–240

Peeling J, Sutherland G. 1993 ^{1}H Magnetic resonance spectroscopy of extracts of human epileptic neocortex and hippocampus. Neurology 43: 589–594

Piatt J H, Hwang P A, Armstrong D C et al. 1988 Chronic focal encephalitis (Rasmussen's syndrome): six cases. Epilepsia 29: 268–279

Power C, Poland S D, Blume W T, Girvin J P, Rice G P A. 1990 Cytomegalovirus and Rasmussen's encephalitis. Lancet 336: 1282–1284

Rasmussen T, Andermann F. 1991 Rasmussen's syndrome: symptomatology of the syndrome of chronic encephalitis and seizures: 35-year experience with 51 cases. In: Lüders HO, ed. Epilepsy surgery. New York: Raven Press, pp 173–182

Rasmussen T, McCann W. 1968 Clinical studies of patients with focal epilepsy due to "chronic encephalitis". Trans Am Neurol Assoc 93: 89–94

Rasmussen T, Olszewski J, Lloyd-Smith D. 1958 Focal seizures due to chronic encephalitis and epilepsy. Neurology 8: 435–445

Robitaille Y. 1991 Neuropathologic aspects of chronic encephalitis. In: Andermann F, ed. Chronic encephalitis and epilepsy: Rasmussen's syndrome. Boston: Butterworth--Heinemann, pp 79–110

Rogers S W, Andrews P I, Gahring L C et al. 1994 Autoantibodies to glutamate receptor GluR3 in Rasmussen's encephalitis. Science 265: 648–651

So N, Gloor P. 1991 Electroencephalography and electrocorticography in chronic encephalitis. In: Andermann F, ed. Chronic encephalitis and epilepsy: Rasmussen's syndrome. Boston: Butterworth-Heinemann, pp 37–45

Spencer S, Spencer D. 1991 Corpus callosotomy in chronic encephalitis. In: Andermann F, ed. Chronic encephalitis and epilepsy: Rasmussen's syndrome. Boston: Butterworth--Heinemann, pp 213–218

Tampieri D, Melanson D, Ethier R. 1991 Imaging of chronic encephalitis. In: Andermann F, ed. Chronic encephalitis and epilepsy: Rasmussen's syndrome. Boston: Butterworth--Heinemann, pp 47–60.

Tien RD, Ashdown BC, Lewis DV, Atkins MR, Burger PC. 1992 Rasmussen's encephalitis: neuroimaging findings in four patients. AJR 158: 1329–1332

Tinuper P, Andermann F, Villemure JG et al. 1988 Functional hemispherectomy for treatment of epilepsy associated with hemiplegia. Ann Neurol 24: 27–34

Vinters HV, Wang R, Wiley CA. 1993 Herpesviruses in chronic encephalitis associated with intractable childhood epilepsy. Hum Pathol 24: 871–879

Walsh PJ. 1991 Treatment of Rasmussen's syndrome with intravenous gammaglobulin. In: Andermann F, ed. Chronic encephalitis and epilepsy: Rasmussen's syndrome. Boston: Butterworth-Heinemann, pp 201–204

Walter GF, Renella RR. 1989 Epstein–Barr virus in brain and Rasmussen's encephalitis. Lancet i: 279–280

11

Language disorders and epilepsy

K. Ballaban-Gil

A number of language disorders have been associated with epilepsy or electroencephalogram (EEG) epileptiform abnormalities. In children, these include the Landau–Kleffner syndrome (acquired epileptic aphasia), electrical status epilepticus in sleep (continuous spikes and waves during slow-wave sleep), developmental dysphasias and, possibly, autism. In adults, aphasia may be an ictal or postictal phenomenon. Nevertheless, the relation between epilepsy and language disorders in patients in whom the two coexist is not always clear. Often, the two conditions may be separate manifestations of a common underlying brain disorder (Deonna 1991). In some cases, however, it has been suggested that the epileptiform discharges may directly lead to the language dysfunction (Tassinari et al 1985, Deonna 1991, Perez et al 1993).

DISORDERS OF HIGHER CORTICAL FUNCTION

Landau–Kleffner syndrome (acquired epileptic aphasia)

Acquired aphasia associated with seizures and epileptiform EEG abormalities was first described by Landau & Kleffner in 1957. This syndrome is characterized by acute or subacute deterioration in language skills in children with previously normal expressive and receptive language development in association with EEG epileptiform abnormalities. It is more common in boys than girls (Msall et al 1986) and usually presents in the preschool years, although it may present as late as 7 years.

Often it begins with receptive difficulties. Parents may report that the child appears deaf and does not respond to verbal language. Later in the course, the child loses expressive language. Initially there are misarticulations, decreased length of sentences and decreased verbal output. Ultimately, the language disorder is usually of verbal auditory agnosia type, in which the children understand little or nothing of what they hear (i.e. cortical deafness) and are essentially mute, although other language disorders, including pure expressive dysphasias, have been reported (Deonna 1991). Language may fluctuate significantly over the course of the illness, with waxing and waning of the language abilities.

Between 70 and 80% of patients with acquired epileptic aphasia have seizures, but these are not mandatory for diagnosis (Hirsch et al 1990, Paquier et al 1992). The seizures may either precede or follow the onset of language regression. If present, seizures are usually easily controlled with antiepileptic medications, including benzodiazepines and valproate. The presence of epileptiform abnormalities on EEG recordings is necessary for the diagnosis of Landau–Kleffner syndrome. The EEG findings are variable and include generalized spike-and-wave (1–3 Hz) discharges, at times maximal over the temporal regions; bitemporal, independent or synchronous spikes; multifocal spikes; or unilateral temporal or central–temporal spikes, often similar in morphology and localization to those seen in benign rolandic epilepsy (Deonna 1991; Fig. 11.1). The background waking rhythms are usually normal (Hirsch et al 1990).

Although the syndrome was initially described as only a disorder of language, it is clear that children may have associated behavioral abnormali-

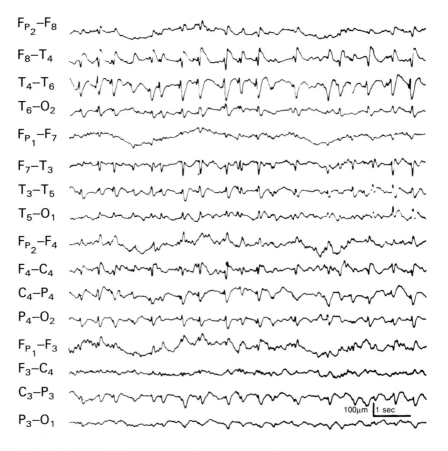

Fig. 11.1   Landau–Kleffner syndrome: Centrotemporal spikes.

ties, including increased activity, decreased attention, distractibility, temper tantrums, aggressiveness, social withdrawal and other social deficits. A few have more global cognitive deterioration (Hirsch et al 1990, Roulet et al 1991). Many of the behavioral abnormalities described in this syndrome are similar to those seen in autistic children (Roulet et al 1991, Perez et al 1993).

Few studies of long-term outcome have been conducted, although there are some reports on small numbers of patients. The course of the illness is variable. The outcomes reported in the literature range from complete recovery to severe aphasia in adult life (Deonna et al 1989, Dugas et al 1991, Paquier et al 1992). Bishop (1985) reported that children with an earlier age of onset had the worst outcomes, although Dugas et al (1991) did not corroborate this. The seizures usually remit during adolescence.

The pathologic basis of this disorder is unknown. Some researchers have suggested an encephalitic etiology (Deonna 1991) but this has not been demonstrated. Cole et al (1988) reported 2 patients with Landau–Kleffner syndrome who underwent temporal lobectomies, 1 for intractable epilepsy, the other for a severe language deficit. In both cases, pathologic examination revealed mild gliosis, without evidence of encephalitis. Otero et al (1989) reported a 7-year-old child with an acquired language disorder and seizures secondary to neurocysticercosis with a lesion in the left Sylvian fissure. However, this was not clearly a case of Landau–Kleffner syndrome because the aphasia may have been a result of the structural lesion. Neuroimaging procedures including computed tomography (CT) and magnetic resonance imaging (MRI), are generally normal. Recently, positron emission tomography (PET) studies have shown unilateral temporal or bitemporal abnormalities manifested either as increased or decreased glucose utilization (Maquet et al 1990).

The relation between the EEG abnormalities and the language dysfunction is not clear. Landau & Kleffner (1957) suggested that persistent discharges in brain regions involved in linguistic communication may result in functional ablation of the areas for normal linguistic activity. Other authors suggested that the epileptiform discharges themselves interfere with language function. Support for this notion comes from reports of transitory cognitive impairments associated with epileptiform discharges (see discussion of transitory cognitive impairment later in this chapter). Further support for a direct relation between epileptiform discharges and language function is found in the results of studies (Marescaux et al 1990, Lerman et al 1991) showing that therapy which successfully treated the EEG abnormalities often improved the language deficit as well. However, other investigators (Holmes et al 1981) have pointed out that there are many patients in whom the clinical seizures improve or resolve and the EEGs normalize, yet the patients have persisting language difficulties. Holmes et al (1981) reported 2 patients with dysphasia in whom there was no correlation between language abnormalities and epileptiform activity; during periods when there was little or no epileptiform activity, speech was still impaired. Others have also reported that there is frequently no correlation between the extent of the EEG abnormality and the degree of language deficit, as well as little correlation among seizure control, EEG improvement and language outcome (Paquier et al 1992). Additionally, many children with epileptiform abnormalities do not have language regression (Deonna 1993). Children with benign rolandic epilepsy, for example, have similar discharges in a similar localization and frequent discharges in sleep. Yet language function in these children does not deteriorate although there are rare reports of speech and oromotor deficits in patients with benign rolandic epilepsy (Roulet 1989,Deonna 1993a).

Unfortunately, there is no definitive treatment for Landau-Kleffner syndrome. In most cases, treatment with conventional antiepileptic drugs has been unsuccessful, or, at best, has temporarily improved language function (Marescaux et al 1990, Paquier et al 1992). As reviewed by Marescaux et al (1990), valproate, ethosuximide and benzodiazepenes are probably the most effective of the antiseizure medications, possibly because they reduce spike frequency. Phenobarbital (phenobarbitone), carbamazepine and phenytoin are either ineffective or said to worsen the electrographic signs and neuropsychological symptoms. A small number of children have been treated with corticosteroids, either oral steroids or adrenocorticotrophic hormone (ACTH), with encouraging improvement in their speech, often associated with normalization of their EEG and improved seizure control (Marescaux et al 1990, Lerman et al 1991). Therapy with corticosteroids appears to be most effective early in the course of the illness (Marescaux et al 1990, Lerman et al 1991). The choice of steroid, either oral or ACTH, is not clearly established. It has been suggested that initial high doses of steroids (hydrocortisone 12 mg/kg per day, prednisone 2 mg/kg per day), which are then tapered, and prolonged duration of treatment (6–12 months) may be most effective (Marescaux et al 1990). Because there are fluctuations in the course of the symptoms even in untreated cases, evaluating the response to treatment must include a temporal assessment of the relationship between treatment and improvements using repeated EEGs and formal neuro-psychological data (Marescaux et al 1990). Morrell and colleagues (1990) have reported improvements in language following subpial transection in a few children, but this remains a controversal treatment.

Developmental language disorders

Children with developmental language disorders, or developmental dysphasia, have delayed, deviant language development from infancy, without a demonstrable regression. Abnormalities may include difficulties in either expressive or receptive language or in both. In some instances, children may have abnormal, delayed language which is followed by a regression and worsening of their already aberrant language. Frequently, language dysfunction in the children with severe developmental dysphasia is similar to that seen in children with acquired aphasia.

Tuchman et al (1991b) reported that the incidence of epilepsy in dysphasic children without associated disabilities was 8%, which is greater than the 1% incidence in the general population. If there was a history of regression, the incidence of epilepsy was 36%. Verbal auditory agnosia, the most frequent language disorder seen in children with Landau–Kleffner syndrome, was associated with the highest risk of epilepsy — 58%. There are a number of reports of epileptiform EEGs in dysphasic children, as well. Sato & Dreifuss (1973) reported a child with developmental expressive aphasia and bitemporal spikes and sharp waves. Maccario and colleagues (1982) reported 7 patients with developmental dysphasia with EEG abnormalities. Two of those patients had previous febrile seizures and none had afebrile seizures. The EEG abnormalities included focal or bilaterally synchronous spike-wave or sharp wave discharges. Tuchman et al (1991b) reported a 9% incidence of epileptiform EEG abnormalities in dysphasic children without a history of seizures. The incidence of epileptiform abnormalities can be state-dependent, and prolonged all-night recordings may be necessary to demonstrate abnormal discharges. Echenne et al (1992) reported epileptiform abnormalities in 30 of 32 dysphasic children in whom all-night EEG recordings were performed. The incidence of epileptiform abnormalities was much lower (10/32) when only routine EEGs were evaluated, and even daytime sleeping records had epileptiform abnormalities in only 13 cases. Documented abnormalities included generalized continuous spikewaves, bursts of generalized spikewaves, generalized spikewaves associated with focal spikes in either right or left temporal occipital or rolandic areas, and bilateral temporal or rolandic spikes and polyspikes.

The EEG abnormalities described in these cases of developmental dysphasia are similar to those reported in acquired epileptic aphasia. Several researchers (Maccario et al 1982, Deonna 1991, 1993, Echenne et al 1992) have postulated that in such cases, the underlying mechanism is identical to that in Landau–Kleffner syndrome, but the dysfunction begins before language has developed. Support for this theory includes a report of homozygous twin girls, one of whom had a developmental dysphasia and the other who had Landau–Kleffner syndrome (Echenne et al 1992).

There are no reports of medical treatment in this population, aside from educational remediation.

Electrical status epilepticus in sleep (continuous spikes and waves during slow sleep)

Electrical status epilepticus in sleep (ESES) is a disorder in which children have developmental regression associated with an epileptiform EEG. This syndrome was first reported by Patry et al in 1971. In it, language and cognitive development before onset are normal or, less frequently, abnormal. The onset of ESES is associated with intellectual regression which is usually global, including behavior and cognition. In some cases, there may be a deterioration in language out of proportion to other abilities (Tassinari et al 1985). Behavioral changes include decreased attention span, hyperactivity, aggressiveness, difficulty in interpersonal interactions, and 'psychotic behavior'. Many of these behaviors are similar to those reported in autistic children.

The majority of children with ESES have seizures which often predate the onset of ESES. New seizure types, particularly absence seizures, may occur at the time the ESES emerges. Tassinari et al (1985) described three groups of patients based on seizure semiology. The first group consisted of children who had only rare nocturnal motor seizures. The second group included patients with a history of nocturnal generalized or partial motor seizures, who developed absence seizures at the time of diagnosis of ESES. The last group was characterized by a history of rare nocturnal seizures, who developed atypical absences, often with atonic or clonic features. Tonic seizures have not been reported in this syndrome, and this can be important in distinguishing between ESES and Lennox–Gastaut syndrome.

The EEG findings in ESES vary according to the state of the patient. According to the strict definition of Patry et al (1971), epileptiform discharges must be present during at least 85% of non-rapid eye movement (REM), or slow-wave, sleep. The percentage of sleep recording during which epileptiform discharges are present is referred to as the spike-wave index. Most authors accept this definition of ESES (Morikawa et al 1985, Tassinari et al 1985), although others include children with a spike-wave index of less than 85% if other clinical features are characteristic (Hirsch et al 1990). During slow-wave sleep, the discharges are usually generalized spike-wave complexes with a frequency of 1.5–2 Hz (Patry et al 1971, Tassinari et al 1985). Less commonly, there may be continuous focal discharges or nearly continuous diffuse bisynchronous sharp waves (Morikawa et al 1985, Jayakar & Seshia 1991; Fig. 11.2). Sleep spindles, K-complexes and vertex waves are often absent. During wakefulness and REM sleep, the record changes abruptly and is characterized by a spike-wave index of less than 25% (Fig. 11.3). The distribution of the discharges also changes, with focal discharges, predominantly frontal, being more common than generalized ones (Tassinari et al 1985, Perez et al 1993). The waking background rhythms are usually normal or near-normal (Morikawa et al 1985). The EEG findings differ from those in benign rolandic epilepsy in that the focal discharges in ESES are more commonly frontocentral, while those in rolandic epilepsy are usually centrotemporal (Tassinari et al 1985). Although sleep increases the discharges in both ESES and benign rolandic epilepsy, in the latter disorder, the discharges are very rarely present in over 85% of the sleep record (Tassinari et al 1985).

Seizures and ESES usually remit in adolescence, and this is often associated with a degree of neuropsychological improvement. As in Landau–Kleffner syndrome, there are few reports of long-term outcome in ESES (Roulet et al 1991). Most patients have persisting cognitive impairments, including verbal

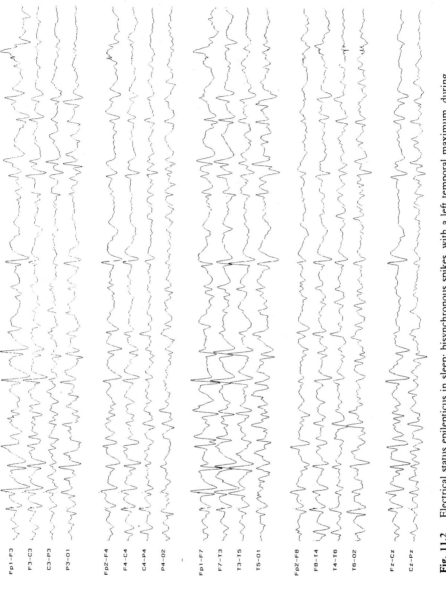

Fig. 11.2 Electrical status epilepticus in sleep: bisynchronous spikes, with a left temporal maximum, during non-rapid eye movement sleep.

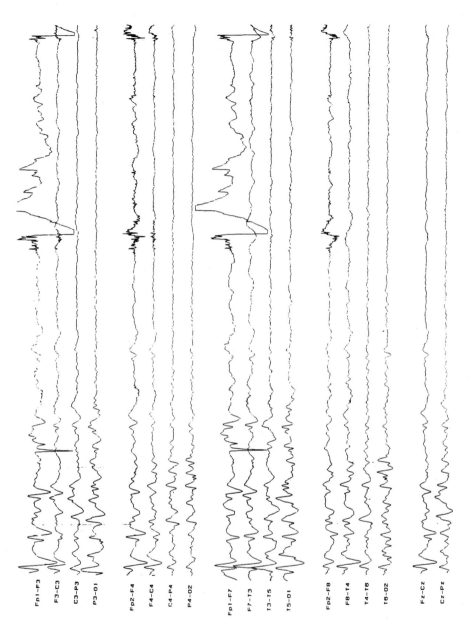

Fig. 11.3 Awakening record in patient with electrical status epilepticus in sleep (same patient as in Fig.11.2). Note the abrupt cessation of spike discharges with arousal.

deficits demonstrable in some instances by a discrepancy between performance and verbal IQs (Boel & Casaer 1989, Roulet et al 1991, Perez et al 1993). EEG abnormalities may also persist. There may be a correlation between the degree of mental deterioration and the spike-wave index and the duration of the EEG abnormalities over time (Tassinari et al 1985). There is no consistently effective treatment for ESES although, as in Landau–Kleffner syndrome, steroids, benzodiazepine, and ethosuximide have been reported to improve both EEG abnormalities and neuropsychological function (Boel & Casaer 1989, Perez et al 1993).

ESES and Landau–Kleffner are classified separately by the Commission on Classification and Terminology of the International League Against Epilepsy (1989). However, as pointed out by some authors (Hirsch et al 1990, Roulet et al 1991), the syndromes have many common features and may represent different manifestations of the same underlying pathology. Both involve a regression in cognitive function in association with an epileptiform EEG. The localization of the discharges may also be similar, although focal discharges in Landau–Kleffner tend to be more centrotemporal, and those in ESES more frontal or frontotemporal. Clinical seizure types are similar, as is the natural history with disappearance of seizures and EEG abnormalities in adolescence. Hirsch et al (1990) reported 5 patients with Landau–Kleffner syndrome, all of whom had continuous spike-wave discharges at some point during their syndrome.

Autism, autistic regression and disintegrative psychosis

Autism is a behavioral syndrome characterized by impaired socialization, impaired communication, language disorder, inadequately modulated affect, and abnormal play. There may be associated symptoms, including stereotyped behaviors, abnormal responses to sensory stimuli, attentional difficulties and cognitive abnormalities (Rapin 1991, Tuchman et al 1991a). Some researchers believe that children must meet all the criteria of autism, as specified by DSM-IIIR (American Psychiatric Association, 1987), to be classified as autistic. Others believe that there is a variable expression of autistic abnormalities (Rapin 1991), with expression ranging from mildly involved through severely impaired. Further elaboration regarding the definition and diagnosis of autism is beyond the scope of the article (for review, see Rapin 1991). However, many of the behavioral, cognitive and language abnormalities described in children with Landau–Kleffner syndrome and ESES are similar to those seen in children with autism (Roulet et al 1991, Perez et al 1993).

While disabilities are present from infancy in many children with autism, in other cases the disabilities are acquired following a period of normal development (Kurita 1985, Rapin 1991). In their study of 314 autistic children, Tuchman et al (1991a) found a history of regression in 39%. Kurita (1985) similarly reported a history of speech loss in 37% of autistic children. Various names have been given to this type of autism, including autistic regression, disintegrative psychosis, Heller's dementia, pervasive disintegrative disorder of development, acquired autistic syndrome, and childhood-onset pervasive developmental disorder. Steffenburg (1991) reported a 38% incidence of epilepsy in autistic or autistic-like children. Tuchman et al (1991b) found that 13% of autistic children without severe mental retardation, but with a history of regression, had epilepsy. Epileptiform EEG abnormalities were present in an additional 8% of autistic but non-epileptic children. Evans-Jones & Rosenbloom (1978) reported paroxysmal abnormalities in 3 of 9 children with disintegrative psychosis. It seems possible that in some cases, particularly those with a history of regression, the mechanism of the dysfunction may be similar to that in Landau–Kleffner syndrome and ESES (Deonna et al 1993b).

TRANSITORY COGNITIVE IMPAIRMENT

The causal relationship between the epileptiform abnormalities and these aforementioned disorders of language has not been clearly established. Studies which have demonstrated brief cognitive deficits, or transitory cognitive impairment, during epileptiform discharges support the notion of a direct cause and effect. Most studies have demonstrated transitory cognitive impairments in approximately 50% of subjects. Simple motor tasks and reaction time measurements are less sensitive in detecting these brief impairments, while tasks involving memory and language function are more sensitive (Aarts et al 1984, Binnie 1993).

Aarts and colleagues (1984) have demonstrated that individuals with generalized or focal discharges have transitory cognitive impairment. Discharges during stimulus presentation were associated with transitory cognitive impairment, while discharges during the patients' responses were not. Individuals with left-sided or dominant hemisphere epileptiform activity had increased errors in verbal tasks, while patients with right-sided discharges had impairment of non-verbal tasks. The selective nature of the impairments based on spike location may suggest that, at least in focal cases, the transient impairment is not due to a general effect on attention. Rather, the focal discharges may disrupt the specific functions for which the particular area is responsible, leaving other psychological functions unimpaired (Aarts et al 1984). Thus, only language function may be impaired while other cognitive functions remain intact. Similarly, Siebelink et al (1988, Kasteleijn-Nolst Trenite et al 1988) demonstrated that subclinical generalized or focal epileptiform discharges ranging in duration from less than 1 second to greater than 3 seconds momentarily interfered with academic skills, including reading and arithmetic. They also found that on IQ testing, certain subtests, particularly those involved with short-term verbal memory, were particularly affected by epileptiform activity. Furthermore, the longer the discharge, the greater the effect on the child's performance. Shewmon & Erwin (1988) demonstrated that this transient impairment may be secondary to the aftercoming slow wave following the spike discharge. They hypothesized that the slow wave results from inhibitory hyperpolarization of the neurons surrounding the spike focus. This inhibition may be responsible for suppressing the normal functions of those neurons, as well as terminating epileptiform activity (Shewmon & Erwin 1988).

APHASIA AND SEIZURES

Ictal and postictal aphasia

In older patients, the occurrence of aphasia and epilepsy (or epileptiform EEGs) is usually the consequence of an underlying cerebral lesion, such as a tumor or a stroke. Such structural lesions may, on the one hand, damage cortical areas responsible for language, resulting in aphasia. Additionally, they may be potentially epileptogenic and lead to seizures. Less frequently, however, aphasia may be a direct consequence of the epileptiform activity, either as an ictal or postictal phenomenon.

Ictal speech arrest, which is a complete cessation of speech, is more common than ictal aphasia. Speech arrest is not necesssarily aphasia; it may be due to transient motor dysfunction secondary to ictal discharges in the motor or supplementary motor area (Rosenbaum et al 1986, Gabr et al 1989, Lüders et al 1991). In these cases, language function may actually be intact. Definite aphasia during seizures is less common. To differentiate between motor impairment of speech versus true aphasia, some authors define ictal aphasia as a state in which the patient has verbal output that is dysphasic — dysfluent, dysnomic or paraphasic (Rosenbaum et al 1986). Some reports of ictal aphasia have been due to impaired consciousness. Both conditions may complicate the evaluation of language function. Hence there are only a few reports of patients with clearly documented aphasia whose onset correlated with the appearance of an electrographic seizure pattern, usually in the left hemisphere (temporal or centroparietal), and which resolved when the seizure discharge ended (Rosenbaum et al 1986, Wells et al 1992). There are also reports of more prolonged periods or aphasia which have been attributed to complex partial status epilepticus, of aphasic status epilepticus (Depasquet et al 1976, Hamilton & Matthews 1979, Racy et al 1980, Dinner et al 1981). However, a temporal relationship between the ictal discharges and the aphasia was not demonstrated. Thus, while the ictal discharges were intermittent, the aphasia persisted between the ictal discharges. Furthermore, in some of these cases, language function did not immediately improve following administration of anti-epileptic drugs (AEDs) which stopped the seizure discharge. In these cases, the aphasia may have been secondary to underlying structural brain disease or post ictal Todd's phenomenon. These cases of aphasic status epilepticus without a clear temporal correlation between the ictal discharges and the aphasia may be similar to some cases of acquired epileptic aphasia in childhood.

Speech disturbances are common during complex partial seizures (Gabr et al 1989). Utilizing surface and subdural electrode recordings, Gabr et al (1989) evaluated the speech manifestations of 100 seizures in 35 patients with temporal lobe epilepsy. They divided speech manifestations into three groups: seizures with vocalization; seizures with normal speech; and seizures with abnormal speech. The abnormal speech was further subdivided into four categories including speech arrest, dysarthria, dysphasia and non-indentifiable speech, defined as monosyllabic utterances and unintelligible words or phrases. They found that the only speech manifestations with localizing value were postictal dysphasia and ictal identifiable speech characterized by spontaneous, linguistically correct speech during the ictus. Postictal dysphasia was associated with seizure onset in the dominant hemisphere, while ictal identifiable speech was associated with seizure onset in the non-dominant temporal lobe. All other ictal speech abnormalities occurred in seizures arising from either dominant or non-dominant hemispheres, and hence had no localizing value.

ELECTRICAL STIMULATION STUDIES AND LANGUAGE

Cortical electrical stimulation studies performed during surgery for epilepsy have also served as useful tools in the study of language. Penfield and colleagues (Penfield & Rasmussen 1949, Penfield & Roberts 1959) were the first to demonstrate language deficits produced by electrical stimulation. They reported several areas of language function, including areas corresponding to Broca's area, Wernicke's area and supplementary motor cortex.

Electrical stimulation can produce both excitatory and inhibitory effects, but it is likely that the effects on language are secondary to the inhibitory effects of temporary depolarization of the neurons (Ojemann et al 1989). As with speech abnormalities associated with seizures, it is important to differentiate between deficits secondary to language impairment and those secondary to motor impairment or impairment in level of responsiveness. Positive motor responses can be excluded as the cause of the deficit by observing for movements of the tongue or facial muscles (Schäffler et al 1993). Negative motor responses or the inability to perform voluntary movements during stimulation may also interfere with verbal output. Some investigators rule out this possibility by having subjects perform oral motor tasks during stimulation (Lüders et al 1991, Schäffler et al 1993). Others point to the ability of the patient to have some verbal output during stimulation to exclude this effect (Ojemann et al 1989). Finally, the possibility of general impairment in responsiveness can be excluded by having the patient perform non-verbal tasks (Lüders et al 1991).

Classic theories regarding the localization of language function have been challenged by recent electrical stimulation studies. Ojemann et al (1989) used intraoperative electrical stimulation to map language abilities in 117 patients. In many of these, language functions were highly localized to small areas, or mosaics, of 1–2 cm^2, usually with one area in the frontal region and one or more in the temporopariental area. There was significant variability in the location of these areas between patients, with relatively few patients having only frontal or only temporoparietal language areas. The area of the individual mosaics, as well as the total area of cortex involved in language function, was found to be much smaller than that associated with Broca's and Wernicke's areas. Lüders et al (1991), utilizing subdural grid electrodes, demonstrated an additional area of cortex involved in language processing in the fusiform (occipitotemporal) gyrus of the basal temporal region of the dominant hemisphere. The deficits produced by stimulation of this area were similar to those observed with stimulation of Wernicke's area. Lesions in Broca's area traditionally involve deficits in expressive language with intact language comprehension. Yet Lüders et al (1991) and Schäffler et al (1993) both reported deficits in language comprehension resulting from electrical stimulation of Broca's area in addition to the expected deficits in language output. It is important to note that all these studies were performed in patients with cerebral pathology and possible compensatory changes. These cases may therefore not represent the areas of language function in normal individuals.

KEY POINTS FOR CLINICAL PRACTICE

- Some language disorders, both acquired or developmental, may be associated with epileptiform EEG abnormalities or epilepsy.
- In many instances, the epileptiform abnormalities are an epiphenomenon of the underlying structural brain pathology. However, in some cases, the epileptiform activity may be directly related to the language deficits.
- In addition to language deficits, there may be abnormalities in behavior and cognition.
- The clinician should consider obtaining EEGs in children with a history of regression in language function. Some studies suggest that prolonged all-night recordings have the highest yield.
- Although there is controversy as to whether the epileptic abnormalities are causally related to the language deficit, the identification of such abnormalities offers some possible therapeutic intervention, such as the option to use antiepileptic medications or corticosteroids.
- In adult patients acute aphasia is most commonly secondary to a structural lesion or metabolic derangements. However, in some instances, the aphasia may be secondary to seizure activity, as well.

ACKNOWLEDGEMENTS

I wish to thank Dr I. Rapin for providing Figure 11.1 and Dr S. Moshé for reviewing the manuscript.

REFERENCES

Aarts J H P, Binnie C D, Smit A M et al. 1984 Selective cognitive impairment during focal and generalized epileptiform EEG activity. Brain 107: 293–308

American Psychiatric Association Committe on Nomenclature and Statistics 1987. Diagnostic and statistical manual of Mental Disorders 3rd edn. Washington: American Psychiatric Association

Binnie C D. 1993 Significance and management of transitory cognitive impairment due to subclinical EEG discharges in children. Brain Dev 15: 23–30

Bishop D V M. 1985 Age of onset and outcome in 'acquired aphasia with convulsive disorder' (Landau–Kleffner syndrome). Dev Med Child Neurol 27: 705–712.

Boel M, Casaer P. 1989 Continuous spikes and waves during slow sleep: a 30 months follow-up study of neuropsychological recovery and EEG findings. Neuropediatrics 20: 176–180

Cole A J, Andermann F, Taylor L et al. 1988 The Landau–Kleffner syndrome of acquired epileptic aphasia: unusual clinical outcome, surgical experience, and absence of encephalitis. Neurology 38: 31–38

Deonna T 1991 Acquired epileptiform aphasia in children (Landau–Kleffner syndrome). J Clin Neurophysiol 8: 288–298

Deonna T 1993 Annotation: Cognitive and behavioral correlates of epileptic activity in children. J Child Psychol Psychiatn 34: 611–620

Deonna T, Peter C, Ziegler A L. 1989 Adult follow-up of the acquired aphasia–epilepsy syndrome in childhood. Report of 7 cases. Neuropediatrics 20: 132–138

Deonna T, Roulet E, Fontan D et al. 1993a Prolonged speech and oromotor deficits of epileptic origin in benign partial epilepsy with rolandic spikes: relationship to acquired epileptic aphasia. Neuropediatrics 24: 83–87

Deonna T, Ziegler A L, Moura-Serra J et al. 1993b Autistic regression in relation to limbic pathology and epilepsy: report of 2 cases. Dev Med Child Neurol 35: 158–176

Depasquet E G, Gaudin E S, Bianchi A et al. 1976 Prolonged and monosymptomatic dysphasic status epilepticus. Neurology 24: 244–247

Dinner D S, Lueders H, Lederman R et al. 1981 Aphasic status epilepticus: a case report. Neurology 31: 888–890

Dugas M, Gerard C L, Franc S et al. 1991 Natural history, course and prognosis of the Landau and Kleffner syndrome. In: Pavao Martins, I, Castro-Caldas, A, van Dongen, H R et al, eds. Acquired aphasia in children. Netherlands: Kluwer Academic Publishers, pp 263–277

Echenne B, Cheminal R, Rivier F et al. 1992 Epileptic electoencephalographic abnormalities and developmental dysphasias: a study of 32 patients. Brain Dev 14: 216–225

Evans-Jones L G, Rosenbloom L. 1978 Disintegrative psychosis in childhood. Dev Med Child Neurol 20: 462–470

Gabr M, Lüders H, Dinner D et al. 1989 Speech manifestations in lateralization of temporal lobe seizures. Ann Neurol 25: 82–87

Hamilton M G, Mattews T. 1979 Aphasia: the sole manifestation of focal status epilepticus. Neurology 29: 745–748

Hirsch E, Marescaux C, Maquet P et al. 1990 Landau–Kleffner syndrome: a clinical and EEG study of five cases. Epilepsia 31: 756–767

Holmes G L, McKeever M, Saunders Z. 1981 Epileptic activity in aphasia of childhood: an epiphenomenon? Epilepsia 22: 631–639

Jayakar P B, Seshia S S. 1991 Electrical status epilepticus during slow wave sleep: a review. J Clin Neurophysiol 8: 299–311

Kasteleijn-Nolst Trenite D G A, Bakker D J, Binnie C D et al. 1988 Psychological effects of subclinical epileptiform EEG discharges. I. Scholastic skills. Epilepsy Res 2: 111–116

Kurita H. 1985 Infantile autism with speech loss before the age of 30 months. J Am Acad Child Psychiatry 24: 191–196

Landau W M, Kleffner F R. 1957 Syndrome of acquired aphasia with convulsive disorder in children. Neurology 7: 523–530

Lerman P, Lerman-Sagie T, Kivity S. 1991 Effect of early corticosteroid therapy for Landau–Kleffner syndrome. Dev Med Child Neurol 33: 257–266

Lüders H, Lesser R P, Hahn J et al. 1991 Basal temporal language area. Brain 114: 743–754

Maccario M, Hefferen S J, Keblusek S J. 1982 Developmental dysphasia and electrographic abnormalities. Dev Med Child Neurol 24: 141–155

Maquet P, Hirsch E, Salmon E et al. 1990 Cerebral glucose utilization during sleep in Landau–Kleffner syndrome: a PET study. Epilepsia 31: 778–783

Marescaux C, Hirsch E, Finck S et al. 1990 Landau–Kleffner syndrome: a pharmacologic study of five cases. Epilepsia 31: 768–777

Morikawa T, Mazakazu S, Osawa T et al. 1985 Five children with continuous spike-wave discharges during sleep. In: Roger J, Dravet C, Bureau M et al, eds. Epileptic syndromes in infancy, childhood and adolescence. Eurotext. London: John Libby, pp 205–212

Morrell F, Cooper M, Ali A et al. 1990 Landau–Kleffner syndrome: metabolic, blood flow and electrographic studies. Epilepsia 31: 672

Msall M, Shapiro B, Balfour P et al. 1986 Acquired epileptic aphasia: diagnostic aspects of progressive language loss in preschool children. Clin Pediatr 25: 248–251

Ojemann G, Ojemann J, Lettich E et al. 1989 Cortical language localization in left, dominant hemisphere: an electrical stimulation mapping investigation in 117 patients. J Neurosurg 71: 316–326

Otero E, Cordova S, Diaz F et al. 1989 Acquired epileptic aphasia (the Landau–Kleffner syndrome) due to neurocysticercosis. Epilepsia 30: 569–572

Paquier P, Van Dongen H R, Loonen C B. 1992 The Landau–Kleffner syndrome or "acquired aphasia with convulsive disorder": long-term follow-up of six children and a review of the recent literature. Arch Neurol 49: 354–359

Patry G, Lyagoubi S, Tassinari C A. 1971 Subclinical "electrical status epilepticus" induced by sleep in children. A clinical and electrographic study of six cases. Arch Neurol 24: 242–252

Penfield W, Rasmussen T. 1949 Vocalization and arrest of speech. Arch Neurol Psychiatry 61: 21–27

Penfield W, Roberts L. 1959 Speech and brain mechanisms. Princeton, NJ: Princeton University Press

Perez E R, Davidoff V, Despland P et al. 1993 Mental and behavioral deterioration of children with epilepsy and CSWS: acquired epileptic frontal syndrome. Dev Med Child Neurol 35: 661–674

Racy A, Osborn M A, Vern B A et al. 1980 Epileptic aphasia: first onset of prolonged monosymptomatic status epilepticus in adults. Arch Neurol 37; 419–422

Rapin I. 1991 Autistic children: diagnosis and clinical features. Pediatrics 87 (suppl 1): 751–760

Rosenbaum D H, Siegel M, Barr W B et al. 1986 Epileptic aphasia. Neurology 36: 822–825

Roulet E, Deonna T, Despland P A. 1989 Prolonged intermittent drooling and oromotor dyspraxia in benign childhood epilepsy with centrotemporal spikes. Epilepsia 30: 564–568

Roulet E, Deonna T, Gaillard F et al. 1991 Acquired aphasia, dementia and behavior disorder with epilepsy and continuous spike and waves during sleep in a child. Epilepsia 32: 495–503

Sato S, Dreifuss F E. 1973 Electroencephalographic findings in a patient with developmental expressive aphasia. Neurology 23: 181–185

Schäffler L, Lüders H O, Dinner D S et al. 1993 Comprehension deficits elicited by electrical stimulation of Broca's area. Brain 116: 695–715

Shewmon D A, Erwin R J. 1988 Focal spike-induced cerebral dysfunction is related to the after-coming slow wave. Ann Neurol 23: 131–137

Siebelink B M, Bakker D J, Binnie C D et al. 1988 Psychological effects of subclinical epileptiform EEG discharges in children. II. General intelligence tests. Epilepsy Res 2: 117–121

Steffenburg S. 1991 Neuropsychiatric asessment of children with autism: a population based study. Dev Med Child Neurol 33: 495–511

Tassinari C A, Bureau M, Dravet C et al. 1985 Epilepsy with continuous spikes and waves during slow sleep. In: Roger J, Dravet C, Bureau M et al, eds. Epileptic syndromes in infancy, childhood and adolescence. Eurotext. London: John Libby, pp 194–204

Tuchman R F, Rapin I, Shinnar S. 1991a Autistic and dysphasic children. I. Clinical characteristics. Pediatrics 88: 1211–1218

Tuchman R F, Rapin I, Shinnar S. 1991b Autistic and dysphasic children. II. Epilepsy. Pediatrics 88: 1219–1225

Wells C R, Labar D R, Solomon G E. 1992 Aphasia as the sole manifestation of simple partial status epilepticus. Epilepsia 33: 84–87

12

Endocrine aspects of epilepsy in women

A. G. Herzog

This chapter proposes the following:

1. There are reciprocal relations between cerebral excitability and reproductive hormonal secretions.
2. There is an association between epilepsy and reproductive endocrine disorders.
3. The interaction between the brain and hormones is important in the pathophysiology and treatment of both epilepsy and reproductive disorders.

The focus is principally clinical and emphasizes complex partial seizures, which are the most common form of epilepsy in adults and which are associated with an unusually high prevalence of reproductive disorders.

EFFECTS OF HORMONES ON EPILEPSY

Experimental data

In most experimental animal models, estrogen lowers the thresholds of seizures induced by electroshock, kindling, pentylenetetrazol, kainic acid, ethyl chloride and other agents and procedures (Spiegel & Wycis 1945, Logothetis & Harner 1960, Woolley & Timiras 1962, Nicoletti et al 1985, Hom & Buterbaugh 1986). In fact, the topical brain application or intravenous systemic administration of estradiol in rabbits produces a significant increase in spontaneous electrically recorded spike discharges (Logothetis & Harner 1960). This increase is more dramatic in animals with pre-existent cortical lesions (Marcus et al 1966). Progesterone, on the other hand, lessens spontaneous induced epileptiform discharges (Spiegel & Wycis 1945, Landgren et al 1978, Nicoletti et al 1985).

Physiological data

Catamenial epilepsy refers to seizure exacerbation in relation to the menstrual cycle (Laidlaw 1956, Newmark & Penry 1980). Three patterns exist.

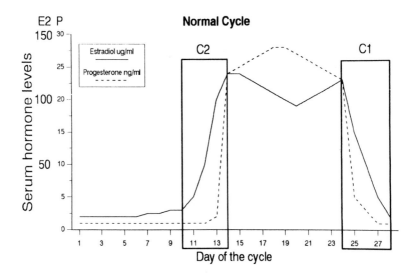

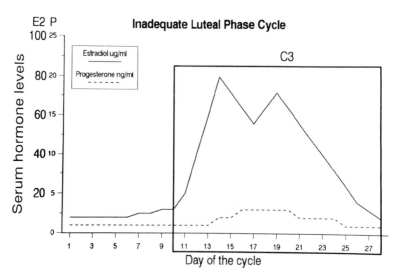

Fig. 12.1   The three patterns of catamenial exacerbation of epilepsy — Cl, C2, C3 — in relation to serum estradiol (E2) and progesterone (P) levels.

1. One-quarter to three-quarters of women with epilepsy describe an increase in seizures during the few days before menstruation and the first 2 or 3 days of menstruation.

2. A predilection for seizure exacerbation may also occur near the middle of the cycle, prior to ovulation, between days 10 and 14.

3. A more difficult pattern to discern is one in which seizures are frequent between day 10 of one cycle and day 2 of the next, relative to the interval between days 3 and 9 (Fig. 12.1).

Physiological variations in endocrine secretion during the menstrual cycle influence the occurrence of seizures. In ovulatory cycles, seizure frequency shows a statistically significant positive correlation with the serum estradiol/progesterone ratio (Backstrom 1976). This ratio is highest during the days prior to ovulation and menstruation, and is lowest during the early and mid luteal phase (Backstrom 1976). Premenstrual exacerbation of seizures has been attributed to the withdrawal of the antiseizure effects of progesterone (Laidlaw 1956). Mid-cycle exacerbations may be due to the preovulatory surge of estrogen unaccompanied by any rise in progesterone until ovulation occurs (Backstrom 1976). Seizures are least common during the mid luteal phase, when progesterone levels are highest (Backstrom 1976).

The premenstrual exacerbation of seizures may be related to a decline in serum antiseizure medication levels as well as to a withdrawal of the anticonvulsant effects of progesterone (Shavit et al 1984, Roscizewska et al 1986). Plasma levels of antiepileptic drug generally decrease several days before menstruation (Shavit et al 1984, Roscizewska et al 1986). Hepatic mechanisms have been implicated (Shavit et al 1984, Roscizewska et al 1986) because antiseizure drugs and gonadal steroids are metabolized by the same microsomal enzyme systems in hepatic cells. The premenstrual decline in gonadal steroid secretion, therefore, may permit increased metabolism of antiepileptic drugs, resulting in lower serum levels.

Pathological data

Inadequate luteal phase refers to less than normal progesterone secretion during the second half of the cycle, regardless of whether ovulation occurs or not (Jones 1976). It can be documented by one or preferably more findings, including:

1. A failure of the basal body temperature to rise by 0.33°C for at least 10 days during the second half of the menstrual cycle;
2. A serum progesterone level of less than 5.0 ng/ml during the mid luteal phase, generally measured between days 20 and 22 of a 28-day cycle;
3. A biopsy which shows underdeveloped secretory endometrium, 8–10 days after ovulation.

During the second half of these cycles serum estradiol/progesterone ratios and seizure frequencies tend to be higher than in normal ovulatory cycles (Backstrom 1976, Mattson et al 1981) and seizure exacerbation may extend from day 10 of one cycle to day 2 of the next.

Pharmacological data

Exogenous hormonal administration also influences human electrical brain-wave activity and epilepsy. Logothetis et al (1959) showed that intravenously administered conjugated estrogen activated epileptiform discharges in 11 of 16 epileptic women and was associated with clinical seizures in 4. Backstrom et al (1984) found that intravenous infusion of progesterone, sufficient to produce luteal-phase serum levels, was associated with a significant decrease in interictal spike frequency in 4 of 7 women with partial epilepsy.

EFFECTS OF EPILEPSY ON HORMONES

Transient postictal effects

Transient endocrine changes may occur following generalized motor and partial seizures. Significant and marked elevation of serum prolactin and cortisol occurs during the first 15 min following a generalized motor seizure and then gradually returns to baseline over the subsequent hour (Trimble 1978, Abbott et al 1980). Simulated generalized seizures, in contrast, are associated with elevation of serum cortisol alone (Abbott et al 1980). Prolactin elevations demonstrate a gradient of occurrence in relation to seizure type. Specifically, Wyllie et al (1984) demonstrated serum prolactin elevations following 80% of grand mal seizures, 45% of complex partial seizures, and only 15% of simple partial seizures. Sperling et al (1986), using depth electrode recordings and video monitoring in human epileptic patients, have reported that prolactin elevation consistently follows seizures which produce intense widespread mesial temporal lobe limbic seizure discharge and does not occur after seizures which do not involve these areas. Transient postictal prolactin elevation has been proposed as a criterion for distinguishing epileptic seizures from pseudoseizures. The absence of prolactin elevation, however, does not rule out the occurrence of epileptic seizures. Furthermore, less than two- to threefold elevation of prolactin above baseline or normal levels may not distinguish epileptic seizures from the mild prolactin elevations that can accompany stress or occur postprandially.

Persistent interictal effects

In an investigation of 50 consecutive women with clinical and electro-encephalographic features of temporal lobe epilepsy (TLE), 28 (56%) had amenorrhea, oligomenorrhea or abnormally long or short menstrual cycle intervals (Herzog et al 1986). Nineteen (38%) of the 28 women with epilepsy and menstrual disorders had readily identifiable reproductive endocrine disorders: polycystic ovarian syndrome (PCO) in 10, hypogonadotropic hypogonadism (HH; hypothalamic amenorrhea) in 6, premature menopause in 2, and functional hyperprolactinemia in 1 (Herzog et al 1986). The numbers of women with clinical and endocrine features of PCO (20%) and of HH (12%) were significantly greater than the estimated frequencies (5 and 1.5%, respectively) in the general female population.

PATHOGENETIC MECHANISMS

Medications

Use of antiepileptic drugs is associated with diminished free/total testosterone ratios in the serum (Herzog et al 1986). The measured free testosterone actually included the entire biologically active portion of testosterone, which means both the large albumin-bound fraction as well as the small entirely free fraction. Furthermore, our data demonstrated an association between use of antiseizure medications and very low serum levels of the adrenal androgen metabolite dehydroepiandrosterone sulfate (Herzog et al 1986, Levesque et al 1986). There was no statistically significant relationship overall, however, between the occurrence of menstrual disorders and the use of antiepileptic drugs (53% among users versus 60% among non-users). Although a recent report demonstrated a relationship between valproate use and PCO (Isojarvi et al 1993), valproate was not yet in common use at the time of our investigation and was not one of the medications taken by any of our subjects. PCO, moreover, was more common among the untreated (30%) than the treated (13%) epileptic women. PCO is characterized by abnormally high androgen levels. Antiseizure medications, such as barbiturates, phenytoin and carbamazepine, induce hepatic enzymes and thereby lower biologically active androgen levels. Valproate does not. It is possible, therefore, that the higher occurrence of PCO among women who take valproate may be related to the failure of this drug to induce hepatic enzymes which lower biologically active fractions of testosterone, although other potential mechanisms of action remain to be assessed. In summary, although antiseizure medications alter reproductive hormone levels, it is unlikely that all of the reproductive endocrine disorders among women with epilepsy can be attributed entirely to drug effects.

Neuroendocrine

Abnormal serum levels of gonadotropins and prolactin, and altered luteinizing hormone (LH) response to gonadotropin-releasing hormone (GnRH) in these women suggested altered function of the hypothalamopituitary axis. Primary structural lesions at the level of the hypothalamus or pituitary, however, were not evident by computed tomography or clinical assessment and follow-up (Herzog et al 1982, 1986).

Abundant data suggest that altered function of temporal lobe structures, a factor common to all patients with TLE who have reproductive dysfunction, may contribute to reproductive and sexual changes (Herzog 1989). TLE most commonly originates from or rapidly involves limbic portions of the temporal lobe. Some of these limbic structures are comprised of anatomically distinct functional divisions that exert opposing modulatory influences on the structure and function of reproductive organs. A notable example is the amygdala, which can be parcelled into corticomedial and basolateral divisions. Each has its largely separate outflow tract, the stria terminalis and ventral amygdalofugal pathway, respectively. Bilateral ablations of the basolateral portion of the amygdala in adult female deer mice can induce anovulatory cycles and polycystic ovarian changes. Stimulation of the corticomedial amygdala in a number of mammalian species induces ovulation and uterine contractions.

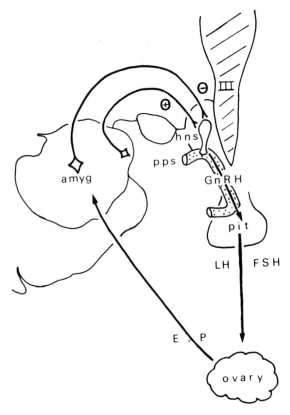

Fig. 12.2   A cross-section of the anterior temporal lobe and diencephalon. It depicts direct projections from the two anatomically distinct functional divisions of the amygdala (amyg) to the same ventromedial hypothalamic neurons. The different influences of these projections on hypothalamic neurosecretory cells (hns) modulate pulsatile gonadotropin-releasing hormone (GnRH) secretion. Releasing hormones enter the pituitary portal system (pps) and regulate the pattern of luteinizing hormone (LH) and follicle-stimulating hormone (FSH) secretion by the pituitary (pit). These gonadotropins induce ovulation and stimulate estradiol (E) and progesterone (P) production. Gonadal steroids, in turn, bind to specific amygdaloid hormone receptors and influence neural activity, including epileptiform discharges.

Transection of the stria terminalis blocks the ovulatory response, whereas a lesion of the ventral amygdalofugal pathway has no such effect. Stimulation and ablation studies in rodents suggest that the corticomedial amygdala promotes sexual activity, while the basolateral amygdala inhibits it. Bilateral amygdalectomy in female monkeys induces amenorrhea and hypogonadal vaginal changes. Temporal lobectomy in men and women with TLE is commonly associated with improved reproductive and sexual function and, less frequently, with the development or exacerbation of reproductive and sexual dysfunction.

Altered temporal lobe function may contribute to reproductive endocrine changes (cf. Herzog 1989). With regard to gonadotropins, the amygdala has extensive, direct anatomic connections with the arcuate and preoptic hypothalamic nuclei, which are involved in the regulation, production, and secretion of GnRH (Fig. 12.2). Alterations in the physiologic frequency or concentration of pulsatile GnRH secretion can induce changes in serum LH and follicle-stimulating hormone (FSH) that resemble patterns found in reproductive endocrine disorders such as PCO and HH. Stimulation of the two major divisions of the amygdala or their outflow tracts can predictably and differentially affect the membrane potentials of the same ventromedial hypothalamic neurons. Stimulation and ablation studies of the amygdala in conjunction with gonadotropin assays, moreover, have shown that the two functional divisions of the amygdala can produce elevations or reductions in pituitary and serum LH levels.

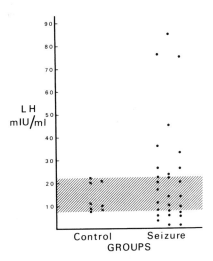

Fig. 12.3 This graph by Herzog et al (1986) shows the much broader range of baseline luteinizing hormone (LH) serum levels as measured during the early follicular phase among 28 women with partial seizures of temporal lobe origin, in comparison to 8 age-matched normal controls. This finding is consistent with the notion that involvement of the limbic system with epileptiform discharges may disrupt normal limbic modulation of hypothalamic regulation of pituitary gonadotropin secretion.

Consistent with these animal data is the finding that women with TLE have a range of early-follicular-phase serum LH levels that extends well above and below normal control values (Fig. 12.3). This has led to the hypothesis that involvement of temporal lobe limbic structures by seizure discharges may disrupt normal limbic modulation of hypothalamic regulation of pituitary secretion and promote the development of reproductive endocrine disorders (Fig. 12.4).

A role for altered temporolimbic electroencephalogram (EEG) activity in the development of some reproductive endocrine disorders among women with epilepsy is supported by finding a significant difference between the EEG laterality distributions associated with PCO and HH (Herzog 1993a; Fig. 12.5). Among 30 women who had reproductive endocrine disorders and complex partial seizures with unilateral TLE discharges, there was a strong predominance of left-sided discharges (15 versus 1) with PCO, and right-sided

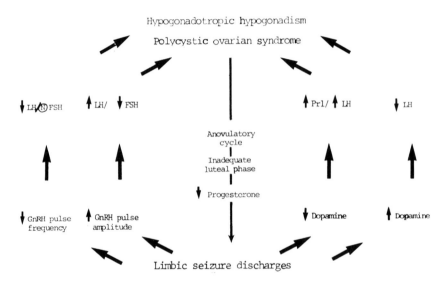

Fig. 12.4   Possible mechanisms by which limbic seizure discharges may promote reproductive endocrine disorders and how abnormal reproductive hormone levels may influence epilepsy. It is based on hypotheses proposed by Herzog et al (1986) which suggest that involvement of limbic structures with epileptiform discharge may disrupt normal limbic modulatory influences on hypothalamic gonadotropin-releasing hormone (GnRH) secretion. Altered frequency or amplitude of GnRH secretion may lead to patterns of pituitary luteinizing hormone (LH) and follicle-stimulating hormone (FSH) secretion which are found in hypogonadotropic hypogonadism and polycystic ovarian syndrome. Kindled limbic seizures alter brain dopamine levels. Hypothalamic dopamine exerts an inhibitory effect on pituitary LH and prolactin (Prl) secretion. Abnormal brain dopamine levels may alter pituitary gonadotropin and prolactin secretion and promote the development of reproductive endocrine disorder. Reproductive endocrine disorders which are associated with partial seizures of temporal lobe origin are characterized by anovulatory cycles and diminished progesterone secretion. An elevated serum estrogen/progesterone ratio may promote the development of seizure discharges in the brain.

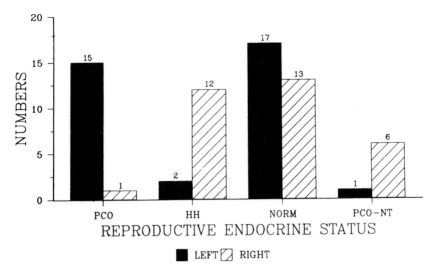

Fig. 12.5 Laterality of epileptiform discharges in epileptic women with unilateral temporal lobe electroencephalogram foci and polycystic ovarian syndrome (PCO), hypogonadotropic hypogonadism (HH) or normal reproductive endocrine function (NORM), as well as unilateral non-temporal lobe foci and polycystic ovarian syndrome (PCO-NT). PCO versus HH: $\chi = 16.1$, d.f. = 1; $P <0.001$. PCO versus NORM: $\chi = 5.1$, d.f. = 1; $P <0.05$. HH versus NORM: $\chi = 5.4$, d.f. = 1; $P <0.02$. PCO versus PCO-NT: $P <0.001$, Fisher's exact test.

discharges (12 versus 2) with HH. Each distribution differed significantly from that of 30 women with epilepsy who had no reproductive endocrine disorder (left/right: 17/13).

Moreover, among women with PCO who had unilateral non-temporal lobe foci, 6 of 7 had right-sided epileptiform discharges. This represents a significant difference from the EEG laterality distribution of women with PCO who had temporal foci. These relationships between altered patterns of reproductive hormonal secretion and the predominant laterality of EEG epileptiform discharges in women with epilepsy are consistent with a lateralized asymmetry in cerebral influences on reproductive endocrine function.

The link between temporal lobe dysfunction and endocrine disorder is further supported by investigations of the pulsatile secretion of LH in women with epilepsy. Untreated women with epilepsy have a higher LH pulse frequency (PF) than normal controls (Bilo et al 1991), while treated women have significantly lower frequencies (Drislane et al 1994). Left temporal epileptiform activity is associated with significantly greater LHPF than right (L/R: 6/3; $P <0.05$) (Herzog et al 1994, Fig. 12.6). The findings suggest that the nature and laterality of temporal lobe EEG activity may be important determinants of LHPF and the development of particular reproductive endocrine disorders.

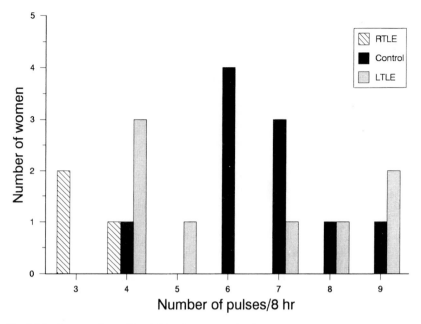

Fig. 12.6 A comparison of luteinizing hormone pulse frequency among epileptic women with unilateral left (LTLE) and right (RTLE)-sided temporal lobe epileptiform discharges and normal controls. Pulse frequency is significantly more variable among epileptic women than among controls (Siegel and Tukey non-parametric test of relative variation in two independent samples, $P < 0.05$). Pulse frequency is significantly greater with LTLE than RTLE (Mann–Whitney U test, $P < 0.05$).

Neurotransmitter

Central dopaminergic mechanisms may also contribute to the relationship between TLE and reproductive endocrine disorders (cf. Herzog 1989, Fig. 12.4). Bromocriptine and dopamine lessen LH and prolactin secretion by the pituitary, and are thought to act in the lateral palisade zone of the median eminence to inhibit GnRH secretion. Clinical studies of PCO syndrome reveal exaggerated suppression of LH levels with dopamine infusion and supranormal elevation of prolactin levels in response to haloperidol. These features and elevated baseline levels of LH and prolactin suggest a decreased level of dopamine activity in the hypothalamus of women with PCO syndrome.

The opposite has been proposed to explain HH. In the absence of hypothyroidism and structural lesions of the pituitary and peripheral endocrine glands, no organic cause is usually demonstrated to explain the low gonadotropin levels in HH. This type of amenorrhea is generally attributed to a functional derangement of the hypothalamopituitary axis, especially excessive dopaminergic tone in the tuberoinfundibular region of the hypothalamus. Altered dopamine and homovanillic acid concentrations in the brains of animals with kindled amygdaloid seizures (Sato & Nakashima 1975) and in the spinal fluid of patients with TLE (Papeschi et al 1972) suggest a relationship between TLE and brain dopamine metabolism. There is reason to consider, therefore, that epileptic discharges in medial temporal limbic structures may influence reproductive endocrine function by modulating dopamine as well as GnRH levels in the hypothalamus.

Neural

Neural innervation of the gonads provides another potential mechanism by which altered brain function may induce reproductive and endocrine changes (Fig. 12.7). This possibility, however, has remained largely unexplored (Herzog 1989). It has been demonstrated that bilateral ovariectomy is followed by unilateral right-sided reduction in hypothalamic GnRH content, while unilateral ovariectomy on either side produces an ipsilateral increase in hypothalamic GnRH content (Gerendai et al 1978a). The findings cannot readily be explained by endocrine factors alone.

The ovary is innervated by both sympathetic noradrenergic fibers originating from neurons in the intermediolateral cell column of the spinal cord, and by parasympathetic cholinergic fibers from the dorsal motor nucleus of the vagus. In rodent models, unilateral ovariectomy is generally associated with contralateral compensatory ovarian hypertrophy. Unilateral ovariectomy, in association with 6-hydroxydopamine application to the remaining ovary, results in decreased compensatory ovarian hypertrophy (Gerandai et al 1978b). This has been attributed to impaired or blocked noradrenergic neural transmission. Unilateral ovariectomy in association with bilateral vagotomy also results in diminished compensatory ovarian hypertrophy, as well as in diminished elevations of serum LH and FSH levels and a prolonged estrus cycle (Burden & Lawrence 1977).

The amygdala has direct efferent projections to both the dorsal motor nucleus of the vagus and the dorsomedial and lateral regions of the hypothalamus (cf. Herzog 1989). The latter regulate sympathetic response through direct projections to the neurons of the intermediolateral cell column of the spinal cord. Temporolimbic stimulation in adrenalectomized and hypophysectomized rats has been shown to increase or decrease estradiol and progesterone concentrations in the contralateral ovarian vein at 105 and 120 min, while ovarian blood flow remains unchanged (Kawakami et al 1981). Thus, there is reason to investigate the possibility that involvement of medial temporal lobe structures with epileptiform discharges may disrupt normal limbic neural as well as neuroendocrine modulation of gonadal vagal fibers from the gonads which terminate in the solitary nucleus of the medulla. The solitary nucleus is directly and extensively connected to the amygdala. The amygdala shows sensitive, short-latency electrophysiologic responses to vagal stimulation. Therefore, sensory input from pelvic reproductive structures may exert modulatory influences on limbic discharges.

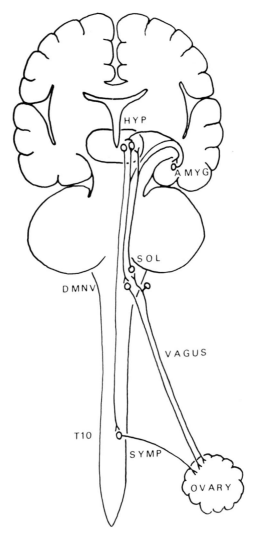

Fig. 12.7 The neural pathways which may mediate limbic influences on gonadal structure and function. The amygdala (AMYG) has direct fiber projections to the dorsomedial and lateral regions of the hypothalamus (HYP). These regions are connected directly to the preganglionic sympathetic neurons in the intermediolateral cell column of the thoracolumbar spinal cord from which originate sympathetic (SYMP) nerve fibers to the gonads. The amygdala also has direct and indirect projections to the dorsal motor nucleus of the vagus (DMNV) from which originate vagal fibers to the gonads. Afferent vagal fibers from the gonads project to the solitary nucleus in the medulla (SOL). The solitary nucleus has direct projections to the amygdala as well as to the hypothalamus.

Hormonal

Reproductive endocrine disorders may favor the development of TLE in women. Medial temporal lobe limbic structures bind hormones (Pfaff &

Keiner 1972, Stumpf 1972) and show sensitive electrophysiologic changes in response to hormonal influence (Sawyer 1972). Animal experimental and human clinical data suggest that estrogen promotes interictal epileptiform brain-wave activity and can precipitate clinical seizures. The antiestrogen clomiphene citrate has been shown significantly to lessen both kainic acid-induced seizures in rats (Nicoletti et al 1985) and seizure frequency in epileptic women with reproductive endocrine disorders (Herzog 1988). Progesterone also lessens the probability of interictal epileptiform activity and has benefited some patients with epilepsy (Zimmerman et al 1973, Mattson et al 1984, Herzog 1986). The anovulatory cycles in PCO and HH, therefore, may expose temporal lobe limbic structures to a constant estrogen effect without the normal progesterone elevation in the luteal phase, and thereby heighten interictal epileptiform activity. In this regard, 56.5% of women with anovulatory cycles or amenorrhea were found to have EEG abnormalities, including some with focal epileptogenic discharges (Sharf et al 1969). Treatment with clomiphene citrate restored EEGs to normal in 54% of them. There was, moreover, an association between correction of the EEG and ovulation and pregnancy. Thus, the hormonal changes associated with anovulatory cycles may favor the development of EEG abnormalities.

PROGESTERONE THERAPY

Progesterone therapy benefits some women with catamenial epilepsy. In our preliminary investigation of 8 women who had complex partial seizures of temporal lobe origin and catamenial exacerbation, natural progesterone, administered in suppository form during the second half of each cycle or just premenstrually, with gradual tapering and discontinuation on day 28, was associated with improvement in 6 and an overall reduction in seizure frequency of 68% (Herzog 1986). We then evaluated the effects of cyclic natural progesterone therapy, in lozenge form, on refractory seizures of temporal lobe origin in 25 women (Herzog 1993b). Eighteen women (72%) experienced a decline in seizure frequency in a 3-month treatment period compared with the 3 months prior to therapy ($P < 0.01$). Average monthly complex partial seizure frequency declined by 54% ($P < 0.01$) and generalized motor seizures by 58% ($P < 0.01$). Two women did not tolerate progesterone because of asthenia and emotional depression. These symptoms resolved within 1 day upon discontinuation of therapy, in both cases. Seizure frequency did not respond by a minimum of 10% in 5 women.

In the absence of an adequate response to conventional antiseizure therapy, treatment may be considered in two settings:

1. women with catamenial epilepsy who have documented inadequate luteal phase

2. women with catamenial epilepsy who have no demonstrable reproductive endocrine abnormality.

The former group may show any of the three previously described patterns of seizure exacerbation, while the latter generally experiences worsening of seizures premenstrually. The pattern should be documented during three cycles using charts which include the days of the month, cycle days and seizure occurrence. Progesterone may be administered throughout the period of seizure exacerbation during the second half of the cycle and then tapered and discontinued over 3 days at the end of the cycle. There are no definite absolute clinical contraindications to the intermittent use of natural progesterone to achieve physiological luteal-range serum levels in a cyclic fashion. It is considered by some to be the treatment of choice for inadequate luteal phase and is regularly used to help induce fertility (Jones 1976). It is yet to be recognized, however, as an approved form of therapy for neurological purposes. Therefore, conventional antiseizure drugs should be considered first and the results of this should be described carefully before resorting to progesterone. Progesterone should be avoided during or in anticipation of pregnancy, unless it is used specifically in conjunction with a gynecologist as part of a fertility program; and in the absence of adequate birth-control measures. It should also be used cautiously in the presence of undiagnosed breast lumps since synthetic progestin administration in experimental animals has been associated with mammary nodule development and, in high doses, malignancy.

Natural progesterone is available as an extract of soy in lozenge, micronized capsule and suppository forms. The usual daily regimen to achieve physiological luteal range serum levels, as measured four hours after administration, ranges from 100 to 200 mg, taken 3 or 4 times daily, with the average daily dose being 600 mg (Herzog 1986, Herzog 1993b). The maintenance dosage and regimen should be individualized and based on a combination of clinical response and serum progesterone levels between 5 and 25 ng/ml. Adverse effects occur with overdosage and include sedation, mental depression and asthenia (Herzog 1986b, Herzog 1993b). Progesterone use may also be associated occasionally with breast tenderness, weight gain and irregular vaginal bleeding. The vehicle used to dissolve progesterone for suppository use may rarely be responsible for the development of an allergic rash. Discontinuation of the hormone or lowering of the dosage resolves these side-effects (Herzog 1986, Herzog 1993b).

Synthetic progestin therapy has also benefited some women with epilepsy (Zimmerman et al 1973, Mattson et al 1984). Parenteral depomedroxy-progesterone significantly lessens seizure frequency when it is given in a dose sufficient to induce amenorrhea (Zimmerman et al 1973, Mattson et al 1984). A regimen of approximately 120–150 mg given intramuscularly every 6–12 weeks generally achieves this goal (Mattson et al 1984). Side-effects include those encountered with natural progesterone. Depot administration, however, is also commonly associated with hot flashes, irregular breakthrough vaginal bleeding and a lengthy delay of 6–12 months in the return of regular ovulatory cycles (Mattson et al 1984). Long-term hypoestrogenic effects on bone density and cardiovascular status need to be considered with chronic use. In our own experience, the weekly intramuscular administration of 400 mg depomedroxyprogesterone to a 44-year-old woman with PCO syndrome and intractable complex partial seizures of left temporal and right frontal origin, despite extensive antiseizure medication trials, was associated with a reduction in average monthly seizure frequency from 22.5 to 2.4. Lower dosages or frequency of administration were less effective.

Oral synthetic progestins administered cyclically or continuously have not proven to be an effective therapy in clinical investigations (Dana Haeri & Richens 1983, Mattson et al 1984), although individual successes with continuous daily oral use of norethistrone and combination pills have been reported (Livingston 1966, Hall 1977).

KEY POINTS FOR CLINICAL PRACTICE

- Seizures do not occur randomly in relation to changes in the physiological reproductive state. They tend to be worse premenstrually; mid-cycle in the late follicular phase; and during the entire second half of the cycle in the setting of inadequate luteal-phase cycles. Exogenous hormonal administration can also affect seizure occurrence.
- In general, estrogens are epileptogenic while progestins have antiseizure properties.
- Epilepsy, especially temporal lobe epilepsy, is commonly associated with menstrual disorders, the majority of which are attributable to reproductive endocrine disorders. PCO and HH are particularly overrepresented.
- Many antiseizure medications alter serum hormone levels but cannot account for all of the reproductive endocrine disorders associated with epilepsy.
- Altered temporolimbic modulation of hypothalamopituitary secretion is implicated as a factor in the development of reproductive endocrine disorders. This is supported by the demonstration of predictable alterations in the pulsatile secretion of LH in relation to the location and laterality of EEG paroxysmal discharges.
- The elevated ratio of serum estrogen/progesterone levels associated with the inadequate luteal-phase cycles which characterize PCO and HH may exacerbate seizure disorders.
- The administration of progesterone during the second half of each cycle to women with a catamenial pattern of seizure exacerbation has been associated with a clinically and statistically significant reduction in the frequency of intractable complex partial and secondary generalized seizures.

REFERENCES

Abbott R J, Browning M C K, Davidson D L W. 1980 Serum prolactin and cortisol
concentrations after grand mal seizures. J Neurol Neurosurg Psychiatry 43: 163–167
Backstrom T. 1976 Epileptic seizures in women related to plasma estrogen and progesterone
during the menstrual cycle. Acta Neurol Scand 54: 321–347
Backstrom T, Zetterlund B, Blum S et al. 1984 Effects of IV progesterone infusions on the
epileptic discharge frequency in women with partial epilepsy. Acta Neurol Scand 69:
240–248
Bilo L, Meo R, Valentino R et al. 1991 Abnormal patterns of luteinizing hormone pulsatility
in women with epilepsy. Fertil Steril 55: 705–711
Burden H W, Lawrence I E. 1977 The effect of denervation on compensatory ovarian
hypertrophy. Neuroendocrinology 23: 368
Dana Haeri J, Richens A. 1983 Effect of noresthisterone on seizures associated with
menstruation. Epilepsia 24: 377–381
Dreifuss J J, Murphy J T, Gloor P. 1986 Contrasting effects of two identified amygdaloid
efferent pathways on single hypothalamic neurons. J Neurophysiol 31: 237
Drislane F W, Coleman A E, Schomer D L et al. 1994 Altered pulsatile secretion of
luteinizing hormone in women with epilepsy. Neurology 44: 306–310
Gerandai I, Rotstejn W H, Marchetti B et al. 1978a Unilateral ovariectomy induced
luteinizing hormone-releasing hormone content changes in the two halves of the
mediobasal hypothalamus. Neurosci Lett 9: 333
Gerandia I, Marchetti B, Maugeri S et al. 1978b Prevention of compensatory ovarian
hypertrophy by local treatment of the ovary with 6-OHDA. Neuroendocrinology 27: 272
Hall S M. 1977 Treatment of menstrual epilepsy with a progesterone-only oral contraceptive.
Epilepsia 18: 235–236
Herzog A G. 1986 Intermittent progesterone therapy and frequency of complex partial
seizures in women with menstrual disorders. Neurology 36: 1607–1610
Herzog A G, Seibel M M, Schomer D L et al. 1986 Reproductive endocrine disorders in
women with partial seizures of temporal lobe origin. Arch Neurol 43: 341–346
Herzog A G. 1989 A hypothesis to integrate partial seizures of temporal lobe origin and
reproductive endocrine disorders. Epilepsy Res 3: 151–159
Herzog A G. 1993a A relationship between particular reproductive endocrine disorders and
the laterality of epileptiform discharges in women with epilepsy. Neurology 43: 1907–1910
Herzog A G. 1993b Progesterone therapy in women with complex partial and secondary
generalized seizures. Ann Neurol 34: 298
Herzog A G, Russell V, Vaitukaitis J L et al. 1982 Neuroendocrine dysfunction in temporal
lobe epilepsy. Arch Neurol 39: 133
Herzog A G. 1988 Clomiphene therapy in epileptic women with menstrual disorders.
Neurology 38: 432–434
Herzog A G, Coleman A E, Drislane F W et al. 1994 Lateralized asymmetry in the
temporolimbic regulation of luteinizing hormone secretion. Neuroendocrinology 60(5): 35
Hom A C, Buterbaugh G G. 1986 Estrogen alters the acquisition of seizures kindled by
repeated amygdala stimulation or pentylenetetrazol administration in ovariectomized female
rats. Epilepsia 27: 103–108
Isojarvi J I T, Laatkainen T J, Pakarinen A J et al. 1993 Polycystic ovaries and hyper-
androgenism in women taking valproate for epilepsy. N Engl J Med 329: 1383–1388
Jones G S. 1976 The luteal phase defect. Fertil Steril 27: 351–356
Kawakami M, Kubo K, Vemura T et al. 1981 Involvement of ovarian innervation in steroid
secretion. Endocrinology 109: 136
Laidlaw J. 1956 Catamenial epilepsy. Lancet 271: 1235–1237
Landgren S, Backstrom T, Kalistratov G. 1978 The effect of progesterone on the spontaneous
interictal spike evoked by the application of penicillin to the cat's cerebral cortex. J Neurol
Sci 36: 119–133
Levesque L A, Herzog A G, Seibel M M. 1986 The effect of phenytoin and carbamazepine
on serum dehydroepiandrosterone sulfate in men and women who have partial seizures
with temporal lobe involvement. J Clin Endocrinol Metab 63: 243
Livingston S. 1966 Drug therapy for epilepsy. Springfield, I L: C C Thomas, pp 1–119
Logothetis J, Harner R. 1960 Electrocortical activation by estrogens. Arch Neurol 3: 290–297
Logothetis J, Harner R, Morrell F et al. 1959 The role of estrogens in catamenial

exacerbation of epilepsy. Neurology (Minneap) 9: 352–360

Marcus E M, Watson C W, Goldman P L. 1966 Effects of steroids on cerebral electrical activity. Arch Neurol 15: 521–532

Mattson R H, Cramer J A, Caldwell B V et al. 1981 Seizure frequency and the menstrual cycle: a clinical study. Epilepsia 22: 242

Mattson R H, Cramer J A, Caldwell B V et al. 1984 Treatment of seizures with medroxyprogesterone acetate: preliminary report. Neurology (Cleveland) 34: 1255–1258.

Newmark N E, Penry J K. 1980 Catamenial epilepsy: a review. Epilepsia 21: 281–300

Nicoletti F, Speciale C, Sortino M A et al. 1985 Comparative effects of estradiol benzoate, the antiestrogen clomiphene citrate, and the progestin medroxyprogesterone acetate on kainic acid-induced seizures in male and female rats. Epilepsia 26: 252–257

Papeschi R, Molina-Negro P, Sourkes T L et al. 1972 The concentration of homovanillic and 5-hydroxyindolaecetic acid in ventricular and lumbar CSF. Neurology 22: 1151

Pfaff D W, Keiner M. 1972 Estradiol-concentrating cells in the rat amygdala as part of a limbic-hypothalamic hormone-sensitive system. In: Eleftheriou BE, ed. The neurobiology of the amygdala. New York: Plenum Press, pp 775–792

Roscizewska D, Buntner B, Guz I et al. 1986 Ovarian hormones, anticonvulsant drugs and seizures during the menstrual cycle in women with epilepsy. J Neurol Neurosurg Psychiatry 49: 47–51

Sato M, Nakashima T. 1975 Kindling: secondary epileptogenesis, sleep and catecholamines. Can J Neurol Sci 2: 439

Sawyer C H. 1972 Functions of the amygdala related to the feedback actions of gonadal steroid hormones. In: Eleftherious BE, ed. The neurobiology of the amygdala. New York: Plenum Press, pp 745–762

Sharf M, Sharf B, Bental E et al. 1969 The electroencephalogram in the investigation of anovulation and its treatment by clomiphene. Lancet 1: 750–753

Shavit G, Lerman P, Korczyn A D et al. 1984 Phenytoin pharmacokinetics in catamenial epilepsy. Neurology 34: 959–961

Sperling M R, Pritchard P B, Engel J Jr et al. 1986 Prolactin in partial epilepsy: an indicator of limbic seizures. Ann Neurol 20: 716–722

Spiegel E, Wycis H. 1945 Anticonvulsant effects of steroids. J Lab Clin Med 30: 947–953

Stumpf W E. 1972 Steroid-concentrating neurons in the amygdala. In: Eleftheriou BE, ed. The neurobiology of the amygdala. New York: Plenum Press, pp 763–774

Trimble M R. 1978 Serum prolactin in epilepsy and hysteria. Br Med J 2: 1682

Woolley D E, Timiras P S. 1962 The gonad–brain relationship: effects of female sex hormones on electroshock convulsions in the rat. Endocrinology 70: 196–209

Wyllie E, Luders H, MacMillan J P et al. 1984 Serum prolactin levels after epileptic seizures. Neurology 34: 1601–1604

Zimmerman A W, Holden K R, Reiter E O et al. 1973 Medroxyprogesterone acetate in the treatment of seizures associated with menstruation. J Pediatr 83: 959–963

13

Endocrine aspects of epilepsy in men

A. G. Herzog

ANDROGENS AND SEXUAL FUNCTION IN MEN WITH EPILEPSY

Reduced potency and hyposexuality occur in 38–71% of men with epilepsy (Gastaut & Collomb 1954, Hierons & Saunders 1966, Kolarsky et al 1967, Taylor 1969, Blumer 1970, Jensen & Larsen 1979, Shukla et al 1979, Fenwick et al 1985). The etiology of these symptoms is likely multifactorial, including psychosocial, epileptic, medicational and hormonal causes (Taylor 1969). Because androgens play an important role in regulating potency and libido (Davidson 1977, Davidson et al 1979), measurement of their serum levels is a regular part of the medical evaluation. The most important androgen is testosterone. Testosterone exists in the serum in three forms: free, albumin-bound and sex hormone-binding globulin (SHBG)-bound (Sodergard et al 1982). Only about 2% occurs in the free form, while 43–45% is bound to SHBG and 53–55% is bound to albumin (Sodergard et al 1982). There is general agreement that the SHBG-bound fraction is not biologically active (Sodergard et al 1982, Cummings & Wall 1985, Manni et al 1985). Considerable evidence exists, however, that the large pool of testosterone that is loosely bound to albumin is available to tissues (Cummings & Wall 1985, Manni et al 1985). Isojarvi et al (1990) have reported three separate measures of serum testosterone in anticonvulsant-treated men with epilepsy. They show how the use of a particular medication or combination of medications can be associated with low free androgen index (a measure of non-SHBG-bound testosterone) despite normal free testosterone and elevated serum levels of total testosterone. Their data highlight an important issue: if androgen deficiency contributes to reproductive and sexual dysfunction in men with epilepsy (Christiansen et al 1975, Toone et al 1983, Rodin et al 1984, Fenwick et al 1986, Herzog et al 1986), which testosterone measurement is most relevant?

Several antiseizure drugs induce hepatic synthesis of increased amounts of SHBG (Barragry et al 1978, Dana-Haeri et al 1982, Toone et al 1983, Connell et al 1984, Macphee et al 1988, Isojarvi et al 1990) that can result in normal or even elevated levels of total testosterone, but reduced concentrations of free and/or non-SHBG-bound testosterone (Barragry et al 1978, Dana-Haeri et al

1982, Toone et al 1983, Connell et al 1984, Macphee et al 1988, Isojarvi et al 1990). Toone et al (1983) found that reductions in free, but not total, testosterone were associated with decreased sexual interest. Fenwick et al (1986) demonstrated a relationship between decreased potency and low free testosterone levels. Isojarvi et al (1990) have shown that the free androgen index, one indicator of the non-SHBG-bound portion of testosterone, may be decreased despite normal free testosterone levels. The clinical significance of this finding is not known. Herzog et al (1986), however, measured abnormally low non-SHBG-bound testosterone levels in 5 of 8 treated epileptic men with diminished sexual interest or reduced potency. Herzog et al (1990), moreover, observed in another investigation that among 13 men with epilepsy, those who were classified as sexually normal had an almost twofold higher average non-SHBG-bound testosterone value than those with reproductive or sexual dysfunction (2.4 versus 1.4 ng/ml). Nevertheless, only 3 of 8 hyposexual men had levels below the normal control range and the average values of both groups were normal. Only one total testosterone value was below the normal control range, and the average total testosterone values were not nearly as disparate (4.8 versus 4.0 ng/ml) between the sexually unaffected and affected groups, respectively. Free testosterone levels were not determined. The demonstration by Isojarvi et al (1990) that the free androgen index may be low when free testosterone levels are normal, and the observations by Herzog et al (1986, 1990) that non-SHBG-bound testosterone may relate to the level of sexual activity, indicate the need for an investigation that compares non-SHBG-bound and free testosterone in terms of their relationships to reproductive and sexual dysfunction. Measures of non-SHBG-bound testosterone rather than free testosterone may provide a more sensitive assessment of biologically and perhaps clinically significant androgen levels.

THE CAUSES OF ANDROGEN DEFICIENCY

Antiseizure medications

Antiseizure medications may reduce biologically active testosterone by directly inhibiting synthesis, as well as by the induction of binding globulin. They act at various levels of testosterone synthesis to inhibit testicular endocrine function (Kuhn-Velten et al 1990). In an in vitro rat Leydig cell model, carbamazepine exhibited potent inhibitory effects at clinically relevant concentrations. High concentrations of phenytoin were required to produce equivalent effect. Valproate had the least effect.

Macphee et al (1988) found a significant inverse correlation between serum carbamazepine and testosterone levels. Consistent correlations between serum hormone levels and antiepileptic drug levels, however, have not been demonstrated (Toone et al 1983, Rodin et al 1984). Other factors, therefore, may also play a role.

Epilepsy

The disruption of normal temporolimbic modulation of hypothalamopituitary function by epileptiform discharges may promote the development of reproductive endocrine disorders (Herzog 1989). Hypogonadism is unusually common among men with epilepsy. In our own series of 20 men with partial seizures of temporal lobe origin (TLE), 11 (55%) had reproductive dysfunction or hyposexuality (Herzog et al 1986). Nine of these 11 (45% overall) had reproductive endocrine disorders, including hypogonadotropic hypogonadism in 25%, hypergonadotropic hypogonadism in 10% and functional hyperprolactinemia in 10%. Hypogonadism and abnormal semen analysis are as common among untreated as among treated men with epilepsy (Taneja et al 1994). Lateralized cerebral and hypothalamic asymmetries, moreover, may be responsible for the association of different patterns of reproductive endocrine secretion with left or right TLE (Herzog et al 1990). We have evaluated pulsatile secretion of luteinizing hormone (LH) over 8 h during concomitant electroencephalogram (EEG) recording in 12 men with unilateral temporal lobe epileptiform discharges and 11 normal controls (Herzog et al 1994). LH pulse frequency was significantly more variable ($P < 0.05$) in

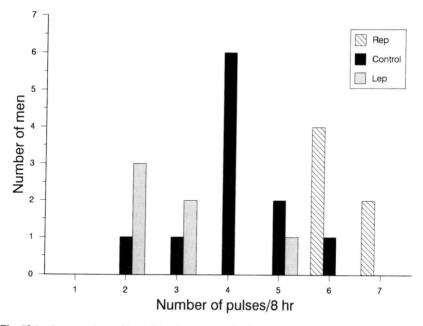

Fig. 13.1 A comparison of luteinizing hormone pulse frequency among epileptic men with unilateral left (Lep) and right (Rep)-sided temporal lobe epileptiform discharges and normal controls. Pulse frequency is significantly more variable among epileptic men than among controls (Siegel and Tukey non-parametric test of relative variation in two independent samples, $P < 0.05$). Pulse frequency is significantly greater with right than left temporal lobe epilepsy (Mann–Whitney U test, $P < 0.05$).

men with TLE than in controls (Fig 13.1). Right temporal epileptiform activity was associated with significantly greater (P <0.05) LH pulse frequency than were left temporal discharges (Fig. 13.1). Paroxysmal unilateral slowing had opposite effects. The findings suggest that the laterality and nature of temporal lobe paroxysmal discharges may be important determinants of LH pulse frequency and the development of particular reproductive endocrine disorders.

Estradiol

In an investigation comparing serum reproductive steroid levels among 20 men who were treated with phenytoin for complex partial seizures, 21 untreated men with complex partial seizures, and 20 age-matched normal controls, total and non-SHBG-bound estradiol levels were significantly higher in the phenytoin group than in either the untreated or normal control groups (Herzog et al 1991). Barbiturates appear to have similar effects. These findings suggest that some antiseizure medications may lower free testosterone levels not only by inducing SHBG synthetase, but perhaps also by the inducing aromatase, which converts free testosterone to estradiol. Estradiol also increases SHBG synthesis. Moreover, it potently inhibits LH secretion and has been suggested to play a major role in negative feedback in men as well as women (Loriaux et al 1977, Winters et al 1979). Suppression of LH secretion results in hypogonadotropic hypogonadism. Chronically low levels of free testosterone lead to testicular failure and hypergonadotropic hypogonadism. This may explain the frequent occurrence of both these reproductive endocrine disorders in men with epilepsy (Herzog et al 1986). Finally, estradiol may produce premature aging of the hypothalamic arcuate nucleus, which secretes gonadotropin-releasing hormone (Finch et al 1984, Brawer et al 1983).

TESTOSTERONE THERAPY

Testosterone replacement is the most common form of therapy for hypogonadism. Its efficacy in men with epilepsy has not been reported. In our own experience with 12 men, intramuscular injections of testosterone enanthate in dosages of 200–400 mg every 3 or 4 weeks has normalized levels of free testosterone and led to moderate improvement in sexual interest and potency scores in all 12 men. Seizure frequency was not changed.

THERAPY WITH TESTOSTERONE AND AROMATASE INHIBITOR

In our experience testosterone therapy has been only moderately effective in restoring reproductive and sexual function. Moreover, testosterone has not lessened seizures despite some reports of anticonvulsant properties in experimental animals (Werboff & Havlena 1963). One possible explanation is that antiseizure drugs which induce increased enzyme synthesis may enhance the conversion of testosterone to estradiol by aromatase (Herzog 1989). Estradiol lowers male sexual interest and function (Beach 1948) and increases the number of seizure discharges (Logothetis & Harner 1960, Longo & Saldana 1966). The addition of testolactone, an aromatase inhibitor, and testosterone to baseline carbamazepine therapy improved sexual questionnaire scores and decreased seizure frequency more than the addition of testosterone alone in a 52-year-old man with intractable seizures (Herzog 1992).

CLOMIPHENE THERAPY

Clomiphene dramatically improved sexual interest, potency and seizure control in 1 man with complex partial seizures and hypogonadotropic hypogonadism (Herzog 1988). Seizures were eliminated during clomiphene use in another case with epilepsy and oligospermia (Check et al 1982). Clomiphene offered no benefit, however, to a man who had complex partial seizures and hypergonadotropic hypogonadism (gonadal failure) (Herzog 1988). Total and free antiepileptic drug levels were not affected. The mechanism of clomiphene's effect on seizure activity is conjectural but may involve either the normalization of the serum testosterone level or direct antiestrogenic effects on epileptogenic limbic structures which have a high density of estradiol receptors.

KEY POINTS FOR CLINICAL PRACTICE

- Diminished sexual function is common among men with epilepsy. Although multifactorial in etiology, it does appear to be related to diminished levels of biologically active testosterone. Non-SHBG testosterone may be a more sensitive measure of biologically active testosterone and may correlate better with sexual function than either free or total testosterone.
- Androgen deficiency in men with epilepsy results from the disruption of normal limbic modulation of hypothalamopituitary function by paroxysmal discharges as well as by the use of antiseizure medications. Antiepileptic drugs decrease biologically active testosterone by inhibiting its synthesis; by increasing the hepatic catabolism of steroids; by inducing SHBG synthesis; and by promoting the conversion of testosterone to estradiol.
- Treatment of hypogonadism in men with epilepsy with testosterone alone appears to be less effective for the management of seizures and hyposexuality than the use of testosterone and an aromatase inhibitor or, in the case of hypogonadotropic hypogonadism, clomiphene.

RECENT ADVANCES IN EPILEPSY

REFERENCES

Barragry J M, Makin H L J, Trafford D J H et al. 1978 Effect of anticonvulsants on plasma testosterone and sex hormone binding globulin levels. J Neurol Neurosurg Psychiatry 41: 913–941

Beach F A. 1948 Hormones and behavior: a survey of interrelationships between endocrine secretions and patterns of overt response. New York: Haber

Blumer D. 1970 Changes of sexual behavior related to temporal lobe disorders in man. J Sex Res 6: 173–180

Brawer J, Schipper H, Robaire B. 1983 Effects of long-term androgen and estradiol exposure on the hypothalamus. Endocrinology 112: 194–199

Check J H, Lublin F D, Mandel M M. 1982 Clomiphene as an anticonvulsant drug. Arch Neurol 39: 784

Christiansen P, Deigaard J, Lund M. 1975 Potens, fertilitet of konshormonudskillelse hos yngre manglige epilepsilidende. Ugeskr Laeger 137: 2402–2405

Connell J M, Rapeport W G, Beastall G H, Brodie M J 1984 Changes in circulating androgens during short-term carbamazepine therapy. Br J Clin Pharmacol 17: 347–351

Cummings D C, Wall S R. 1985 Non-sex hormone binding globulin and bound testosterone as a marker for hypogonadism. J Clin Endocrinol Metab 61: 873–876

Dana-Haeri J, Oxley J, Richens A. 1982 Reduction of free testosterone by antiepileptic drugs. Br Med J 284: 85–86

Davidson J M. 1977 Neurohormonal basis of sexual behavior. In: Greep RP, ed. Reproductive physiology II. Baltimore, MD: University Park Press p 225

Davidson J M, Camargo C A, Smith E R. 1979 Effects of androgen on sexual behavior in hypogonadal men. J Clin Endocrinol Metab 48: 955

Fenwick P B C, Toone B K, Wheeler M J et al. 1985 Sexual behavior in a centre for epilepsy. Acta Neurol Scand 71: 428–435

Fenwick P B C, Mercer C, Grant R et al. 1986 Nocturnal penile tumescence and serum testosterone levels. Arch Sex Behav 15: 13–21

Finch C E, Felicio L S, Mobbs C V, Nelson J F. 1984 Ovarian and steroidal influences on neuroendocrine aging processes in female rodents. Endocrinol Rev 5: 467–497

Gastaut H, Collomb H. 1954 Etude du comportement sexuel chez les epileptiques psychomoteurs. Ann Med Psychol 112: 657–696

Herzog A G. 1988 Seizure control with clomiphene therapy: a case report. Arch Neurol 45: 209–210

Herzog A G. 1989 A hypothesis to integrate partial seizures of temporal lobe origin and reproductive endocrine disorders. Epilepsy Res 3: 151–159

Herzog A G. 1992 The effects of aromatase inhibitor therapy on sexual function and seizure frequency in a man with epilepsy. Neurology 42 (suppl 3): 400

Herzog A G, Drislane F W, Schomer D L et al. 1990 Abnormal pulsatile secretion of luteinizing hormone in men with epilepsy: relationship to laterality and nature of paroxysmal discharges. Neurology 40: 1557–1561

Herzog A G, Levesque L, Drislane F et al. 1991 Phenytoin-induced elevation of serum estradiol and reproductive dysfunction in men with epilepsy. Epilepsia 32: 550–553

Herzog A G, Seibel M M, Schomer D L et al. 1986 Reproductive endocrine disorders in men with partial seizures of temporal lobe origin. Arch Neurol 43: 347–350

Herzog A G, Coleman A E, Drislane F W, Schomer D S. 1994 Asymmetric temporal lobe modulation of luteinizing hormone secretion. Neuroendocrinology, 60(S): 35

Hierons R, Saunders M. 1966 Impotence in patients with temporal lobe lesions. Lancet ii: 761–764

Isojarvi J I T, Pakarinen A J, Ylipalosaari P J, Myllyla V V. 1990 Serum hormones in male epileptic patients receiving anticonvulsant medication. Arch Neurol 47: 670–676

Jensen I, Larsen J K. 1979 Mental aspects of temporal lobe epilepsy. J Neurol Neurosurg Psychiatry 42: 256–265

Kolarsky A, Freund K, Machek J et al. 1967 Association with early temporal lobe damage. Arch Gen Psychiatry 17: 735–743

Kuhn-Velten W N, Herzog A G, Muller M R. 1990 Acute effects of anticonvulsant drugs on gonadotropin-stimulated and precursor-supported testicular androgen production. Eur J Pharmacol 181: 151–155

Logothetis J, Harner R. 1960 Electrocortical activation by estrogens. Arch Neurol 3: 290–297

Longo L P S, Saldana L E G. 1966 Hormones and their influence in epilepsy. Acta Neurol Latinoam 12: 29–47

Loriaux D, Vigersky S, Marynick S et al. 1977 Androgen and estrogen effects in the regulation of LH in man. In: Troen P, Nankin H, eds. The testis in normal and infertile men. New York: Raven Press, p 213

Macphee G J A, Larkin J G, Butler E et al. 1988 Circulating hormones and pituitary responsiveness in young epileptic men receiving long-term antiepileptic medication. Epilepsia 29: 468–475

Manni A, Partridge W M, Cefalu W et al. 1985 Bioavailability of albumin-bound testosterone. J Clin Endocrinol Metab 61: 705–710

Rodin E, Subramanian M G, Gilroy J. 1984 Investigation of sex hormones in male epileptic patients. Epilepsia 25: 690–694

Shukla G E, Srivastava O N, Katiyar B C. 1979 Sexual disturbances in temporal lobe epilepsy: a controlled study. Br J Psychiatry 134: 288–292

Sodergard R, Backstrom T, Shanbhag V, Carstensen H. 1982 Calculation of free and bound fractions of testosterone and estradiol-17 beta to plasma proteins at body temperature. J Steroid Biochem 16: 801–810

Taneja N, Kucheria K, Jain S, Maheshwari M C. 1994 Effect of phenytoin on semen. Epilepsia 35: 136–140

Taylor D C. 1969 Sexual behavior and temporal lobe epilepsy. Arch Neurol 21: 510–516

Toone B K, Wheeler M, Nanjee M et al. 1983 Sex hormones, sexual activity and plasma anticonvulsant levels in male epileptics. J Neurol Neurosurg Psychiatry 46: 824–826

Werboff L H, Havlena J. 1963 Audiogenic seizures in adult male rats treated with various hormones. Gen Comp Endocrinol 3: 389–397

Winters S, Janick J, Loriaux L, Sherins R. 1979 Studies on the role of sex steroids in the feedback control of gonadotropin concentrations in men. II. Use of the estrogen antagonist clomiphene citrate. J Clin Endocrinol Metab 48: 222–227

14

Seizures and epilepsy in the elderly

M. L. Scheuer

Until recently we believed that epilepsy was most likely to develop in young children, and that the onset of epilepsy in old age was atypical. Over the past decade, however, an enlarging body of epidemiologic data accrued from community-based studies has led to the conclusion that the peak risk for epilepsy onset may occur in old age (Luhdorf et al 1986b, Forsgren 1990, Loiseau et al 1990, Hauser et al 1993). Recognition of a second incidence peak raises important questions regarding the causes and treatment of epilepsy in the elderly. Can epilepsy in the elderly be prevented through reduction of risk factors? Is the natural history of epilepsy in the elderly substantially different than that in younger adults? Are the effects of epilepsy, and of the treatment of seizures with drugs, substantially different in an older person? How can unwanted complications caused by the concurrence of epilepsy and other medical disorders be minimized? Efforts to answer some of these questions have only recently begun, and so current therapeutic decisions must be based on limited information and clinical extrapolation.

EPIDEMIOLOGY

The number of elderly (here defined as age 65 or older) people in the world is rapidly increasing. A disproportionate increase in the elderly segment of the population is occurring, and this is expected to accelerate over the next two to three decades. Whereas only 9.5% of the population of the USA was 65 or older in 1965, in 1990 this group comprised 12.6% of the population. By 2025 this number is expected to rise to 19.5%. By then 8.5% of the population will be age 75 and older (Torrey et al 1987). Demographers project that 20% of the world's population, or at least 2.5 billion people, will be aged 65 or older by the year 2050 (Olshansky et al 1993).

Several epidemiologic studies have indicated that the incidence of seizures and epilepsy rises significantly following age 60 (Luhdorf et al 1986b, Forsgren 1990, Loiseau et al 1990, Hauser et al 1993). The extensive community-based study of epilepsy in Rochester, Minnesota by Hauser and his colleagues (1993) documented the annual incidence of epilepsy at 134/100 000 in persons aged 65 and older (1935–1984). Luhdorf et al (1986b) found an annual epilepsy incidence rate of 77/100 000 in persons aged 60 and older in Denmark. In south-west France, Loiseau and colleagues (1990) found an annual incidence of 33/100 000 in those aged 60 and older. The latter study may have underestimated the incidence of epilepsy due to its reliance on neurologists' reports and electroencephalogram records. Forsgren's study (1990), which documented first seizure cases in a Swedish county, found the greatest incidence in those aged 60 or older.

Of the available studies, that of Hauser and colleagues (1993) contains the most extensive and detailed data set. These data document a progressive increase in the incidence of epilepsy following age 60 (Fig 14.1). In the 1975–1984 data set, including 16 600 persons aged 80 or older, the annual incidence of epilepsy was about 250/100 000 following age 80. This rate is substantially higher than the 79/100 000 per year rate seen in the first year of life (the incidence peak in infancy). Data collected by Hauser & Olafsson during a recent study of the age-specific incidence of seizures and epilepsy in Iceland reportedly closely mirror the rates documented in the Rochester, Minnesota population (Hauser 1994).

Using incidence rates from the Rochester, Minnesota population and data from the 1990 US census, about 41 700 persons aged 65 and older develop epilepsy each year in the USA (US Bureau of the Census 1992, Hauser et al 1993). Using prevalence data from the same population (Hauser et al 1991), there were 331 000 elderly individuals with epilepsy in the USA in 1990. Based on current projections, these figures will double by 2025. Thus, epilepsy in the elderly currently represents a substantial public health problem. This problem will certainly enlarge over the next several decades. Only a reduction in the incidence of elderly-onset epilepsy will forestall the projected increase.

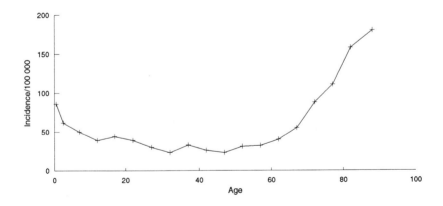

Fig.14.1 Age-specific annual epilepsy incidence data (1935–1984) for Rochester, Minnesota. Data from Hauser et al (1993).

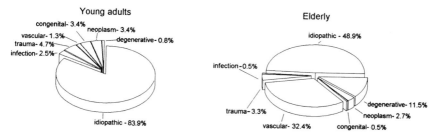

Fig.14.2   Etiology of epilepsy in young adults (onset between ages 15 and 34 years) and the elderly (onset above age 64) in Rochester, Minnesota, 1935–1984. Data from Hauser (1992).

ETIOLOGY AND SEIZURE TYPES

In comparison to younger individuals, isolated seizures in the elderly are more likely the result of an acute metabolic disturbance or structural injury to the brain. Published reports regarding the etiology of seizures and epilepsy in the elderly usually fail to distinguish between epilepsy and isolated seizures, and between acute symptomatic and unprovoked seizures. In addition, most have been retrospective studies subject to substantial sources of bias. Despite these limitations, seizures and epilepsy related to cerebrovascular disease (17–69%), and seizures of unknown cause (9–68%), dominate as etiologies (White et al 1953, Juul-Jensen 1964, Woodcock and Cosgrove 1964, Carney et al 1969, Courjon et al 1970, Fuerstein et al 1970, Schold et al 1977, Gupta 1983, Luhdorf et al 1986c, Sundaram 1989, Henny et al 1990, Loiseau et al 1990, Sung & Chu 1990, Cohen & Scheuer 1991, Hauser et al 1991, Hauser 1992). The best data regarding the etiology of new-onset epilepsy in the elderly derive from the Rochester, Minnesota community-based studies of Hauser and colleagues. Between 1935 and 1984, they found that, 49% of cases were of idiopathic or cryptogenic origin, and 32% were related to cerebrovascular disease (Hauser 1992, Hauser et al 1993). Neurodegenerative disorders accounted for an additional 11.5% of cases (Fig. 14.2).

Few studies have addressed the relative frequencies of various seizure types in the elderly. In general, partial-onset seizures appear to predominate, occurring in 45–80% of elderly patients. Convulsive seizures (most reports did not distinguish between generalized tonic–clonic and partial seizures with secondary generalization) are also common, affecting 9–50% (Woodcock & Cosgrove 1964, Carney et al 1969, Schold et al 1977, Sundaram 1989, Henny et al 1990, Sung & Chu 1990, Cohen & Scheuer 1991, Hauser 1992). In a recent study of first seizures and epilepsy in south-west France, virtually all elderly patients with new-onset epilepsy were diagnosed as having sympto-matic localization-related epilepsies (Loiseau et al 1990). In Rochester, Minnesota, partial-onset seizures accounted for 68% of elderly incident cases, whereas generalized major motor seizures occurred in 27%. The latter classifications were based on clinical data alone and do not permit clear distinction between primary and secondarily generalized seizures. In summary, available data suggest that the majority of new epilepsy cases in older persons present with partial-onset seizures. However, uncertainty exists as to whether true idiopathic generalized forms of epilepsy can present in old age.

PATHOGENESIS

The major identifiable cause of elderly-onset epilepsy is stroke. This accounts for 32–55% of cases in recent studies (Loiseau et al 1990; Hauser et al 1993). Estimates of the incidence of epilepsy following stroke range from 5 to 19% (Hauser et al 1984, Olsen et al 1987, Viitancen et al 1988, Walczak et al 1991). Seizures as a late sequela of stroke occurred in 32% of those who had seizures during the acute peri-infarction period, compared to 10% of those who did not (Kilpatrick et al 1992). Both cortical and subcortical strokes have been associated with development of epilepsy (Gupta et al 1988, Roberts et al 1988, Shinton et al 1988, Kilpatrick et al 1992). The relation between epilepsy and lacunar infarcts is currently unclear. Lacunar infarcts seen on brain imaging examinations could represent a marker for additional small-vessel disease affecting cortical regions, or they could play a direct permissive role in seizure occurrence through alterations in input and feedback to susceptible populations of cortical neurons.

Between 8 and 49% of elderly-onset epilepsy is still classified as idiopathic or cryptogenic (Loiseau et al 1990, Hauser et al 1993). If the latter figure is correct, then the dramatic rise in the incidence of epilepsy in the elderly could reflect a fundamental change in the brain's susceptibility to epileptogenesis. The occurrence and causes of such a putative change are, at present, purely speculative. Recent work, however, suggests that such changes might indeed occur with aging. Aged rats, compared to younger animals, have earlier and more frequent seizures following intraperitoneal or subcutaneous administration of kainic acid. In addition, kainate induced greater releases of glutamate, aspartate and norepinephrine (noradrenaline) in the brains of aged as compared to control rats (Dawson & Wallace 1992). Another study of kainate effects in young, middle-aged and old rats showed that kainate-induced status epilepticus occurred much more frequently in old rats, even at doses which appeared to be non-toxic in young rats (Wozniak et al 1991).

A possible cause of age-related changes in seizure susceptibility could be abnormalities of neuronal oxidative phosphorylation induced by neuronal mitochondrial DNA mutations accumulated over a lifetime. Human brain and muscle cells increasingly accumulate deletions of mitochondrial DNA with age, forming a possible basis for diffuse but subtle alterations in mitochondrial bioenergetic functions (Linnane et al 1989, Beal et al 1993 Cortopassie et al 1992, Wallace 1992). This, in turn, could affect neuronal membrane potential, transmitter synthesis, receptor synthesis or receptor function. As a result the aged brain might be more likely to express seizures. Seizures induced by such a mechanism could conceivably be of either focal or generalized onset.

DIFFERENTIAL DIAGNOSIS

The evaluation of an elderly patient with a seizure or epilepsy is similar to that undertaken in a younger patient (Scheuer & Pedley 1990). However, it must emphasize age-related changes in the differential diagnosis of paroxysmal events. Perhaps even more than in younger persons, the nature of paroxysmal spells in the elderly is often unclear at initial presentation. Syncopal events due to cardiac arrhythmia or medication-induced orthostatic hypotension become more common with increasing age, but clinical history usually allows ready distinction between these and complex partial or clearcut convulsive seizures (McIntosh et al 1993). Brief tonic stiffening and tonic jerks sometimes accompany syncopal events of cardiac origin, though, and may cloud the diagnosis (Aminoff et al 1988). Migraine headache in the elderly is rare, although migraine auras without associated headache must sometimes be distinguished from simple partial seizures. The appearance of psychogenic non-epileptic seizures (pseudoseizures) in old age is rare.

Transient ischemic attacks (TIAs) usually present as loss of neurological function, that is, as negative signs and symptoms, and can therefore generally be distinguished from seizures, which typically present with positive phenomena (e.g. jerking, automatisms, increased tone). Consciousness is rarely lost during a TIA. Sensory symptoms may occur during either seizures or TIAs, but are generally more prolonged and widespread during ischemic events. Of note, prolonged episodes of Todd's paralysis occasionally follow seizures in elderly persons, creating further difficulties in distinguishing seizures from TIA or stroke.

Episodes of nocturnal confusion sometimes punctuate the early course of dementia, and may prompt initial medical evaluation. Such episodes can be confused with complex partial seizures. However, episodic confusion associated with dementia typically occurs in the evening hours and lacks the paroxysmal onset and termination associated with seizures. Confusional spells generally last hours, not minutes. This distinction is not always clear, however, and some seizures in elderly patients are accompanied by prolonged postictal confusion, even in individuals with normal baseline neurological function (Godfrey et al 1982, Gallassi et al 1988, 1992).

Episodes of excessive daytime somnolence, sometimes accompanied by automatic behavior resembling the automatisms of complex partial seizures, occur in some elderly patients with sleep deprivation secondary to sleep apnea. Stimulation generally arouses such patients to normal mentation, in contradistinction to complex partial seizures. Excessive snoring, daytime somnolence and clinical examination usually allow differentiation between a sleep disorder and epilepsy.

DIAGNOSTIC EVALUATION

A thorough history should be obtained, including interview of family members or caretakers. A careful medication history should be elicited, because multiple prescription drugs are commonly used by elderly patients; some of these medications occasionally cause seizures (Messing et al 1984, Burke et al 1992). Other drugs may exert a permissive effect by unmasking potentially epileptogenic foci in an elderly brain. Trauma should always be considered, even if a history is lacking. Subdural hematomas in the elderly, for example, sometimes follow minor and poorly recalled head injury. Physical examination, serum electrolyte determination, electrocardiogram (ECG), magnetic resonance imaging (MRI) and electroencephalogram (EEG) should be performed in all patients. An erythrocyte sedimentation rate may be helpful in screening for a possible vasculitic origin of seizures. Because elderly persons often recover more slowly than younger individuals following a seizure, spinal fluid examination may be necessary to exclude a central nervous system infection as the etiology of new-onset seizures. Additional studies should not be considered routine and should be performed only when indicated by the outcome of prior examinations. Such studies might include elective lumbar puncture, bacterial or viral cultures, toxicologic screens, or studies for the evaluation of possible cerebrovascular disease. At present, available data do not support routine evaluation for stroke (e.g. carotid Doppler studies, echocardiogram, procoagulant studies) unless evidence of possible cerebrovascular disease has been obtained during the initial evaluation.

Electroencephalography

The EEG remains the primary laboratory tool for evaluating the young or elderly patient with known or suspected seizures. Several EEG changes become evident with increasing age, and must be considered when interpreting the EEG. Brief runs of temporal 8–10 Hz activity and episodic temporal θ activities often present predominantly or only on the left, become increasingly common after 50 years of age (Kellaway 1990). Temporal region α activity, when fragmentary and sharply contoured, is sometimes misinterpreted as epileptiform patterns. Although some clinicians consider these findings normal age-related variants, others suggest that these patterns may be markers for undiagnosed cerebrovascular insufficiency. Kellaway (1990) noted that in patients with cerebrovascular insufficiency, temporal slow activity developed at an earlier age and higher incidence than in age-matched controls. However, these findings have not been systematically studied, and their significance remains uncertain. There is no evidence that such findings are related to epilepsy.

Small sharp spikes (benign epileptiform transients of sleep or benign sporadic sleep spikes) become more frequent with increasing age. These benign transients are generally of maximal amplitude over the temporal regions, last less that 50 ms and have a characteristic diphasic morphology with approximately equal positive and negative components. Small sharp spikes usually occur sporadically during drowsiness and typically occur independently in either temporal region. They are exceedingly rare during wakefulness and abate during deeper sleep stages. They must be distinguished from typical spikes and sharp waves which are, in distinction to small sharp spikes, strongly associated with epilepsy.

A rare and unusual pattern of somewhat paroxysmal evolving θ range temporal-parietal activities occurs in persons over age 50. This pattern, called subclinical rhythmic electrographic discharge in adults (SREDA), typically evolves over 1 to several minutes from slower to faster rhythmic θ activities and from higher to lower amplitude. Such a pattern of evolution would be uncommon during an epileptic seizure. SREDA has not been associated with seizures or epilepsy (Kellaway 1990).

To date, EEG has provided little help in determining which stroke patients are at risk of developing seizures or epilepsy (Holmes 1980, Gupta et al 1980, Dam et al 1985, Kilpatrick et al 1990). In a retrospective study of post stroke seizures, periodic lateralized epileptiform discharges (PLEDs) appearing within 1 week of stroke were always associated with seizures (Holmes 1980). The early appearance of sharp waves or other epileptiform abnormalities also indicated a greater risk of seizures. However, non-epileptiform EEG patterns (e.g. normal, diffuse slowing, or focal slowing) remained the most common finding among patients who developed poststroke seizures. The latter observation has been typical of the limited published data on the role of EEG in the evaluation of patients with stroke.

No prospective studies have evaluated the role of EEG findings in predicting recurrence risk following a first unprovoked seizure in an elderly person. Neither have EEG data been studied as a predictor of relapse risk following antiepileptic drug withdrawal in successfully treated elderly patients.

PROGNOSIS

Only a limited amount is known about the prognosis of patients developing seizures or epilepsy in old age. Most data regarding prognosis following late-onset seizures derive from hospital-based series, and thus are subject to multiple biases. For instance, Luhdorf and colleagues (1986a) retrospectively studied the prognosis of seizures and epilepsy in a hospitalized population of patients aged 60 or older. The group included 151 patients with new-onset seizures and 88 patients with established epilepsy. At least 12 months of follow-up were available for most patients. At least one seizure recurrence occurred in 75% of patients and was treated with antiepileptic drugs. Of those previously untreated patients observed for at least 12 months, 62% became seizure-free and 26% had fewer than 3 seizures per year. Patients with seizure recurrence in the first year following initial hospital admission tended to have more seizures in comparison with patients who were seizure-free in the first year. Only 47% with established epilepsy remained seizure-free in the study period. They also found that there was an increased mortality rate in seizure patients older than 60 years. This was true for several subgroups: those with brain tumors or strokes; those with established epilepsy (described as institutionalized patients with chronic epilepsy); and those not previously treated with antiepileptic drugs (mainly those with new-onset seizures). The number of deaths in patients with seizures of unknown cause did not exceed that seen in a control population (Luhdorf et al 1987).

In another recent series, Ettinger & Shinnar (1993) studied 80 hospitalized patients presenting at age 60 or older with new-onset seizures or epilepsy. A slight majority of such seizures were due to acute disorders, including stroke (14%), toxic–metabolic derangements (16%) and hypotension (10%). Seizures related to pre-existing illnesses were primarily the result of earlier strokes (40%), and far less frequently from neoplasms (7%) or dementing illnesses (4%). Idiopathic seizures accounted for only 8% of cases. Morbidity and mortality were highly correlated with the underlying cause of the seizures rather than with seizures themselves. Idiopathic seizures reportedly carried no morbidity or mortality.

These data suggest that the increased risk of death in patients with late-onset seizures is primarily related to seizure etiology. Whether seizures alone represent a threat to certain vulnerable groups, such as those with coronary artery disease, remains unknown. In the extreme case of status epilepticus, age has been documented as one of the primary determinants of mortality, along with etiology and duration of status epilepticus (Towne et al 1994). Prospective controlled studies are needed to evaluate the effect of typical seizures and epilepsy on morbidity and mortality in the elderly.

It is unclear whether seizure control is more easily attained in older or younger individuals. Some have suggested that seizures are more readily controlled in old age. Our experience in the Columbia-Presbyterian Medical Center's neurology clinic suggests that this is not necessarily so. Of actively treated persons aged 75 or older with epilepsy, 15% had more than 10 seizures per year, 40% had 1–10 seizures per year and 45% were seizure-free. This question merits further study, as initial treatment might be altered if seizure control is possible, for example, at lower serum antiepileptic drug concentrations.

No prospective studies have evaluated recurrence risk following a first unprovoked seizure in an elderly person. Because a far greater fraction of epilepsies in the elderly are related to remote symptomatic etiologies (primarily stroke), the recurrence risk following a first unprovoked seizure is probably in general significantly greater than that of younger cohorts. Such a presumption, however, assumes equal likelihood of recurrence in elderly versus young patients for a particular etiology. Selected data from experimental animals suggest that the elderly brain may be more likely to generate seizures (see section on pathogenesis above), but the applicability of such findings to humans is uncertain. Prospective studies of recurrence risk in the elderly are greatly needed, as rational decisions regarding initiation of drug therapy rest primarily on a risk–benefit assessment of recurrence probability versus antiepileptic drug-associated adverse effects.

Relapse risk upon antiepileptic drug withdrawal following a prolonged period of freedom from seizures, and the safety of such withdrawal, have also not been systematically studied. If study results from younger cohorts can be extrapolated to the elderly, then perhaps 30–50% might be expected to relapse following drug withdrawal. Given the high incidence of symptomatic epilepsies in this group, the relapse rate might be even greater. Some elderly persons (for instance, those with significant cardiovascular disease) might be at increased risk for complications at the time of seizure recurrence. On the other hand, the risks of prolonged antiepileptic drug therapy (see below) could outweigh the risks associated with seizure relapse, and so favor drug withdrawal in appropriate patients. This issue warrants prospective controlled clinical studies.

ANTIEPILEPTIC DRUG PHARMACOLOGY IN THE ELDERLY

General considerations

Many reports have described age-related changes in drug disposition and sensitivity in the elderly. However, these reports have usually been single cases, or have failed to document important pharmacokinetic data (Greenblatt et al 1982, Schmucker 1985, Loi & Vestal 1987, Montamat et al 1989, Tregaskis & Stevenson 1990). Methods utilizing drug half-life ($t_{1/2}$) as the major indicator of age-related alterations in metabolism might fail to reflect true drug metabolism, since $t_{1/2}$ is both inversely proportional to drug clearance and proportional to volume of distribution (see below). Meaningful assessments of age-related changes in drug effect must ultimately account for alterations in pharmacokinetics (absorption, distribution, metabolism and excretion) and pharmacodynamic (site of action) effects (Schmucker 1985). A recent pharmacokinetic and pharmacodynamic study of age-related changes in thiopental's (thiopentone's) anesthetic effect exemplifies the issues and complexities inherent in studies of age-related pharmacologic changes (Stanski & Maitre 1990). Elderly patients are clearly more sensitive than younger patients to the anesthetic effects of thiopental. Non-linear mixed effects modeling of data from 64 subjects, however, revealed that this increased sensitivity was not due to a change in the brain's responsiveness to drug. Rather, age-related changes were found to be due to changes in early intracompartment movement of drug (i.e. drug distribution within the body) resulting in an increased early effect of a thiopental dose.

An individual's ability to eliminate drug can be represented by drug clearance. Drug clearance reflects the ability to eliminate a drug completely from a volume of body fluid per unit time. Total body drug clearance (Cl_T) determines the steady-state total serum concentration (C_T) of a drug, because:

$$C_T = \frac{F \cdot D}{Cl_T}$$

(eqn 1)

where D = dose per time interval and F = bioavailability. When the free (non-protein-bound) fraction of a drug is altered by aging or disease, the clearance of free drug (Cl_F) may more accurately describe drug elimination. Because the steady-state concentration of free drug (C_F) is determined by:

$$C_F = C_T. \text{ (free fraction)}$$

(eqn 2)

and

$$C_F = \frac{F \cdot D}{Cl_F}$$

(eqn 3)

rearranging and solving for total clearance yields (Greenblatt et al 1982, Levy & Unadkat 1989):

$$Cl_T = Cl_F. \text{ (free fraction)}.$$

(eqn 4)

Drug clearance is a meaningful parameter of drug elimination for those drugs which follow first-order kinetics at clinically useful concentrations. For such drugs, clearance is independent of concentration. However, some drugs exhibit capacity-limited (saturation) kinetics at clinically useful concentrations (e.g. phenytoin, theophylline). Other models must be used to describe the metabolism of such compounds (see below).

The elimination $t_{1/2}$ of a drug provides a useful number for estimating time to steady state following a dosage change, but it is not necessarily a good longitudinal index of drug elimination rate in an individual or population. This is because:

$$t_{1/2} = \frac{0.693 \cdot V_d}{Cl_T}$$

(eqn 5)

where V_d = volume of distribution. $t_{1/2}$ is thus affected by both V_d and Cl_T. Age-related changes in the V_d of many drugs are well-documented, often resulting from an increase in the proportion of adipose to lean tissue mass with age. A significant change in $t_{1/2}$ might be due to a change in V_d alone. Since V_d is often difficult to calculate accurately, measurement of total drug clearance provides a better index of drug elimination (Greenblatt et al 1982, Schmucker 1985).

The occurrence of significant age-related changes in the pharmacokinetics of some drugs is supported by a substantial amount of animal and human data. However, the relative contributions of various phases of drug disposition (absorption, distribution, hepatic and renal metabolism, renal and biliary excretion) to age-related alterations in pharmacokinetics are usually unknown (Greenblatt et al 1982, Schmucker 1985, Loi & Vestal 1987, Tregaskis & Stevenson 1990, Woodhouse & James 1990, Yuen 1990). Altered pharmacokinetics in old age, and the inherent difficulties in assessing human receptor and intracellular responses to a drug, have particularly vexed pharmacodynamic studies in the elderly. The extent and significance of altered drug pharmacodynamics in the elderly are currently largely unknown (Feely & Coakley 1990, Swift 1990).

Unfortunately, our limited understanding of age-related alterations in drug pharmacology provides us with little basis for rational dosing of most drugs, including antiepileptic drugs, in the elderly.

Phenytoin

Elderly persons with epilepsy commonly receive phenytoin (Oles et al 1987). A recent review of epilepsy patients aged 75 or older seen at Columbia-Presbyterian Medical Center's neurology clinic revealed that 71% were taking phenytoin, usually as monotherapy (Cohen & Scheuer 1991). About 6% of nursing home residents may be receiving phenytoin (Drinka et al 1993, Cloyed et al 1994).

Phenytoin is one of the few drugs which exhibits capacity-limited, or saturable, kinetics at clinically useful serum concentrations. Its clearance is thus concentration-dependent. It is hepatically metabolized by microsomal P-450 enzymes. Thus, age-related declines in hepatic size and function might be of real significance in patients receiving phenytoin. The ability to eliminate phenytoin can be expressed by an equation comparable to the Michaelis–Menten relationship for enzyme kinetics:

$$D = \frac{V_{max} \cdot C_T}{K_m + C_T} \qquad \text{(eqn 6)}$$

where V_{max} equals the maximal rate at which the drug can be metabolized and K_m is the drug concentration at which one-half the maximal metabolic rate is achieved (Bauer & Blouin 1982, Winter & Tozer 1986, Levy & Unadkat 1989, Hudson et al 1990). Free drug elimination could be represented by a similar equation incorporating free drug concentration.

Early reports suggested that phenytoin concentrations were weakly but positively correlated with age in patients on a fixed dose of 300 mg/day (Houghton et al 1975), and that phenytoin plasma concentration per unit dose was significantly greater in elderly (65–85 years) compared to younger (25–45 years) women (Sherwin et al 1974). Hayes and colleagues (1975) evaluated phenytoin clearance in young and elderly (greater than 65 years) volunteers receiving a single oral or intravenous dose of phenytoin. Because only low plasma phenytoin concentrations were seen in this study, phenytoin elimi-

nation followed a log-linear decay curve and so allowed meaningful calculation of clearance. They found that phenytoin clearance increased markedly in
the elderly, and they attributed this to decreased albumin concentrations with
corresponding increased phenytoin free fraction. Because phenytoin is highly
bound to serum albumin and its free fraction is inversely correlated with
serum albumin concentration (Porter & Layzer 1975, Patterson et al 1982,
Tiula & Elfving 1987, Barre et al 1988), age-related changes in total
phenytoin clearance might be expected if age- or disease-related declines in
serum albumin concentration occur (Greenblatt et al 1982, Patterson et al
1982). However, total phenytoin clearance does not necessarily reflect free
phenytoin clearance (see equation 4). If the free fraction of drug increases,
then total clearance increases (assuming that zero-order kinetics are not in
effect) despite unchanged free clearance.

Studies evaluating age-related changes in phenytoin's elimination parameters have generated conflicting results (Fig. 14.3). One report, based on a
small number of elderly patients, found no important difference between V_{max}
and K_m in younger and older patients; phenytoin free fraction was not
assessed, and V_{max} and K_m estimates were apparently based on data from 4
patients (Lambie & Caird 1977). Bauer & Blouin (1982) noted a significant
decrease in V_{max} (6.0 versus 7.5 mg/kg per day) but not K_m (5.8 versus 5.7

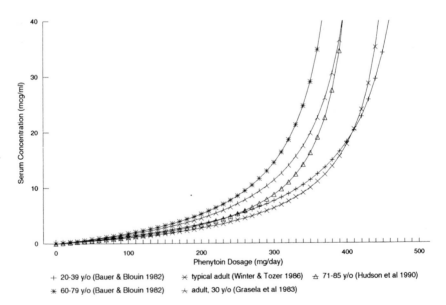

+ 20-39 y/o (Bauer & Blouin 1982)   ✳ typical adult (Winter & Tozer 1986)   △ 71-85 y/o (Hudson et al 1990)

✳ 60-79 y/o (Bauer & Blouin 1982)   ✦ adult, 30 y/o (Grasela et al 1983)

Fig.14.3 Sample phenytoin sodium dose–concentration relationships for young and elderly
70 kg adults, based on data derived from various sources (note that the data from Grasela et
al 1983 were corrected to reflect V_{max} for phenytoin sodium). Although data from the studies
of Bauer & Blouin (1982) and Hudson et al (1990) suggest that the curve for the elderly is
shifted towards the left, the northern European young adult population of Grasela et al
(1983) has a similar dose–concentration relationship.

µg/ml) in patients aged 60–79 versus 20–39 years. They suggested that 200 mg/day of phenytoin might be an appropriate starting dosage for elderly patients. Hudson and colleagues (1990) found that several methods utilizing population data for V_{max} or both K_m and V_{max} yielded similarly good precision in predicting phenytoin dosage requirements in the elderly. Their study data list a mean V_{max} of 6.2 mg/kg per day and mean K_m of 3.9 µg/ml in 9 patients aged 71–85 years.

The above studies did not address the potentially important issue of changes in the metabolism of free phenytoin in the elderly. At least one study (Hayes et al 1975) suggested that this may be an important consideration. Although the decline in serum albumin concentration expected in healthy elderly persons would produce only clinically insignificant changes in free phenytoin fraction (Porter & Layzer 1975, Campion et al 1988), elderly persons with epilepsy often suffer from concurrent illnesses which may cause greater declines in albumin concentration. This in turn could increase the free phenytoin fraction and total clearance and result in the appearance of dose-related side-effects at relatively low total serum phenytoin concentrations. Any associated decline in free phenytoin clearance would further complicate the dose–toxicity relationship. Such a decline in free phenytoin clearance, corrected for liver volume, was documented by Bach et al (1981). Additional clinical studies are needed to define better possible changes in phenytoin kinetics with age. For now, conservative initiation of therapy with 200 mg of phenytoin per day, followed by 30 mg per day dose increments as clinically indicated, seems prudent. Occasional determination of free phenytoin concentration, especially in ill or debilitated elderly patients, may be useful.

Carbamazepine

Despite the increasing use of carbamazepine in the elderly, only two studies have addressed age-related changes in its pharmacokinetics, and none has considered its efficacy or tolerability.

Cloyd and colleagues (1994) estimated carbamazepine's clearance in 7 elderly patients based on daily drug dose and steady-state serum concentrations, and compared this to clearance data from 11 younger patients. They found a 40% reduction in clearance in the elderly.

Another study compared pharmacokinetic parameters following single oral carbamazepine doses in two groups: 5 healthy volunteers aged 65–75, and six aged 20–25 years. This study utilized limited plasma and saliva samples to determine pharmacokinetic parameters. No significant age-related changes occurred in area under the concentration–time curve or terminal elimination rate constant. No significant changes in carbamazepine 10, 11 epoxide concentrations occurred (Hockings et al 1986). Due to the small number of subjects evaluated, this study's statistical power to detect potentially significant differences was very limited. In addition, patients treated with carbamazepine develop substantial autoinduction of carbamazepine metabolism following several weeks of treatment. This effect could not be evaluated in a single dose study. These results thus shed little light on age-related changes in carbamazepine metabolism.

Given Cloyd et al's preliminary data, which are in general agreement with my own observations regarding carbamazepine's metabolism in elderly persons, initiation of carbamazepine therapy should proceed slowly in people over age 65. An initial dose might be 100 mg/day followed by upward titration in 100 mg increments every 4–7 days as tolerated and clinically necessary. Given the uncertainties regarding the drug's side-effect profile in the elderly, an initial target trough serum concentration of 5–7 µg/ml may be reasonable. This concentration should be attained gradually, if clinically appropriate, and subsequent dose adjustments should be based on the clinical response.

Phenobarbital and primidone

There is little information about barbiturate pharmacokinetics in the elderly. Phenobarbital and primidone are partly eliminated by the kidney, and renal excretion tends to decline with age (Schmucker 1985, Scheuer 1992). Furlanut and colleagues (1978) suggested a positive correlation between age and the serum concentration of phenobarbital attained per mg/kg dose. This correlation was only statistically significant for women. Another study evaluated primidone steady-state pharmacokinetics in the elderly and found no change in primidone clearance or half-life, but a statistically significant increase in the concentration of phenylethylmalonamide (PEMA), as well as decreased renal excretion of PEMA in 10 elderly subjects compared with 8 young controls (Martines et al 1990). The study's authors concluded that these changes were probably of little clinical significance.

Controlled studies evaluating adverse effects of barbiturates in the elderly have not been performed. However, many physicians believe that barbiturates are more likely to produce sedation and mental dulling in elderly patients. Because of the uncertainties regarding barbiturate pharmacokinetics and adverse effects in older people, phenobarbital and primidone cannot be viewed as first-line therapy. If barbiturate use becomes necessary, then starting doses of one-third to one-half those used in younger adults should be prescribed. Patients should then be screened frequently for subtle or overt adverse effects.

Valproic acid

An early study comparing single-dose valproate pharmacokinetics in young and elderly healthy volunteers found that valproate's volume of distribution and half-life were increased in the elderly; there was no change in total clearance, however (Bryson et al 1983). The investigators concluded that changes in valproate's metabolism with aging were probably insignificant.

However, this study looked only at total valproate clearance. Subsequent studies have evaluated free valproate pharmacokinetics and have demonstrated changes that are potentially clinically important. A single-dose study using healthy volunteers demonstrated that the half-life, volume of distribution and total clearance of valproate were little changed in the elderly. However, free valproate concentration was significantly increased, and free clearance decreased, in old age (Perucca et al 1984). A multidose study subsequently confirmed these findings. Elderly persons showed a 65% decrease in free valproate clearance and a 67% increase in free valproate concentration (Bauer et al 1985). Thus, in old age less valproate circulates bound to albumin, and the liver's ability to metabolize valproate decreases.

Although valproate is increasingly used in the elderly for a variety of indications, there has been only one published study of its adverse effect profile in this age group (see below). As valproate generally has fewer effects than other antiepileptic drugs on the hepatic metabolism of concurrently administered drugs, and because elderly persons typically receive multiple drugs (see below), there are potential advantages to using valproate in older patients with epilepsy. Recent clinical trial data indicate that valproate is effective against secondarily generalized seizures, and to a lesser extent against complex partial seizures (Mattson et al 1992). These are the primary seizure types seen in the elderly.

Felbamate, gabapentin and lamotrigine

Most clinical trials of the newly approved antiepileptic drugs specifically excluded patients over age 70 from participation. Thus, virtually no data are available regarding the efficacy, pharmacokinetics or adverse effects of these drugs in the elderly.

Approximately 50% of felbamate, a dicarbamate compound, undergoes hepatic metabolism. The remainder is largely excreted unchanged in the urine. Felbamate circulates primarily as free drug; only about 25% is bound to plasma proteins. Its half-life is about 20 h when it is used as monotherapy in adults, and its metabolism is linear at clinically useful dosages. Some age-related alterations in the component of hepatic metabolism could well occur in the elderly, but this effect may not be of major importance given the large component of renal excretion. Felbamate's long half-life might allow infrequent dosing and so improve compliance, but gastrointestinal discomfort often limits the amount which can be tolerated in a single dose. Side-effects such as anorexia, gastrointestinal distress and insomnia, first noted during clinical trials, limit felbamate's tolerability in the elderly (Palmer 1993). Concern about the development of aplastic anaemia, currently estimated to occur in about 1 in 5000 cases, may further restrict felbamate's use. It is not known if this serious complication is more apt to occur in older people. Finally, drug interactions also complicate felbamate's use.

Gabapentin, originally synthesized as an analogue of the inhibitory neurotransmitter γ- aminobutyric acid (GABA), does not act as an agonist at any known GABA receptor subtype in the brain, nor does it undergo conversion to GABA or affect GABA metabolism. Gabapentin is absorbed by a saturable transport mechanism in the intestine. It is not metabolized, but rather excreted almost completely in the urine as unchanged drug. Less than 5% circulates bound to plasma proteins. Its serum half-life ranges from 5 to 8 h, but the duration of its effect may be longer. Gabapentin has no known significant interactions with other drugs. In the USA it is currently only approved for use as an adjunct to therapy with other antiepileptic drugs. Side-effects have usually been mild and well tolerated. No significant adverse cognitive effects have been documented to date, but this issue has not been well studied (Goa & Sorkin 1993). A single abstract reported that decreasing renal clearance of gabapentin with age paralleled declining creatinine clearance (Boyd et al 1990). The manufacturer recommends that gabapentin dosage be adjusted according to creatinine clearance. With the exception of a short half-life (which appears to necessitate multiple daily doses), available clinical and pharmacokinetic data suggest that gabapentin monotherapy might be a good treatment option in the elderly. However, since adequate monotherapy trials have not yet been completed, we do not know whether gabapentin is an effective and safe drug when used as sole therapy in adults. Pending such data, and additional clinical experience specifically in the elderly, gabapentin's role in the treatment of elderly persons with epilepsy remains uncertain.

Lamotrigine's disposition and efficacy in the elderly have not been studied. It is widely used in Europe for the treatment of partial-onset seizures, and it will probably be available for use as adjunctive therapy in the USA before publication of this volume. Lamotrigine's mechanism of action is unknown. About 55% circulates bound to plasma proteins. It undergoes extensive hepatic metabolism, and 90–95% of the drug is excreted as a glucuronide conjugate in the urine. It appears to have little ability to induce hepatic microsomal enzymes or alter the metabolism of other drugs, although other drugs can produce major changes in lamotrigine's metabolism. As monotherapy, its half-life is about 24 h. Elimination kinetics remain linear at clinically useful dosages. Adverse effects have generally been mild, although about 10% of subjects in clinical trials developed rash. However, only 1–2% discontinued lamotrigine due to rash (Goa et al 1993). If ongoing clinical trials support the safety and efficacy of lamotrigine as monotherapy, then it, too, may be a good drug for use in the elderly.

The advent of these and several other new antiepilepitic drugs highlights our paucity of knowledge regarding the use of this class of drugs, new or old, in the elderly. The foundation of rational antiepileptic drug therapy in the elderly must be laid before the projected rapid increase in the size of the elderly population.

Adverse effects of antiepileptic drugs in the elderly

Despite the high incidence of epilepsy in the elderly, and the possibly greater sensitivity of elderly persons to the dose-related neurotoxic side effects of antiepileptic drugs (e.g. ataxia, mental dulling, impaired memory, behavioral disturbance, or visual complaints), there has been only one systematic study of adverse effects published to date (Craig & Tallis 1994). In this single-blind trial, 38 elderly patients with new onset unprovoked seizures or epilepsy were randomized to receive phenytoin or valproate. Initial daily target doses for phenytoin and valproate were 225 and 600 mg respectively. Antiepileptic drug dosages were thereafter adjusted as clinically indicated. Patients received, on average, 247 mg/day of phenytoin and 688 mg/day of valproate, resulting in respective mean serum concentrations of 15.5 µg/ml (31 µmol/ml) and 57 µg/ml (396 µmol/ml). A battery of neuropsychological tests revealed only slight changes due to either drug, some for the better. Only a few minor differences in cognitive effects were found between the phenytoin and valproate-treated groups (valproate was associated with slightly worse choice reaction time during the first 3 months of therapy but not thereafter). Unsteadiness and sleepiness occurred more often in patients on phenytoin, and tremor and edema more often in those receiving valproate. Although the study was not designed to assess drug efficacy, most patients experienced complete seizure control, and no substantial differences were seen between the two treatment groups. Approximately 25% of patients followed beyond 3 months continued to have seizures, but these were generally infrequent.

Cognitive side-effects related to treatment can develop insidiously in the elderly. The evaluation may be confounded by perceptions of expected gradual cognitive impairments with aging. Although systematic data are lacking, clinicians generally believe that such effects are more likely to occur in patients receiving barbiturates. Phenobarbital has been identified as an independent risk factor for falls in the elderly, resulting in hip fractures (Grisso et al 1991). Other studies have found sedative use a major risk factor for falls or hip fracture in elderly persons (Ray et al 1987, Tinetti et al 1988).

Phenytoin, carbamazepine, phenobarbital or primidone could accelerate loss of bone mass in elderly persons (Reynolds 1975, Hoikka et al 1984, Hunt et al 1986, Takeshita et al 1989), and this potential adverse effect might be especially important in older women. Postmenopausal women are, in general, at greater risk of age-related fractures due to a progressive loss of skeletal mass (Riggs et al 1982, Riggs & Melton 1986, Hall et al 1987, Cummings et al 1993). There is substantial evidence supporting a chronic adverse effect of antiepileptic drugs on skeletal metabolism, manifest as abnormalities of bone metabolic markers, abnormally low bone density and histologically proven osteomalacia (Richens & Rowe 1970, Hunter et al 1971, Christiansen et al 1972, 1973, Hahn 1976, Hahn 1980, Hoikka et al 1982, 1984, Wolschendorf et al 1983, Takeshita et al 1989, Collins et al 1991). Thus, postmenopausal women taking antiepileptic drugs may represent a high-risk group for age-related fractures.

Carbamazepine and phenytoin pose potential cardiac risks to elderly persons with cardiac conduction system disease. Administration of the intravenous formulation of phenytoin to patients over 40–50 years of age is associated with a relatively high risk of hypotension and arrhythmias (Ramsey 1989, Donovan & Cline 1991). These undesirable effects can generally be avoided by slowing infusion rates to 5–25 mg/min (Donovan & Cline 1991, Scheuer 1992). Adverse cardiac effects due to orally administered phenytoin have been rare (Durelli et al 1985). Recent reports implicate orally administered carbamazepine as a precipitant of arrhythmias in some middle-aged and elderly persons with underlying conduction system disease. Reported arrhythmias include sinus arrest, bundle branch block, fascicular block, sinus bradycardia and bradycardia–tachycardia syndrome (Takayanagi et al 1990, Kenneback et al 1991). The incidence of this side-effect, and primary risk factors for its occurrence, are unknown. However, a recent study found no difference in the incidence of bradyarrhythmias between a group of carbamazepine-treated patients (mean age 59) and an age-matched reference population (Kenneback al 1992). Given the high prevalence of cardiac disease in the elderly, baseline ECGs should probably be obtained prior to initiation of carbamazepine therapy. If an ECG reveals a significant cardiac conduction abnormality, then another antiepileptic drug should be used or consideration given to hospital admission for cardiac telemetry during introduction of carbamazepine (Kenneback et al 1991).

There have been several cases of carbamazepine-induced urinary retention. These occurred in the setting of presumed dysfunction of the peripheral autonomic nervous system associated with long-standing diabetes mellitus or Fabry's disease (Steiner & Birmanns 1993). A possible anticholinergic effect was postulated as the cause of the urinary retention. Carbamazepine should be introduced cautiously in individuals who might have autonomic dysfunction (such as those with long-standing diabetes); such patients should be advised to call their physician should urinary difficulties occur.

The high incidence and prevalence of medical disease in elderly persons invariably result in interactions among epilepsy, its treatment, concurrent medical diseases and their treatment. Drug interactions are most frequent, but these may also be the unfavorable effects of antiepileptic drugs or other medications on either the medical illness or epilepsy. For instance, carbamazepine can precipitate arrhythmias. Theophylline, phenylpropanolamine and some psychotropic agents can lower seizure threshold in occasional susceptible individuals. The problems posed by the occurrence of medical illness with epilepsy were recently reviewed (Scheuer 1992).

Although persons aged 65 and older comprise only 12.6% of the population of the USA, they receive about 25–32% of prescribed medications (Schmucker 1985, Burke et al 1992, Vestal et al 1992). Epilepsy patients aged 75 and older treated at Columbia-Presbyterian Medical Center took a mean of 3.1 medications (range 0–10) in addition to prescribed antiepileptic drugs (Cohen & Scheuer 1991). Due to the substantial effects of many antiepileptic drugs on hepatic metabolism, there is great potential for significant drug interactions in the population of elderly persons with epilepsy (see Kutt 1989, Scheuer 1992 for reviews).

The patient and patient's family or caretakers should be alerted to the manifestations of possible antiepileptic drug side-effects and drug interactions. Serum antiepileptic drug concentrations should be obtained in patients presenting with possible drug-related symptoms. Free drug concentration should probably be measured in symptomatic elderly patients taking highly protein-bound drugs such as phenytoin or valproate because total drug concentration may not reflect pharmacologically available drug in such cases.

KEY POINTS FOR CLINICAL PRACTICE

- The incidence of epilepsy rises rapidly following age 60. The greatest risk of developing epilepsy occurs in old age. Stroke is the most common identifiable etiology, but many cases are still of idiopathic or cryptogenic origin.
- The recurrence risk following a first unprovoked seizure in old age is unknown, as are the age-specific efficacy, pharmacokinetic and side-effect profiles of most antiepileptic drugs. The likelihood of successful antiepileptic drug withdrawal, and the advisability of an attempt at drug withdrawal, from a well-controlled elderly patient is currently unknown.
- Treatment following a first *unprovoked* convulsive seizure in an elderly person may be reasonable but could potentially be deferred if the patient is in good health, has a normal or only mildly and non-specifically abnormal EEG, and no history of a previous cerebral injury which would increase the relative risk of seizure recurrence. Treatment of acute symptomatic seizures (e.g. those triggered by acute infection, metabolic disarray or drugs) is best accomplished by treatment of the underlying disorder; chronic antiepileptic drug therapy is rarely necessary following resolution of the acute precipitant.
- Recurrent unprovoked seizures (epilepsy) necessitate antiepileptic drug treatment. Current drugs of first choice include phenytoin, valproate and carbamazepine. The role of newer antiepileptic drugs in treatment of the elderly remains to be defined. In choosing a first antiepileptic drug, weigh the patient's existing medical disorders against the adverse-effect profiles of available drugs. Choose the drug which seems least likely to exacerbate coexisting problems, while effectively treating the patient's seizure type.
- Initiate antiepileptic drug therapy conservatively whenever possible. Titrate drug dose to the desired clinical effect while observing carefully for side-effects. Exercise great care when treating patients over age 75, because clinical experience in this group is lacking. In general, depend most on clinical response (seizure control and symptoms of toxicity) to

guide therapeutic changes. The customarily reported therapeutic concentrations of antiepileptic drugs cannot automatically be extrapolated to the elderly.

- Antiepileptic drug withdrawal should be considered in those elderly persons with a history of only a few seizures who have remained completely seizure-free on medication for 2 years. However, drug withdrawal should only be considered when the patient is deemed healthy enough to survive the potential morbidity of a convulsive seizure, and has appropriate observers at home.

REFERENCES

Aminoff M J, Scheinman M M, Griffin J C, Herre J M. 1988 Electrocerebral accompaniments of syncope associated with malignant ventricular arrhythmias. Ann Intern Med 108: 791–796

Bach B, Hansen J M, Kampmann J P, Rasmussen S N, Skovsted L. 1981 Disposition of antipyrine and phenytoin correlated with age and liver volume in man. Clin Pharmacokin 6: 389–396

Barre J, Didey F, Delion F et al. 1988 Problems in therapeutic drug monitoring: free drug level monitoring. Ther Drug Monit 10: 133–143

Bauer L A, Blouin R A. 1982 Age and phenytoin kinetics in adult epileptics. Clin Pharmacol Ther 31: 301–304

Bauer L A, Davis R, Wilensky A et al. 1985 Valproic acid clearance: Unbound fraction and diurnal variation in young and elderly adults. Clin Pharmacol Ther 37: 697–700

Beal M F, Hyman T, Koroshetz W. 1993 Do defects in mitochondrial energy metabolism underline the pathology of neurodegenerative diseases? TINS 16: 125–131

Boyd R A, Bockbrader D, Turck A J et al. 1990 Effect of subject age on the single dose pharmacokinetics of orally administered gabapentin. Pharmacol Res 207: S215

Bryson S M, Verma N, Scott P J W et al. 1983 Pharmacokinetics of valproic acid in young and elderly subjects. Br J Clin Pharmacol 16: 104–105

Burke L B, Jolson H M, Goetsch R A, Ahronheim J C. 1992 Geriatric drug use and adverse drug event reporting in 1990: a descriptive analysis of two national data bases. Annu Rev Geronto Geriatrics 12: 1–28

Campion E W, deLabry L O, Glynn R J. 1988 The effect of age on serum albumin in healthy males: report from the normative aging study. J Gerontolo 43: M18–M20

Carney L R, Hudgins R L, Espinosa R E, Klass D W. 1969 Seizures beginning after the age of 60. Arch Intern Med 124: 707–709

Christiansen C, Kristensen M, Rødbro P. 1972 Latent osteomalacia in epileptic patients on anticonvulsants. Br Med J 3: 738

Christiansen C, Rødbro P, Lund M. 1973 Incidence of anticonvulsant osteomalacia and effect of vitamin D: controlled therapeutic trial. Br Med J 4: 695–701

Cloyd J C, Lackner T E, Leppik I E. 1994 Antiepileptic drugs in the elderly: pharmaco-epidemiology and pharmacokinetics. Arch Family Med 3: 589–598

Cohen J, Scheuer M I. 1991 Antiepileptic drug use in elderly patients with epilepsy. Epilepsia 32 (suppl 3): 53

Collins N, Maher J, Cole M et al. 1991 A prospective study to evaluate the dose of vitamin D required to correct low 25-hyroxyvitamin D levels, calcium, and alkaline phosphatase in patients at risk of developing antiepileptic drug-induced osteomalacia. Q J Med 78: 113

Cortopassi G A, Shibata D, Soong N-W, Arnheim N. 1992 A pattern of accumulation of a somatic deletion of mitochondrial DNA in aging human tissues. Proc Natl Acad Sci 89: 7370–7374

Courjon J, Artru F, Zeskov P. 1970 A propos des crises d'epilepsie apparaissant apres 60 ans observees en clientele de neurolgie dans un service de neuro-chirurgie. Semin Hop Paris 46: 3129–3132

Craig I, Tallis R. 1994 Impact of valproate and phenytoin on cognitive function in elderly patients: results of a single-blind randomized comparative study. Epilepsia 35: 381–390

Cummings S R, Black D M, Nevitt M C et al. 1993 Bone density at various sites for prediction of hip fractures. Lancet 341: 72

Dam A M, Fuglsnag-Frederiksen A, Svarre-Olsen U et al. 1985 Late-onset epilepsy: etiologies, types of seizure, and value of clinical investigation, EEG, and computerized tomography scan. Epilepsia 26: 227–231

Dawson R, Wallace D R. 1992 Kainic acid-induced seizures in aged rats: neurochemical correlates. Brain Res Bull 29: 459–468

Donovan P J, Cline D. 1991 Phenytoin administration by constant intravenous infusion: selective rates of administration. Ann Emerg Med 20: 139–142

Drinka P J, Langer E H, Voeks S K, Goodwin J S. 1993 Low serum folic acid in a nursing home population: a clinical experience. J Am Coll Nutr 12: 186–189

Durelli L, Mutani R, Sechi G P et al. 1985 Cardiac side effects of phenytoin and carbamazepine: a dose-related phenomenon? Arch Neurol 42: 1067–1068

Ettinger A B, Shinnar S. 1993 New-onset seizures in an elderly hospitalized population. Neurology 43: 489–492

Feely J, Coakley D. 1990 Altered pharmacodynamics in the elderly. Clin Geriatr Med 6: 269–283

Forsgren L. 1990 Prospective incidence study and clinical characterization of seizures in newly referred adults. Epilepsia 31: 292–301

Fuerstein J, Wever M, Kurtz D et al. 1970 Etude statistique des crises epileptiques apparaissant apres l'age de 60 ans. Semin Hop Paris 46: 3125–3128

Furlanut M, Benetello P, Testa G et al. 1978 The effect of dose, age, and sex on the serum levels of phenobarbital and diphenylhydantoin in epileptic patients. Pharmacol Res Commun 10: 85–89

Gallassi R, Morreale A, Lorusso S et al. 1988 Epilepsy presenting as memory disturbances. Epilepsia 29: 624–629

Gallassi R, Morreale A, DiSarro R, Lugaresi E. 1992 Epileptic amnesic syndrome. Epilepsia 33 (suppl 6): S21–S25

Goa K L, Sorkin E M. 1993 Gabapentin: a review of its pharmacological properties and clinical potential in epilepsy. Drugs 46: 409–427

Goa K L, Ross S R, Chrisp P. 1993 Lamotrigine: a review of its pharmacological properties and clinical efficacy in epilepsy. Drugs 46: 152–176

Godfrey J W, Roberts M A, Caird F I. 1982 Epileptic seizures in the elderly: II. Diagnostic problems. Age Ageing 11: 29–34

Grasela T H, Sheiner L B, Rambeck B et al. 1983 Steady-state pharmacokinetics of phenytoin from routinely collected patient data. Clin Pharmacokin 8: 355–364

Greenblatt D J, Sellers E M, Shader R I. 1982 Medical intelligence. N Engl J Med 306: 1081–1088

Grisso J A, Kelsey J L, Strom B L et al. 1991 Risk factors for falls as a cause of hip fracture in women. N Eng J Med 324: 1326–1331

Gupta K. 1983 Epilepsy in the elderly: how far to investigate? Br J Clin Pract 37: 249–252

Gupta S R, Naheedy M H, Elias D et al. 1988 Postinfarction seizures: a clinical study. Stroke 19: 1477–1481

Hahn T J. 1976 Bone complications of anticonvulsants. Drugs 12: 201

Hahn T J. 1980 Drug-induced disorders of vitamin D and mineral metabolism. Clin Endocrinol Metab 9: 107

Hall F M, Davis M A, Baran D T. 1987 Bone mineral screening for osteoporosis. N Engl J Med 316: 212

Hauser W A. 1992 Seizure disorders: the changes with age. Epilepsia 33 (suppl 4): S6–S14

Hauser W A. 1994 Personal communication

Hauser W A, Ramirez-Lassepas M, Rosenstein R. 1984 Risk for seizures and epilepsy following cerebrovascular insults. Epilepsia 25: 666

Hauser W A, Annegers J F, Kurland L T. 1991 Prevalence of epilepsy in Rochester, Minnesota: 1940–1980. Epilepsia 32: 429–445

Hauser W A, Annegers J F, Kurland L T. 1993 Incidence of epilepsy and unprovoked seizures in Rochester, Minnesota: 1935–1984. Epilepsia 34: 453–468

Hayes M J, Langman M J S, Short A H. 1975 Changes in drug metabolism with increase in age: 2. Phenytoin clearance and protein binding. Br J Clin Pharmacol 2: 73–79

Henny C, Despland P-A, Regli F. 1990 Premiere crise epileptique apres l'age de 60 ans: etiologie, presentation clinique et EEG. Schweiz Med Wochenschr 120: 787–792

Hockings N, Pall A, Moody J et al. 1986 The effects of age on carbamazepine pharmacokinetics and adverse effects. Br J Clin Pharmacol 22: 725–728

Hoikka V, Savolainen K, Alhava E M et al. 1982 Anticonvulsant osteomalacia in epileptic outpatients. Ann Clin Res 14: 129

Hoikka V, Alhava E M, Karjalainen P et al. 1984 Carbamazepine and bone mineral metabolism. Acta Neurol Scand 70: 77–80

Holmes G L. 1980 The electroencephalogram as a predictor of seizures following cerebral infarction. Clin Electroencephalogr 11: 83–86

Houghton G W, Richens A, Leighton M. 1975 Effect of age, height, weight and sex on serum phenytoin concentration in epileptic patients. Br J Clin Pharmacol 2: 251–256

Hudson S A, Farquhar D L, Thompson D et al. 1990 Phenytoin dosage individualization – five methods compared in the elderly. J Clin Pharm Ther 15: 25–34

Hunt P A, Wu-Chen M L, Handal N J et al. 1986 Bone disease induced by anticonvulsant therapy and treatment with calcitriol (1,25-dihydroxyvitamin D3). Am J Dis Child 140: 715–718

Hunter J, Maxwell J, Stewart D, Parsons V, Williams R. 1971 Altered calcium metabolism in epileptic children on anticonvulsants. Br Med J ii: 202

Juul-Jensen. P. 1964 Pathogenesis and prognosis. Acta Neurol Scand 40 (suppl 5): 26–42

Kellaway P. 1990 An orderly approach to visual analysis. In: Daly DD, Pedley TA eds. Current practice of clinical electroencephalography, 2nd edn. New York: Raven Press, pp 139–199

Kenneback G, Bergefeldt L, Vallin H et al. 1991 Electrophysiologic effects and clinical hazards of carbamazepine treatment for neurologic disorders in patients with abnormalities of the cardiac conduction system. Am Heart J 121: 1421–1429

Kenneback G, Bergfeldt L, Tomson T et al. 1992 Carbamazepine induced bradycardia – a problem in general or only in susceptible patients? A 24-h long-term electrocardiogram study. Epilepsy Res 13: 141–145

Kilpatrick C J, Davis S M, Tress B M et al. 1990 Epileptic seizures in acute stroke. Arch Neurol 47: 157–160

Kilpatrick C J, Davis S M, Hopper J L et al. 1992 Early seizures after acute stroke: risk of late seizures. Arch Neurol 49: 509–511

Kutt H. 1989 Interactions between antiepileptic and other drugs. In: Pitlick WH, ed. Antiepileptic drug interactions. New York: Demos, pp 39–63

Lambie D C, Caird F I. 1977 Phenytoin dosage in the elderly. Age Ageing 6: 133–137

Levy R H, Unadkat J D. 1989 General principles: drug absorption, distribution and elimination. In: Levy R, Mattson R, Meldrum B, Penry J K, Dreifuss F E, eds. Antiepileptic drugs, 3rd edn. New York: Raven Press, pp 1–22

Linnane A W, Ozawa T, Marzuki S, Tanaka M. 1989 Mitochondrial DNA mutations as an important contributor to ageing and degenerative diseases. Lancet 1: 642–645

Loi C M, Vestal R E. 1987 Drug metabolism in the elderly. Pharmacol Ther 36: 131–149

Loiseau J, Loiseau P, Duche B et al. 1990 A survey of epilipetic disorders in southwest France: seizures in elderly patients. Ann Neurol 27: 232–237

Luhdorf K, Jensen L D, Plesner A M. 1986a Epilepsy in the elderly: prognosis. Acta Neurol Scand 74: 409–415

Luhdorf K, Jensen L D, Plesner A M. 1986b Epilepsy in the elderly: incidence, social function, and disability. Epilepsia 27: 135–141

Luhdorf K, Jensen L D, Plesner A M. 1986c Etiology of seizures in the elderly. Epilepsia 27: 458–463

Luhdorf K, Jensen L D, Plesner A M. 1987 Epilepsy in the elderly: life expectancy and causes of death. Acta Neurol Scand 76: 183–190

McIntosh S, Dacosta D, Kenny L A. 1993 Outcome of an integrated approach to the investigation of dizziness, falls, and syncope in elderly patients referred to a syncope clinic. Age Ageing 22: 53–58

Martines C, Gatti G, Sasso E et al. 1990 The disposition of primidone in elderly patients. Br J Clin Pharmacol 30: 607–611

Mattson R H, Carmer J A, Collins J F et al. 1992 A comparison of valproate with carbamazepine for the treatment of complex partial seizures and secondarily generalized tonic–clonic seizures in adults. N Engl J Med 327: 765–771

Messing R O, Closson R G, Simon R P. 1984 Drug-induced seizures: a 10-year experience. Neurology 34: 1582–1586

Montamat S C, Cusack B J, Vestal R E. 1989 Management of drug therapy in the elderly. N Engl J Med 321: 303–309

Oles K S, Gal P, Kiffin Penry J et al. 1987 Use of antiepileptic drugs in the elderly population. Public Health Rep 102: 335–337

Olsen T S, Hogenhaven H, Thage O. 1987 Epilepsy after stroke. Neurology 37: 1209–1211

Olshansky S J, Carnes B A, Cassel C K. 1993 The aging of the human species. Sci Am (April): 46–52

Palmer K J. 1993 Felbamate: a review of its pharmacodynamic and pharmacokinetic properties, and therapeutic efficacy in epilepsy. Drugs 45: 1041–1065

Patterson M, Heazelwood R, Smithurst B et al. 1982 Plasma protein binding of phenytoin in the aged: in vivo studies. Br J Clin Pharmacol 13: 423–425

Perucca E, Grimaldi R, Gatti G et al. 1984 Pharmacokinetics of valproic acid in the elderly. Br J Clin Pharmacol 17: 665–669

Porter R J, Layzer R B. 1975 Plasma albumin concentration and diphenylhydantoin binding in man. Arch Neurol 32: 298–303

Ramsey R E. 1989 Pharmacokinetics and clinical use of parenteral phenytoin, phenobarbital, and paraldehyde. Epilepsia 30: S1–S3

Ray W A, Griffin M R, Schaffner W et al. 1987 Psychotropic drug use and the risk of hip fracture. N Engl J Med 316: 363–369

Reynolds E H. 1975 Chronic antiepileptic toxicity: A review. Epilepsia 16: 319–352

Richens A, Rowe D J F. 1970 Disturbance of calcium metabolism by anticonvulsant drugs. Br Med J 3: 73

Riggs B L, Melton L J. 1986 Involutional osteoporosis. N Engl J Med 314: 1676

Riggs B L, Wahner H W, Seeman E et al. 1982 Changes in bone mineral density of the proximal femur and spine with aging. Differences between the postmenopausal and senile osteoporosis syndromes. J Clin Invest 70: 716

Ritschel W A. 1988 Gerontokinetics. The pharmacokinetics of drugs in the elderly. New Jersey: Telford Press

Roberts R C, Shorvon S D, Cox T C S et al. 1988 Clinically unsuspected cerebral infarction revealed by computed tomography scanning in late onset epilepsy. Epilepsia 29: 190–194

Scheuer M L. 1992 Medical aspects of treating epilepsy. In: Pedley TA, Meldrum BS, eds Recent advances in epilepsy, 5. London: Churchhill Livingstone, pp 127–157

Scheuer M L, Pedley T A. 1990 The evaluation and treatment of seizures. N Engl J Med 323: 1468–1474

Schmucker D L. 1985 Aging and drug disposition: an update. Pharmacol Rev 37: 133–148

Schold C, Yarnell P R, Earnest M R. 1977 Origin of seizures in elderly patients. JAMA 238: 1177–1178

Sherwin A L, Loynd J S, Bock G W et al. 1974 Effects of age, sex, obesity, and pregnancy on plasma diphenylhydantoin levels. Epilepsia 15: 507–521

Shinton R A, Gill J S, Melnick S C et al. 1988 The frequency, characteristics and prognosis of epileptic seizures at the onset of stroke. J Neurol Neurosurg Psychiatry 51: 273–276

Stanski D R, Maitre P O. 1990 Population pharmacokinetics and pharmacodynamics of thiopental: the effect of age revisited. Anesthesiology 72: 412–422

Steiner I, Birmanns B. 1993 Carbamazepine-induced urinary retention in long-standing diabetes mellitus. Neurology 43: 1855–1856

Sundaram M B M. 1989 Etiology and patterns of seizures in the elderly. Neuroepidemiology 8: 234–238

Sung C Y, Chu N S. 1990 Epileptic seizures in elderly people: aetiology and seizure type. Age Aging 19: 25–30

Swift C G. 1990 Pharmacodynamics: changes in homeostatic mechanisms, receptor and target organ sensitivity in the elderly. Br Med Bull 46: 36–52

Takayanagi K, Yamaguchi H, Hayashi T et al. 1990 Carbamazepine-induced bradycardia–tachycardia syndrome with pharmacological analysis and concurrent ECG monitoring. J Electrocardiol 23: 85–88

Takeshita N, Seino Y, Ishida H et al. 1989 Increased circulating levels of α-carboxyglutamic acid-containing protein and decreased bone mass in children on anticonvulsant therapy. Calcif Tissue Int 44: 80–85

Tinetti M E, Speechley M. Ginter S F. 1988 Risk factors for falls among elderly persons living in the community. N Engl J Med 319: 1701–1707

Tiula E, Elfving S. 1987 Serum protein binding of phenytoin, diazepam and propranolol in age-related decrease in renal function. Ann Clin Res 19: 163–169

Torrey B B, Kinsella K, Taeuber C M. 1987 An aging world. Washington, DC: US Department of Commerce, Bureau of the Census

Towne A R, Pellock J M, Ko D, DeLorenzo R J. 1994 Determinants of mortality in status epilepticus. Epilepsia 35: 27–34

Tregaskis B F, Stevenson I H. 1990 Pharmacokinetics in old age. Br Med Bull 46: 9–21

US Bureau of the Census 1992 Statistical abstract of the United States: 1992, 112th edn Washington, DC: US Bureau of the Census, p 14

Vestal R E, Montamat S C, Nielson C P. 1992 Drugs in special patient groups: the elderly. In: Melmon K L, Morrelli H F, Hoffman B B et al. eds. Clinical pharmacology: basic principles in therapeutics, 3rd edn. New York: McGraw-Hill, 851–874

Viitanen M, Eriksson S, Asplund K. 1988 Risk of recurrent stroke, myocardial infarction and epilepsy during long-term follow-up after stroke. Eur Neurol 28: 227–231

Walczak T S, Sacco R L, Mohr J P. 1991 Prevalence and features of stroke-related seizures analyzed according to stroke subtype. Epilepsia 32: 62–63

Wallace D C. 1992 Mitochondrial genetics: a paradigm for aging and degenerative diseases? Science 256: 628–632

White P T, Bailey A A, Bickford R G. 1953 Epileptic disorders in the aged. Neurology 3: 674–678

Winter M E, Tozer T N. 1986 Phenytoin. In: Evans WE, eds. Applied pharmacokinetics: principles of therapeutic drug monitoring, 2nd edn. Vancouver: Applied Therapeutics, pp 493–539

Wolschendorf K, Vanselow K, Möller W D et al. 1983 A quantitative determination of anticonvulsant-induced bone demineralization by an improved x-ray densitometry technique. Neuroradiology 25: 315

Woodcock S, Cosgrove J B R. 1964 Epilepsy after the age of 50. Neurology 14: 34–40

Woodhouse K W, James O F W. 1990 Hepatic drug metabolism and ageing. Br Med Bull 46: 22–35

Wozniak D F, Stewart G R, Miller J P, Olney J W. 1991 Age-related sensitivity to kainate neurotoxicity. Exp Neurol 114: 250–253

Yuen G J. 1990 Altered pharmacokinetics in the elderly. Clin Geriatr Med 6: 257–267

15

Mortality in epilepsy

L. Nashef   J. W. A. S. Sander   S. D. Shorvon

In writing his textbook on prognosis, Rodin (1968) expressed misgivings in addressing outcome. Given that epilepsy was not considered a disease but a symptom of a variety of illnesses, what was the sense in writing about prognosis? Yet, epilepsy has its own consequences; it is both a symptom and a disease, and seizures have implications beyond those of their underlying cause. With advances in treatment, and in an attempt to minimize restrictions, epilepsy has come to be regarded as benign, with consequences of seizures underplayed. The pendulum may have swung too far. Mortality in patients with epilepsy is increased two to three times that of the general population, with both underlying disease and epilepsy contributing to this excess. Acknowledgement of this increased risk, while keeping it in perspective, is necessary both in terms of better clinical management and strategies for prevention.

In this chapter, we show that in recent-onset epilepsy mortality is mainly that of underlying disease, and in chronic cases, excess deaths are primarily epilepsy-related. We address the possible contribution of mortality to prevalence and outline causes of death, including the rediscovered entity of sudden unexpected death in epilepsy.

MORTALITY OF EPILEPSY IN THE POPULATION

Overall national mortality data

G. Mackenzie Bacon (1868) suggested that once cases with known secondary epilepsy were excluded, causes of death may be categorized as follows: '1. Those arising from the long continued effects of the disease on the body; 2. Deaths after a rapid succession of fits; 3. Sudden deaths in a fit; 4. Accidents due to fits.' He added that 'if practitioners would adopt some such system . . . we should not have to lament such a meaningless blank as the word now represents in lists of mortality'.

The situation is similar today. National mortality data have made but small contribution to the study of mortality in epilepsy. A total of 906 deaths in 1991 in England and Wales (1.78/100 000 of population) were listed as due to epilepsy (Office of Population Censuses and Surveys 1991). Apart from the subheading of status epilepticus, this figure is not usefully subdivided. Based on the *International Classification of Diseases* code, listed causes of death are entirely dependent on death certificate completion and inconsistencies thereof. Epilepsy was recorded in only 74% of certificates in Warsaw where death was due to epilepsy (Zielinski 1974).

Similar gross national figures have been obtained from other countries (Chandra et al 1984, Jallon et al 1989) and compared between different countries and different epochs (Massey & Schoenberg 1985). Reported rates range from 0.6 to 4.0 deaths/100 000 per year. Inaccuracies in death certification coupled with doubt about the way cases are ascertained and causes ascribed render these figures fairly meaningless.

Influence of underlying disease and epilepsy on mortality

Mortality in epilepsy has been shown in most studies (Henriksen et al 1970, Hauser et al 1980) to be increased compared with the general population. The subject has been reviewed by Hauser & Hesdorffer (1990) who, in contrast to earlier writers (Bacon 1868, Munson 1910), emphasize the excess mortality due to underlying disease. They state that: 'Studies suggest that the underlying conditions, rather than the epilepsy itself may explain most of the increased relative risk in younger patients'.

In support of this view, and reflecting the fact that epilepsy is secondary to a number of disease processes, is the observation, in longitudinal studies, that mortality is highest in the first few years after diagnosis (Hauser et al 1980, Cockerell et al 1994). However, mortality is also elevated when patients with idiopathic epilepsy are considered separately (Henriksen et al 1970, Hauser et al 1980). Excess mortality is likely to be related not only to underlying disease but also to epilepsy per se.

The impact of mortality on prevalence of epilepsy

The prevalence of epilepsy (approximately 0.5%) depends on incidence (approximately 0.05% annually), remission and mortality. Remission has been considered the significant factor in accounting for the difference between cumulative incidence and prevalence. A significant contribution of excess mortality has been discounted (Juul-Jensen & Foldspang 1983) except with reference to developing countries (Sander 1993). However, in the ongoing most recent comprehensive population-based longitudinal study (Sander et al 1990), of 564 definite cases 114 have already died with an all-cause standardized mortality ratio (SMR; Table 15.1) of 3.0 (confidence intervals (CI) 2.5–3.7) and a mean follow-up of 6.9 years (Cockerell et al 1994).

It is of interest to consider briefly the developing world in this context. Incidence rates may be higher owing to a higher risk of symptomatic epilepsy and the age-structure of the population (Shorvon & Bharucha 1993). Treatment rates, on the other hand, based on drug supply figures and field

Table 15.1 Definitions

Standardized mortality ratio
The ratio of deaths observed in a group to the number of deaths that would be expected to have occurred during a follow-up period if the group in question had experienced the same age- and sex-specific death rates as in the control population

Proportional mortality ratio
The proportion of deaths due to a specific cause amongst a study population compared with a control group

---

surveys are very low, at 1.6–20% (Shorvon & Bharucha 1993). Although spontaneous remission does occur, rates are lower in untreated groups (Sander 1993). Thus, in developing countries, lower remission and higher incidence may be expected to lead to higher prevalence. Yet, except in selected populations, prevalence rates remain comparable at around 0.5% (Sander 1993, Shorvon & Bharucha 1993), and although these may only be gross estimates with uncertainty about complete case-ascertainment, mortality is likely to be a factor in accounting for the discrepancy.

Selected and unselected studies

Table 15.2 lists and classifies some of the studies reported on mortality. Different approaches have made difficult comparisons between different studies. Problems of definition and limitations of epidemiological studies in epilepsy have been reviewed (Sander & Shorvon 1987). Death certificate-based studies may underestimate mortality from or related to epilepsy, although false positives may also occur (Hauser et al 1980). Similarly, conclusions from selected cohorts cannot be extrapolated to the majority with epilepsy or to other selected groups.

Population-based series have thus far been widely considered to be the most informative. Calculations based on deaths per person-years are compared to national all-cause mortality data. The assumption is made that cases lost to observation have the same experience as those remaining. Whether this is justified in mortality studies is unknown and not all studies clearly report on patient years lost to follow-up.

Furthermore, while invaluable in defining the overall problem, population studies give limited information in terms of defining prognosis in individual cases. Broad categories (cryptogenic/idiopathic, remote symptomatic, acute symptomatic, or associated with congenital/perinatal neurological abnormality) are used in surveys in view of the inevitably incomplete clinical information in such studies. Nevertheless, even though the categories are based on presumed causation, they do not reflect conceptual developments in the classification of epilepsy syndromes, nor indeed improved imaging techniques which allow for more accurate diagnosis. It is with reference to

Table 15.2 Mortality series in epilepsy

Some mortality series based on cohorts with epilepsy
General population
    National General Practice Study of Epilepsy (NGPSE), UK — Cockerell et al (1994)
    Rochester, USA — Hauser et al (1980)
    Warsaw, Poland — Zielinski (1974)
Residents in institutions
    Finland — Iivanainen & Lehtinen (1979)
    Chalfont, UK — Klenerman et al (1993)
    Craig Colony, USA — Munson (1910)
    Chalfont, UK — White et al (1979)
    Warsaw, Poland — Zielinski (1974)
Clinical series
    Denmark — Henriksen et al (1970)
    Lausanne, Switzerland — Penning et al (1969)
    Sweden — Brorson & Wranne (1987)
    France — Chevrie & Aicardi (1978)*
Insurance company series[†]

Some mortality series based on deaths in epilepsy
National mortality data/based on death certificates
    USA — Chandra et al (1984)
    France — Jallon et al (1989)
    USA — Satisahandra (1988)
    International — Massey & Schoenberg (1985)
Coroner's postmortem series
    USA — Freytag & Lindenberg (1964)
    Denmark — Lund & Gormsen (1985)
Clinical series
    Norway — Krohn (1963)
    Japan — Hashimoto et al (1989)

---

*Series based on cases with convulsions during the first year of life.
[†]As quoted by Hauser & Hesdorffer (1990) for a number of countries.

cases with cryptogenic/idiopathic epilepsies, which constitute the largest single category in general population-based studies, that this is most relevant.

Future investigators need to narrow inclusion criteria rather than widen them. Prospective population-based studies of selected cohorts with well-defined diagnostic categories are needed. The importance of tracing each individual registered need hardly be emphasized. It may then be possible to address the relative contributions to seizure type, severity, duration and frequency as well as treatment options within a diagnostic category.

VARIABLES AFFECTING EXCESS MORTALITY

Within the often quoted SMR of 2–3 in patients with epilepsy is a wide range from no increased risk to an SMR of 8 or more. Studies to date suggest that the following factors may influence mortality.

Age

The excess observed mortality in patients with epilepsy decreases with increasing age, remaining above that of the general population (Zielinski 1974, Luhdorf et al 1987, Hauser & Hesdorffer 1990). This may simply reflect epilepsy deaths being lost within much higher mortalities from other causes. Luhdorf et al (1987) studied mortality in a cohort with epilepsy over the age of 60 and found an increased mortality in patients with established epilepsy, in patients with new-onset secondary epilepsy, but not in patients with new-onset epilepsy and no identified cause. In young age-groups increased mortality in epilepsy when associated with neurological abnormalities also needs to be considered.

Sex

Excess mortality in epilepsy is reportedly higher in males (Henriksen et al 1970, Hauser et al 1980). The contribution of accidental deaths, generally more common among males (Office of Population Censuses and Surveys 1991), is unknown. Occasional higher SMRs are quoted in young females (Zielinski 1974), probably reflecting the particularly low mortality for females aged 1–34 in the general population in the developed world.

Race

A higher mortality is reported in the USA for the non-white as compared to the white population with epilepsy (Chandra et al 1984). This needs to be considered in the context of lower socioeconomic status and possible higher prevalence rates of epilepsy among Afro-Americans (Haerer et al 1986, Sander & Shorvon 1987).

Seizure characteristics and diagnostic category

Absence seizures are not reported to be associated with higher mortality, while generalized tonic–clonic and myoclonic seizures are. Complex partial seizures do not appear to carry an additional risk (Henriksen et al 1970, Hauser et al 1980). Henriksen et al (1970) reported that patients who at follow-up had severe and moderately severe epilepsy (in terms of fit frequency) showed a statistically significant higher mortality as compared to seizure-free and slight cases. Patients with remote symptomatic epilepsy have a higher excess risk compared to patients with cryptogenic/idiopathic epilepsy (Hauser et al 1980, Luhdorf et al 1987).

Mental handicap

It is generally considered that mortality is higher in epilepsy when associated with mental handicap; however, there are often coexisting neurological signs and the two are usually combined (Brorson & Wranne 1987). Mental handicap in general is also associated with a higher risk of accidents.

CAUSES OF DEATH IN EPILEPSY: STUDIES OF PROPORTIONAL MORTALITY

Difficulty in assigning cases

Death in epilepsy may be apparently unrelated, related to underlying disease, or related directly or indirectly to epilepsy, as outlined in Table 15.3. There

Table 15.3   Causes of death in epilepsy

Apparently unrelated
Malignancy outside the central nervous system
Accidents not as a consequence to seizures

Related to underlying disease
Brain tumours
Cerebrovascular disease
Cerebral infection

Related directly or indirectly to epilepsy
Non-accidental deaths in the context of a witnessed seizure
Sudden unexpected deaths
Deaths related to status epilepticus
Accidental deaths as a consequence of seizures
Deaths as a consequence of treatment of epilepsy
Suicides
Respiratory deaths

is overlap between the three categories and cases need to be judged individually, although it is not always possible to assign a death appropriately. Clearly not all accidents, suicides, sudden deaths or pneumonias are epilepsy-related. Similarly, most deaths from status epilepticus in hospital series have been judged to be related to underlying disease (Oxbury & Whitty 1971). However, the presence of status may influence mortality related to the underlying condition, as found by Goulon in bacterial meningitis, where mortality was 82% in cases complicated by status, compared with 33% without (Shorvon 1994).

Both population-based studies and those with known deaths (Table 15.2) as their starting point provide data on proportional mortality. Wannamaker (1990) quotes different studies with deaths attributed to epilepsy accounting for 24–62% of the total, although some of these exclude deaths due to tumour or cerebrovascular disease.

Accidental deaths

Drowning

Drowning is a danger for the patient with epilepsy. Diekema et al (1993) observed a relative risk of drowning for children (0–19) with epilepsy compared to those without of 13.8 (CI 7.0–27) and a relative risk of drowning in the bathtub of 96 (95% CI 33–275). Patients with epilepsy constitute some 0–8% of drowning series (Orlowski et al 1982, Diekema et al 1993, Ryan & Dowling 1993) and deaths from non-intentional drowning constitute 1.8–10% of deaths in epilepsy (Krohn 1963, Freytag & Lindenberg 1964, Iivanainen & Lehtinen 1979, Klenerman et al 1993). Drowning may occur in the bath or while swimming but also if a seizure occurs by the waterside. The risk is greater in the absence of supervision and in association with other handicap. The relative risks of drowning in different circumstances have been addressed; however, the merit of such comparisons is doubtful as differences are more likely to be exposure-dependent.

In 1991, in England and Wales there were 231 unintentional deaths by drowning (35 bath deaths) and a further 285 were unclassified as to whether they were accidental or purposefully inflicted (Office of Population Censuses and Surveys 1991). How many of those had epilepsy is not stated. Although absolute numbers may not be large, their importance lies in the potential for prevention. Showering while seated with good ventilation and thermostat-controlled water temperature poses a much smaller risk than the bath (Ryan & Dowling 1993). A shallow bath with adequate supervision is an alternative, although difficult to provide without invading privacy. Relatives who find an older child or an adult fitting may be unable to lift them out of the bath (Ryan & Dowling 1993) and the advice should be immediately to pull the plug while maintaining the head above water. Similarly, advice given to patients regarding heights is not usually extended to unprotected waterfronts where patients with epilepsy would be well-advised to keep a safe distance. Personal flotation devices during supervised watersports and informed supervision while swimming are essential (Ryan & Dowling 1993).

Other accidents

Epilepsy patients are usually advised to avoid situations where the occurrence of a fit may be particularly dangerous. The magnitude of accidental mortality is unknown as epilepsy is often not recorded when death certificates are issued in seizure-related fatal accidents. According to Zielinski (1974), epilepsy was cited in only 43% of such accidents. In proportional mortality studies accidental deaths (excluding drowning) constitute 0.8–18% of total deaths from epilepsy (Krohn 1963, Freytag & Lindenberg 1964, Iivanainen & Lehtinen 1979, Klenerman et al 1993). Other studies do not separate drowning cases (Hauser et al 1980, Henriksen et al 1970) and quote accidental fatalities at 6.4–11% of total deaths, while some (Zielinski 1974, Hashimoto et al 1989) separate accidental fatalities due to seizures from those not due to seizures, a distinction not always possible to make.

In addition to circumstance-dependent fatalities such as those due to road traffic accidents or burns, seizures associated with falls have their own risk. They may result in potentially fatal head injuries, cervical trauma or fractures of limbs. Russell-Jones & Shorvon (1989) addressed the risk of head injury associated with seizures based on the number sustained relative to total recorded seizures among long-term residents with epilepsy. Of all seizures, 2.7% (6.1% if associated with falling) resulted in head injury requiring medical attention, but only 1 in every 4208 seizures associated with falls resulted in skull fracture, extradural or subdural haemorrhage. They concluded that while minor seizure-related head injury was common, severe head injury was rare. It is not clear how many seizures may have occurred with protective helmets worn or on soft surfaces. It is interesting that non-drowning accidents in a mortality study at the same centre only constituted 0.8% of total deaths (Klenerman et al 1993), emphasizing that accidental deaths in epilepsy are potentially preventable.

One specific area regulated by legislation is that of epilepsy and driving. Legislation first introduced in the UK in the 1930s was absolute, barring altogether a person 'suffering from epilepsy' from holding a driving licence. The law has relaxed over the years and now requires a one year seizure-free period. This is in marked contrast, for example, to legislation in the State of Wisconsin where only a 3-month fit-free period is required. Hansotia & Broste (1991) conclude on the basis of Wisconsin data that 'drivers with epilepsy or diabetes mellitus have slightly increased risks of traffic accidents' and state their view that the increases in risk do not justify 'further restrictions on driving privileges'. Yet according to Taylor (1989), driver-collapse accounts for approximately 4 per 1000 serious road traffic accidents, of which some 50% are due to epilepsy. While the majority of such cases are undeclared, how many would have satisfied the British, or indeed the Wisconsin, guidelines is unknown.

Pneumonia and other respiratory diseases

The susceptibility of patients with epilepsy to respiratory infections was highlighted by Munson (1910), and confirmed by other reports (Krohn 1963, Iivananen & Lehtinen 1979). In Krohn's view (1963), such patients were not dying of pneumonia, but getting pneumonia because they were dying. Patients who are debilitated or have uncontrolled disease are more at risk and in more recent series tended to be elderly (Klenerman et al 1993). Aspiration during seizures, however, is another possible mechanism, although this has not been formally tested.

Status epilepticus

Prognosis and outcome have recently been reviewed (Shorvon 1994). Although status epilepticus is more common in children, mortality is higher in adults and appears to have declined in recent hospital series (18% of total cases, 7% of children and 28% of adults in combined results from 12 case-series after 1970 — Shorvon 1994). In most cases death is considered mainly due to underlying disease, with some 2% of deaths being directly attributable to status. Population-based data are not available, and most hospital series reported are from specialized centres. Whether higher death rates occur in patients without severe underlying pathology when treated in less specialized units is unknown, nor is the proportion with iatrogenic deaths. The contribution at the present time of antiepileptic drug withdrawal, emphasized by Hunter in 1959 in precipitating status (Shorvon 1994), is unknown.

Status epilepticus in proportional mortality data is listed as the cause in some 10% or less of epilepsy deaths (Krohn 1963, Zielinski 1974, Iivanainen & Lehtinen 1979). Klenerman et al (1993) reported 0.8% death from status in a recent study of institutionalized patients as compared to 11% in the same centre two decades previously. Prompt treatment of the serial seizures/pre-status stage was felt to be partly responsible for the decrease, although more accurate certification may also have contributed, as previous unwitnessed sudden deaths were more likely to be attributed to status. Munson (1910) reported that 59 deaths (10% of total) at the Craig Colony were due to status epilepticus — 'much fewer' from 'status and series' than in the earlier years of the colony. He felt that these were 'conditions which permit no temporizing and must be stopped as soon as possible' — a view strongly held today (Shorvon 1994).

Seizure-related deaths and sudden deaths in epilepsy

Seizure-related and sudden unexpected deaths in epilepsy were previously well-documented by medical attendants at 'epilepsy colonies' (Bacon 1868, Munson 1910, Spratling 1904). Currently they are familiar to both pathologists and coroners (Freytag & Lindenberg 1964, Hirsch & Martin 1971, Leetsma et al 1989) as well as at residential institutions (Brown 1992, Klenerman et al 1993). Yet they remain generally underrecognized, and, indeed, until recently the message has been that, short of an accident consequent to a seizure, epilepsy is not fatal. The general lack of awareness has meant that bereaved relatives have felt particularly isolated in their unexplained loss and only recently has a self-help group been formed in the UK (Epilepsy Bereaved? PO Box 1777, Bournemouth BH5 1YR).

The subject has been reviewed by Jay & Leetsma in 1981. In such deaths postmortem examination fails to reveal an anatomical or toxicological cause. Some witnessed deaths occur during or shortly after a seizure and a few occur with no clear convulsive movements. The majority, however, are unwitnessed and the person is usually found dead, often in or off the bed. Evidence for an associated seizure is found in some 50% of cases (Leetsma et al 1989), and a past history of generalized tonic–clonic seizures is reported in most (Leetsma et al 1989, Earnest et al 1992). Male Afro-Americans with excess alcohol intake are reported to be more at risk (Leetsma et al 1989). It may be that unwitnessed seizures are more likely to be fatal.

In proportional mortality series, between 7.5 and 17% of deaths in people who have epilepsy fall into this category (Wannamaker 1990). These deaths occur whether seizures are moderately or poorly controlled, although cohorts with more severe epilepsy appear to be at higher risk. The influence of epilepsy diagnosis as opposed to seizure type and frequency is still uncertain, but it has been suggested that sudden deaths are more likely in remote symptomatic epilepsy, with a higher percentage of anatomical lesions found on neuropathology than in epilepsy patients dying in other circumstances (Leetsma 1990). However, such deaths do occur in primary generalized epilepsy, including juvenile myoclonic. It has also been suggested, on the basis of postmortem antiepileptic drug levels, that withdrawal/non-compliance may be a precipitating factor (Lund & Gormsen 1985). Apart from the questionable reliability of post-mortem samples (Brown et al 1990), the value of drug levels, once overdose is excluded, is open to debate, as subtherapeutic levels are adequate for many patients. Furthermore, sudden unexpected death in epilepsy was recorded (Munson 1910) before the introduction of modern antiepileptic therapy. Nevertheless, the potential contribution of improved seizure control in reducing the risk of sudden death, and the dangers inherent in non-compliance and drug withdrawal should not be dismissed. Comparisons of incidence in treated and untreated population-based-cohorts are not available.

Incidence of sudden death in a general population with epilepsy has been estimated at between $1:370$ and $1:1110$/year (Leetsma et al 1989). Jick et al (1992) reported an estimated incidence of 1.3/1000 years at risk among individuals aged 15–49 years. Certain selected populations, however, have a much higher risk. Seven out of 151 cases over a 5-year period were reported among patients enrolled in an adult epilepsy surgery programme (Dasheiff 1991). An incidence of $1:260$/year was reported for combined sudden unexpected and seizure-related deaths among long-term residents with epilepsy (Klenerman et al 1993). In a study of an outpatient cohort with epilepsy seen at a tertiary referral centre (Nashef et al 1994), an incidence of $1:200$/year was found, with a mean duration of epilepsy of 21 years and mean age at death of 29 years (mean age for the cohort 32.5 years). In the Cook County series of 60 cases (Leetsma et al 1989), in 51/51 cases where the information was available, duration of epilepsy was 10 years or less with a mean age at death of 35 years, suggesting that it may be more the age of the patient (young adult) rather than duration of epilepsy that defines risk. At the other end of the spectrum, in terms of frequency of seizures, only 2 such deaths were reported by the Medical Research Council antiepileptic drug withdrawal study group (1991) involving 1013 patients and up to 5-year follow-up.

Information on other age groups is limited. Such deaths in an elderly population are difficult to separate from deaths due to ischaemic heart disease (IHD). However, Luhdorf et al (1987) found a higher incidence of sudden death in general than expected in an elderly population with epilepsy. Annegers et al (1984), based on mortality findings in an unselected population with epilepsy, reported an excess of IHD in persons under 65. However, 13/48 'cardiac deaths' at all ages were sudden in previously healthy individuals, 8 in the remote symptomatic group, 4 the idiopathic group and 1 in the neurodeficit group. The increased SMRs reached statistical significance only in the remote symptomatic group, the other numbers being too small to exclude an increased risk. Ages and postmortem findings were not detailed but all sudden deaths were attributed to IHD. There were three mutually exclusive categories of IHD, depending on presentation. SMR was highest for the sudden death group at 2.29 (95% CI 1.22–3.93), intermediate for myocardial infarction and comparable to the general population for angina pectoris. Some 5.5% (13) of deaths in the study were directly attributed to epilepsy. Given close to 10 000 person-years and an approximate incidence of 1:1000 of sudden death (unrelated to IHD) in an unselected cohort, 10 such cases only may be expected. These data may not therefore be at variance with other sources.

Sudden deaths in epilepsy do occur in children, and constituted in one study 10% of total sudden deaths among children aged 2–20 years (Keeling & Knowles 1989). In another study, 11/93 deaths among children with epilepsy were probable 'sudden unexplained deaths' (Harvey et al 1991). In one clinical series, 3 of 120 children with epilepsy and no neurological deficit followed for up to 12 years (total years of follow-up not stated) died a sudden unexpected death (Brorson & Wranne 1987). It remains uncertain whether the incidence is lower in children than young adults and whether children with mental handicap and/or neurological deficit are at an increased risk.

Although a lifelong assessment of risk per individual of seizure-related and sudden death cannot be estimated on the basis of currently available data, cumulative risk in patients with chronic epilepsy is likely to be below the '3 to 4 percent' stated by Spratling for non-accidental seizure-related deaths (1904), an experience predating the introduction of modern antiepileptic therapy.

Causes of deaths stated in death certificates in such cases vary and include status epilepticus, epileptic seizure, asphyxia, anoxia, respiratory arrest, suffocation and unascertained. Except where they occur in residential institutions or in hospitals, they are likely, in the UK, to be referred to the coroner and thus circumstances of death are recorded.

Pulmonary oedema, well-documented in seizures, with or without congestion of other organs, is a frequent postmortem finding in sudden death cases (Terrence et al 1981, Leetsma et al 1989). Mechanisms put forward have recently concentrated on the possible role of cardiac arrhythmias as the primary event. Although changes in cardiac rate are common (Blumhardt et al 1986), malignant arrhythmias appear to be relatively rare in seizures. They are, however, reported and include bradycardia and sinus arrest (Joske & Davis 1991, Fincham et al 1992). Hypoxia secondary to central or obstructive apnoea or pulmonary oedema is an alternative hypothesis. Changes in respiratory pattern, including apnoea, occur during seizures (Schraeder & Lathers 1990). Both cardiac and respiratory disturbances or other as yet unknown mechanisms may play a part. The release of endogenous opioids peri-ictally, for example, may aggravate autonomic disturbances already present. It has been suggested that in cases where no clear convulsive movements occur the deaths may still be in the context of a paroxysmal epileptiform electroencephalogram discharge (Brown 1992).

The question has arisen as to whether suffocation due to external factors plays an important role, as argued by Wilson (1978), who advocated smother-proof pillows. Although many sudden death cases are nocturnal, the number found in a position suggestive of suffocation due to soft bedding is small. In our own ongoing study of circumstances surrounding sudden death in epilepsy, 19 self-referred bereaved relatives have so far been interviewed with medical details substantiated from previous physicians, death certificates, coroner's and postmortem reports. Only 2/19 were found face down into a pillow.

Although much remains to be learnt about seizure-related and sudden deaths, implications based on current evidence can be summarized as follows: control of epilepsy may influence rates of sudden death and, although deaths do occur with relatively few seizures, intractable cases appear to be at higher risk. The relatively high incidence in selected groups needs to be taken into consideration in clinical management.

Suicides

The subject of suicide and epilepsy has been reviewed by Barraclough (1987), with both self-poisoning and suicides apparently increased in patients with epilepsy. In proportional mortality series, suicides have constituted some 2–10% of total deaths. An exceptionally high 20% was reported from Denmark (Henriksen et al 1970), where suicide rates in general are particularly high. Suicide, however, was not reported to be increased in the population-based Rochester study, with only 3 suicides reported in 8233 person-years. Zielinski (1974) reported a higher incidence among patients with epilepsy in the community as compared to institutionalized patients. An increased number of suicides has also been reported in posttemporal lobectomy patients, particularly in the first few years of follow-up (Marsh

& Taylor). Force et al (1989) found a younger age at suicide than in the general population and an association with more severe epilepsy. Mendez & Doss (1992), partly on the basis of their experience with 4 patients, suggest a greater association with psychotic behaviours and psychic symptoms than with major depression or the psychosocial burden of being epileptic. This would appear to be supported by the observation that the excess risk has been estimated at 25 times that of the general population for patients with temporal lobe epilepsy (Barraclough 1987). While it may be that only selected groups are at particular risk early after diagnosis, this is clearly another area where deaths are potentially preventable.

Mortality related to treatment of epilepsy

Cancer and antiepileptic medication

It has been suggested that some antiepileptic drugs are associated with a small increased long-term risk of secondary neoplasia. Associations between phenytoin and lymphomas, barbiturates with liver tumours, and barbiturates and lung cancer have been considered. Excess lung cancer was reported in more than one study either within the first few years of diagnosis (Shirts et al 1986) or where smoking history was not available (Klenerman et al 1993). An excess of pancreatic and hepatobiliary cancer (carcinoma of the gallbladder and cholangiocarcinoma) has also been reported (Klenerman et al 1993) but numbers were small. In a study of over 2000 residents with epilepsy, White et al (1979) defined the limits of an overall increase in risk for cancer (excluding the central nervous system) at between 1.1 and 1.8 times the average. Clemmesen et al (1974) and Shirts et al (1986) found no such overall increase. A large study of 8004 patients with epilepsy from Denmark (Olsen et al 1989) showed no overall increased risk when brain cancers were excluded, a significant decrease in bladder cancer and melanomas, a non-significant increase of non-Hodgkin's lymphomas, and a significant but small increase in lung cancers (relative risk 1.4, 95% CI 1.2–1.7). The lack of associated increase in bladder cancer did not support the hypothesis that the increase was smoking-related.

In summary, once central nervous system neoplasms are excluded, any reported excess of cancers is small or borderline, although doubt remains regarding neoplasms of the lung and non-Hodgkin's lymphomas. At present these findings do not influence clinical decisions.

Deaths attributed to antiepileptic therapy

Deaths may sometimes occur as a direct consequence of an adverse reaction to antiepileptic therapy. Idiosyncratic reactions such as blood dyscrasia may be life-threatening. Hepatic failure fatalities with phenytoin, phenobarbitone and sodium valproate, for example, have been well-documented. In the case of valproate (Dreifuss et al 1987), such fatalities were most likely to occur in children with neurodeficit aged 0–2 years on polytherapy. Other examples include sinus arrest with carbamazepine (Jacome 1987) and liver failure as part of an allergic reaction with lamotrigine (Duncan 1994). Comparative estimates of rates of occurrence of such deaths per treatment years are not available, and it is difficult to estimate the magnitude of risk.

Mortality postsurgery for epilepsy

It may be expected that mortality after surgery for epilepsy would decline towards that of the normal population. However, as reported by Polkey (1989), whereas low perioperative mortality has continued to decline, long-term mortality after surgery is elevated. Two series (Jensen 1975, Taylor & Marsh 1977) report excess long-term mortality with some one-half to two-thirds of deaths related to seizures or suicides. Although, as concluded by Jensen, this may be less than expected in a non-operated group (a proposition not directly tested), it remains above that of the general population, and is thus a cause for concern.

CONCLUSIONS

Despite all that has been achieved, there remains much to understand regarding mortality in epilepsy. Rodin (1968) pointed out that 'general statements covering all epileptics are likely to be an oversimplification'. Studies looking at prognosis in well-defined diagnostic groups are required. The influence of mortality on prevalence in the developed and developing world (where treatment rates are lower), the incidence and mechanisms of sudden and seizure-related deaths, and long-term mortality after epilepsy surgery are but a few examples of areas for future research.

Contrary to the experience of early physicians, epilepsy has, in recent years, been perceived as a benign condition. Yet the available evidence, particularly in chronic cases, argues against this view. Treatment has concentrated on achieving seizure control and more recently improving quality of life. Better survival in chronic epilepsy should also be one of the goals.

KEY POINTS FOR CLINICAL PRACTICE

- Epilepsy is not always a benign condition: underlying disease and epilepsy both contribute to reported excess mortality.
- Deaths from status epilepticus in hospitals have fallen and early treatment is strongly advocated.
- Patients with generalized seizures, particularly young adults, are at risk of unexpected death at an incidence of 1:200 to 1:100/year. Physicians need to acknowledge this entity and ensure that bereaved relatives are

given adequate support with referral to self-help groups and counselling where appropriate.

- Accidental deaths, including drowning, occur more frequently among patients with epilepsy and are potentially preventable, as are suicides.
- Deaths directly attributable to antiepileptic therapy can occur. Constant vigilance is required, particularly when an agent is first prescribed.
- Long-term mortality after epilepsy surgery has been reported to be raised, with deaths mainly due to suicides or continuing epilepsy. Given the revival of surgical treatment for epilepsy, this has significant implications for patient management and follow-up.
- Every effort should be made to control epilepsy, as improved control is likely to influence mortality.

REFERENCES

Annegers J F, Hauser W A, Shirts S B. 1984 Heart disease mortality and morbidity in patients with epilepsy. Epilepsia 25: 699–704

Bacon G M. 1868 On the modes of death in epilepsy. Lancet 1: 555–556

Barraclough B M. 1987 The suicide rate of epilepsy. Acta Psychiatr Scand 76: 339–345

Blumhardt L D, Smith P E M, Owen L. 1986 Electrographic accompaniments of temporal lobe epileptic seizures. Lancet 1: 1051–1055

Brorson L O, Wranne L. 1987 Long-term prognosis in childhood epilepsy: survival and seizure prognosis. Epilepsia 28: 324–330

Brown S W. 1992 Sudden death and epilepsy: clinical review. Seizure 1: 71–73

Brown S W, Mawer G E, Lawler W et al. 1990 Sudden death in epilepsy (letter). Lancet 335: 606–607

Chandra V, Barucha N E, Schoenberg B S, Feskanich D. 1984 National mortality data for deaths due to and all deaths related to epilepsy in the United States. In: Porter R J, ed. Advances in epileptology. New York: Raven Press, pp 531–534

Chevrie J J, Aicardi J. 1978 Convulsive disorders in the first year of life. Neurological and mental outcome and mortality. Epilepsia 19: 67–74

Clemmesen J, Fuglsang-Frederiksen V, Plum C. 1974. Are anticonvulsants oncogenic? Lancet i: 705–707

Cockerell O C, Johnson A L, Hart Y M et al. 1994 Personal communication

Dasheiff R M. 1991 Sudden unexpected death in epilepsy: a series from an epilepsy surgery programme and speculation on the relationship to sudden cardiac death. J Clin Neurophys 8: 216–222

Diekema D S, Quan L, Holt V L. 1993 Epilepsy as a risk factor for submersion injury in children. Pediatrics 91: 612–616

Dreifuss F E, Santilli N, Langer D H, Sweeney K P, Moline K A, Menander K B. 1987 Valproic acid hepatic fatalities: a retrospective review. Neurology 37: 379–385

Duncan J S. 1994 Personal communication

Earnest M P, Thomas G E, Randall A E, Kenneth F H. 1992 The sudden unexplained death syndrome in epilepsy. Epilepsia 33: 310–316

Fincham R W, Shivapour E T, Leis A A, Martins J B. 1992 Ictal bradycardia with syncope: a case report. Neurology 42: 2222–2223

Force L, Jallon P, Hoffman J J. 1989 Suicide and epilepsy. Adv Epileptol 17: 356–358

Freytag E, Lindenberg R. 1964 Medicolegal autopsies on epileptics. Arch Pathol 78: 274–286

Haerer A F, Anderson D W, Schoenberg B S. 1986 Prevalence and clinical features of epilepsy in a biracial United States population. Epilepsia 27: 66–75

Hansotia P, Broste S K. 1991 The effect of epilepsy or diabetes mellitus on the risk of automobile accidents. N Engl J Med 324: 22–26

Harvey A S, Hopkins I J, Nolan T M, Carlin J B. 1991 Mortality in children with epilepsy: an epidemiological study. AES proceedings. Epilepsia 32 (suppl 3): 54

Hashimoto K, Fukushima Y, Saito F, Wada K. 1989 Mortality and causes of death in patients with epilepsy over 16 years of age. Jpn J Psychiatry Neurol 43: 546–547

Hauser W A, Hesdorffer D C. 1990 Mortality. In: Epilepsy: frequency, causes and consequences. Maryland: Epilepsy Foundation of USA pp 297–326

Hauser A W, Annegers J F, Elveback L R. 1980 Mortality in patients with epilepsy. Epilepsia 21: 399–412

Henriksen B, Juul-Jensen P, Lund M. 1970 The mortality of epileptics. In: Brackenridge R D C, ed. Proceedings of the 10th International Congress of Life Assurance Medicine. London: Putman, pp 139–148

Hirsch C S, Martin D L. 1971 Unexpected death in young epileptics. Neurology 21: 682–690

Iivanainen M, Lehtinen J. 1979 Causes of death in institutionalized epileptics. Epilepsia 20: 485–492

Jacome D E. 1987 Syncope and sudden death attributed to carbamazepine. J Neurol Neurosurg Psychiatry 50: 1245

Jallon P, Haton F, Maguin P. 1989 Death among epileptics. Adv Epileptol 17: 351–355

Jay G W, Leetsma J E. 1981 Sudden death in epilepsy. A comprehensive review of the literature and proposed mechanisms. Acta Neurol Scand 63 (suppl 82): 5–66

Jensen I. 1975 Temporal lobe epilepsy. Late mortality in patients treated with unilateral temporal lobe resections. Acta Neurol Scand 52: 374–380

Jick S S, Cole T B, Mesher R A, Tennis P, Jick H. 1992 Sudden unexplained death in young persons with primary epilepsy. Pharmcoepidemiol Drug Safety 1: 59–64

Juul-Jensen P, Foldspang A. 1983 Natural history of epileptic seizures. Epilepsia 24: 297–312

Joske D J L, Davis M J E. 1991 Sino-atrial arrest due to temporal lobe epilepsy. Aust NZJ Med 21: 62–64

Keeling J W, Knowles S A S. 1989 Sudden death in childhood and adolescence. J Pathol 159: 221–224

Klenerman P, Sander J W A S, Shorvon S D. 1993 Mortality in patients with epilepsy: a study of patients in long term residential care. J Neurol Neurosurg Psychiatry 56: 149–152

Krohn W. 1963 Causes of death among epileptics. Epilepsia 4: 315–321

Leetsma J E. 1990 A pathological review. In: Lathers C M, Schraeder P L, eds. Epilepsy and sudden death. New York: Marcel Dekker, 61–88

Leetsma J E, Walczak T, Hughes J R, Kalelkar M B, Teas S S. 1989 A prospective study on sudden unexpected death in epilepsy. Ann Neurol 26: 195–203

Luhdorf K, Jensen L K, Plesner A M. 1987 Epilepsy in the elderly: life expectancy and causes of death. Acta Neurol Scand 76: 183–190

Lund A, Gormsen H. 1985 The role of antiepileptics in sudden death in epilepsy. Acta Neurol Scand 72: 444–446

Massey E W, Schoenberg B S. 1985 Mortality from epilepsy. International patterns and changes over time. Neuroepidemiology 4: 65–70

Medical Research Council antiepileptic drug withdrawal study group. 1991 Randomized study of antiepileptic drug withdrawal in patients in remission. Lancet 337: 1175–1180

Mendez M F, Doss R C. 1992 Ictal and suicidal aspects of suicide in epileptic patients. Int J Psychiatry Med 22: 231–237

Munson J F. 1910 Death in epilepsy. Med Record. Jan 8; 77: 58–62

Nashef L, Fish D F, Sander J W A S, Shorvon S D. 1994 Incidence of sudden unexpected death in an outpatient cohort with epilepsy at a tertiary referral centre (in press)

Office of Population Censuses. 1991 Mortality Statistics. Cause, England and Wales. Series DH 2: 18

Olsen J H, Boice J D, Jensen J P A, Fraumeni J F. 1989 Cancer among epileptic patients exposed to antiepileptic drugs. J Natl Cancer Inst 81: 803–809

Orlowski J P, Rothner D A, Lueders H. 1982 Submersion accidents in children with epilepsy. Am J Dis Child 136: 777–780

Oxbury J M, Whitty C W M. 1971 Causes and consequences of status epilepticus in adults: a study of 86 cases. Brain 94: 735–744

Penning R, Muller C, Ciompi L. 1969 Mortalite et cause de deces des epileptiques. Psychiatr Clin 2: 85–94

Polkey C E. 1989 Surgical treatment of chronic epilepsy. In: Trimble M eR, ed. Chronic epilepsy: its prognosis and management. Chichester: John Wiley, pp 189–207

Rodin E A. 1968 The prognosis of patients with epilepsy. Illinois: Charles C Thomas, pp 156–171

Russell-Jones D L, Shorvon S D. 1989 The frequency and consequences of head injury in epileptic seizures. JH Neurol Neurosurg Psychiatry. 52: 659–662

Ryan C A, Dowling G. 1993 Drowning deaths in people with epilepsy. Can Med Assoc J 148: 781–784

Sander J W A S. 1993 Some aspects of prognosis in the epilepsies: a review. Epilepsia 34: 1007–1016

Sander J W A S, Shorvon S D. 1987 Incidence and prevalence studies in epilepsy and their methodological problems: a review. JNNP 50: 829–839

Sander J W A S, Hart Y M, Johnson A L, Shorvon S D. 1990 National general practice study of epilepsy: newly diagnosed epileptic seizures in a general population. Lancet 336: 1267–1271

Satishchandra P, Chandra V, Schoenberg B S. 1988 Case control study of associated conditions at the time of death in patients with epilepsy. Neuroepidemiology 7: 109–114

Schraeder P L, Lathers C M. 1990 The relation of paroxysmal autonomic dysfunction and epileptogenic activity. In: Epilepsy and sudden death. New York: Marcel Dekker, pp 121–197

Shirts S B, Naaegers J F, Hauser A W, Kurland L T. 1986 Cancer incidence in a cohort of patients with seizure disorders. J Natl Cancer Inst 77: 83–87

Shorvon S D. 1994 Prognosis and outcome of status epilepticus. In: Status epilepticus. Cambridge, Cambridge University Press: pp 293–301

Shorvon S D, Bharucha N E. 1993 Epilepsy in developing countries: epidemiology, aetiology and health care. In: Laidlaw J, Richens A, Chadwick D, eds. A textbook of epilepsy. Edinburgh: Churchill Livingstone, pp 23–45

Spratling W P. 1904 Prognosis. In: Epilepsy and its treatment. Philadelphia PA: WB Saunders, p 304

Taylor J. 1989 Driving and epilepsy: new draft EEC directive for a common community driving license. In: Chadwick D, ed. Fourth international symposium on sodium valproate and epilepsy. London: Royal Society of Medicine

Taylor D C, Marsh S M. 1977 Implications of long-term follow-up studies in epilepsy: with a note on the cause of death. In: Penry JK, ed. Epilepsy, the Eighth International Symposium. New York: Raven Press, pp 27–34

Terrence C F, Rao G R, Perper J A 1981 Neurogenic pulmonary edema in unexpected unexplained death of epileptic patients. Ann Neurol 9: 458–464

Wannamaker B B. 1990 A perspective of death of persons with epilepsy. In: Lathers CM, Schraeder P L, eds. Epilepsy and sudden death. New York: Marcel Dekker, pp 27–37

White S J, McLean A E M, Howland C. 1979 Anticonvulsant drugs and cancer. A cohort study in patients with severe epilepsy. Lancet ii: 458–460

Wilson J B. 1978 Hazards of epilepsy. Br Med J 2: 200

Zielinski J J. 1974 Epilepsy and mortality rate and cause of death. Epilepsia 15: 191–201

Index